Nutritional Factors in the Induction and Maintenance of Malignancy

Bristol-Myers

Nutrition

Symposia

Series Editor
JERRY L. MOORE
Nutritional Division
Mead Johnson & Company

1   R. W. Winters and H. L. Greene (Editors):
    Nutritional Support of the Seriously Ill Patient, 1983

2   C. E. Butterworth, Jr., and Martha L. Hutchinson (Editors):
    Nutritional Factors in the Induction and Maintenance of
    Malignancy, 1983

In Preparation 3   Morris Green and H. L. Greene (Editors):
    The Role of the Gastrointestinal Tract in Nutrient Delivery
    (tentative)

Nutritional Factors in the Induction and Maintenance of Malignancy

Edited by

C. E. BUTTERWORTH, JR.

Department of Nutrition Sciences
Medical Center
University of Alabama in Birmingham
Birmingham, Alabama

MARTHA L. HUTCHINSON

Nutrition Research
Division of Oncology
Fred Hutchinson Cancer Research Center
Seattle, Washington

1983

ACADEMIC PRESS

A Subsidiary of Harcourt Brace Jovanovich, Publishers

New York   London

Paris   San Diego   San Francisco   São Paulo   Sydney   Tokyo   Toronto

ACADEMIC PRESS, INC.
111 Fifth Avenue, New York, New York 10003

United Kingdom Edition published by
ACADEMIC PRESS, INC. (LONDON) LTD.
24/28 Oval Road, London NW1   7DX

Library of Congress Cataloging in Publication Data
Main entry under title:

Nutritional factors in the induction and maintenance of
    malignancy.

    (The Bristol-Myers nutrition symposia ; 2)
    Includes index.
    1. Carcinogenesis--Congresses. 2. Cancer--Nutritional
aspects--Congresses. 3. Vitamins--Physiological effect--
Congresses. I. Butterworth, C. E. (Charles Edwin)
II. Hutchinson, Martha L. III. Series. [DNLM:
1. Neoplasms--Diet therapy--Congresses. 2. Neoplasms--
Prevention and control--Congresses. QZ 200 N9766 1982]
RC268.5.N87   1983   616.99'4071   83—5020
ISBN 0—12—147520—4

PRINTED IN THE UNITED STATES OF AMERICA

83 84 85 86   9 8 7 6 5 4 3 2 1

Contents

1   Why Isolate Cancer?

DENIS BURKITT

2   Nutritional Considerations in the Epidemiology of Lymphoma

DAVID T. PURTILO

3   Viral-Induced Changes in Metabolic Function and Nutritional Requirements of Cultured Human Cells

FRED RAPP

4   Lectin-Induced Changes in Metabolic Function and Nutritional Requirements of Cultured Human Lymphocytes

PETER B. ROWE

5 Fragile Chromosomes

GRANT R. SUTHERLAND

6 Variations in Chromatin Structure and Nucleosomal DNA Repeat Length with Nutritional Manipulation

C. ELIZABETH CASTRO AND J. SANDERS SEVALL

7 Cytogenetic Studies of a Family with a Hereditary Defect of Cellular Folate Uptake and High Incidence of Hematologic Disease

DIANE C. ARTHUR, THOMAS J. DANZL, AND
RICHARD F. BRANDA

8 Virus-Induced Folates and Folate Enzymes: Formation and Incorporation into Viral Particles

LLOYD M. KOZLOFF

9 Growth-Regulating Effects of Naturally Occurring Metabolites of Folate and Ascorbate on Malignant Cells

CECILE LEUCHTENBERGER AND RUDOLF
LEUCHTENBERGER

10 The Metabolism of Vitamin A and Its Functions

H. F. DELUCA

11 Effects of Supplemental Dietary Vitamin A and β-Carotene on Experimental Tumors, Local Tumor Excision, Chemotherapy, Radiation Injury, and Radiotherapy

STANLEY M. LEVENSON, GIUSEPPE RETTURA, AND ELI SEIFTER

Contributors

Numbers in parentheses indicate the pages on which the authors' contributions begin.

Diane C. Arthur (101), Departments of Laboratory Medicine/Pathology and Pediatrics, University of Minnesota Hospitals, Minneapolis, Minnesota 55455

Richard F. Branda[1] (101), Department of Medicine, Division of Hematology, University of Minnesota Hospitals, Minneapolis, Minnesota 55455

Elizabeth Bright-See (217), Ludwig Institute for Cancer Research, Toronto Branch for Human Cancer Prevention, Toronto, Ontario M4Y 1M4, Canada

Denis Burkitt (1), Unit of Geographical Pathology, St. Thomas's Hospital Medical School, London S.E.1, England

C. Elizabeth Castro (75), Department of Cellular and Molecular Biology, Southwest Foundation for Research and Education, San Antonio, Texas 78284

Thomas J. Danzl (101), Department of Laboratory Medicine/Pathology, University of Minnesota Hospitals, Minneapolis, Minnesota 55455

H. F. DeLuca (149), Department of Biochemistry, University of Wisconsin, Madison, Wisconsin 53706

Victor Herbert (273), Hematology and Nutrition Laboratory, Veterans Administration Medical Center, Bronx, New York 10468, and State University of New York Downstate Medical Center, Brooklyn, New York 11203

Lloyd M. Kozloff (113), Department of Microbiology, University of California, San Francisco, California 94143

[1]Present address: Department of Medicine, University of Vermont, Burlington, Vermont 05401.

Carlos L. Krumdieck (225), Department of Nutrition Sciences, University of Alabama in Birmingham, Birmingham, Alabama 35294

Cecile Leuchtenberger[2] (131), Department of Cytochemistry, Swiss Institute for Experimental Cancer Research, 1066 Epalinges, Switzerland

Rudolf Leuchtenberger[2] (131), Department of Cytochemistry, Swiss Institute for Experimental Cancer Research, 1066 Epalinges, Switzerland

Stanley M. Levenson (169), Department of Surgery, Albert Einstein College of Medicine, and Montefiore Hospital and Medical Center, Bronx, New York 10461

Frank L. Meyskens, Jr. (205), Department of Internal Medicine and Cancer Center Division, University of Arizona Health Sciences Center, Tucson, Arizona 85724

Kathleen M. Nauss (247), Laboratory of Nutritional Pathology, Massachusetts Institute of Technology, Cambridge, Massachusetts 02139

Paul M. Newberne (247), Laboratory of Nutritional Pathology, Massachusetts Institute of Technology, Cambridge, Massachusetts 02139

David T. Purtilo (11), Department of Pathology and Laboratory Medicine, University of Nebraska Medical Center, Omaha, Nebraska 68105

Fred Rapp (29), Department of Microbiology, The Milton S. Hershey Medical Center, The Pennsylvania State University, Hershey, Pennsylvania 17033

Giuseppe Rettura (169), Department of Surgery, Albert Einstein College of Medicine, and Montefiore Hospital and Medical Center, Bronx, New York 10461

Adrianne E. Rogers (247), Department of Nutrition and Food Science, Massachusetts Institute of Technology, Cambridge, Massachusetts 02139

Peter B. Rowe (51), Children's Medical Research Foundation, The University of Sydney, Camperdown, New South Wales, Australia 2050

Eli Seifter (169), Departments of Biochemistry and Surgery, Albert Einstein College of Medicine, Bronx, New York 10461

J. Sanders Sevall (75), Department of Cellular and Molecular Biology, Southwest Foundation for Research and Education, San Antonio, Texas 78284

Grant R. Sutherland (63), Cytogenetics Unit, Department of Histopathology, The Adelaide Children's Hospital, North Adelaide, South Australia, Australia 5006

Sylvia Wassertheil-Smoller (289), Department of Community Health, Division of Epidemiology and Biostatistics, Albert Einstein College of Medicine, Bronx, New York 10461

---

[2]Present address: Hirzbodenpark 18, 4052 Basel, Switzerland.

Editor's Foreword

The role of nutrients in initiating and promoting (or in resisting) oncogenic transformation in living cells is of prime importance to our management and understanding of cancer in humans. The impact of valid epidemiological observations on diet and cancer, of sound animal model experimentation, and of *in vitro* findings on the clinical management of specific human malignancies is increasing rapidly. Data presented in this symposium relating dietary components, especially vitamins, to neoplastic induction are of great potential value for understanding human cancer etiology and for formulating improved therapy.

The second annual Bristol-Myers Symposium on Nutrition Research, held December 9–10, 1982, in Washington, D.C., served as a unique interdisciplinary forum for experts in the field of nutrition, molecular biology, epidemiology, and biochemistry to discuss this timely topic of nutritional factors in the induction and maintenance of malignancy. As cochairpersons of the symposium and as editors of this volume, Dr. Charles E. Butterworth, Jr., and Dr. Martha L. Hutchinson are to be congratulated on planning the program, on securing the participation of world-renowned experts in this difficult and challenging field, and now on completing preparation of these valuable proceedings of the symposium.

On behalf of the symposium's sponsor, Bristol-Myers, on behalf of the readers and the scientific community whose professional efforts will be enhanced by the symposium and its proceedings, and most importantly on behalf of present and future patients whose lives and health may be aided by these efforts, I extend to Dr. Butterworth, Dr. Hutchinson, and all the participants a hearty thanks for a job well done!

Jerry L. Moore
Series Editor

Foreword

The knowledge gained from nutrition research is being increasingly applied toward finding new ways to improve and extend human life. And few areas of research present such challenges as those involved with unraveling the riddles of cancer.

Nutrition researchers and cancer researchers have not often met together. Yet there is an increasing body of evidence to support the belief that nutrition is closely associated with both preventing and treating cancer. Nutrition research has thus begun to take its rightful place among the many disciplines that contribute to our understanding and control of cancer.

The progress achieved by those studying the nutritional aspects of cancer is the subject of these proceedings of the second annual Bristol-Myers Symposium on Nutrition Research.

For more than 70 years, our Mead Johnson & Company subsidiary has pioneered in nutrition research and development to meet the special dietary needs of infants, children, and adults.

This long-standing involvement in nutrition research has made us acutely conscious of an ongoing need among academic investigators: the ever-present necessity for funding. Particularly in these difficult economic times, it is imperative that academic researchers have funds available to support their most vital, creative, and innovative programs.

That is why, in 1980, Bristol-Myers and Mead Johnson established a major corporate nutrition grant and award program designed to encourage the finest and most innovative nutrition research at the academic level.

This program includes three major elements:

• First, an unrestricted grant program totaling more than $1 million for nutrition research at major American and foreign institutions.

• Second, an annual prize of $25,000 to an individual scientist for distinguished achievement in nutrition research.

• Third, an annual symposium on nutrition research. Last year's symposium, the first in this series, focused on nutritional management of the seriously ill patient and was organized by the Columbia University College of Physicians & Surgeons. The 1983 meeting, organized by the University of Indiana School of Medicine, will look at the role of the gastrointestinal tract in nutrient delivery.

The symposium entitled "Nutritional Factors in the Induction and Maintenance of Malignancy" reported in this volume has special significance for us because it combines two of our company's major medical research interests. In addition to our nutrition research program, we have since 1977 sponsored a major program of unrestricted cancer research grants that now involves 13 institutions in the United States and abroad. Annual symposia and an annual award for distinguished achievement in cancer research are also elements of the cancer grant program.

Early in 1983, Bristol-Myers increased its unrestricted support of innovative research at medical schools and universities throughout the world with the addition of a new program of grants and symposia in orthopaedic research. The company's commitment to unrestricted medical research now exceeds $8 million, and we expect that figure to become even higher in the years ahead.

We hope that symposia such as the one reported here, with the opportunities they provide for important interaction among scientists, will lead to a growing body of knowledge that can be used in the prevention and treatment of cancer and of other diseases.

Richard L. Gelb
Chairman of the Board
Bristol-Myers Company

Preface

The last decade has witnessed some rather remarkable changes in basic concepts and attitudes toward cancer. Faced with limited therapeutic success (if not downright dismal failure) after nearly 40 years of "destructive" therapy, as exemplified by the nonspecific alkylating agents and ionizing radiation (each of which can be mutagenic in itself), emphasis seems to be shifting toward (a) primary prevention and (b) physiologic regulation of cellular proliferation. In each of these two approaches, new attention is now being given to the *positive* contribution that can occur with manipulation of nutritional factors and improvement of the repair process.

Epidemiologists are beginning to explore the association of dietary patterns with certain forms of cancer, leading to hope for *primary prevention* of cancer through dietary modification and supplementation. Physicians are beginning to think in terms of *localized* nutritional deficiency, and of heritable defects of nutrient metabolism that may lend themselves to specific supplementation as a means to prevent cancer. We also seem to be moving in the direction of accepting the concept of *reversibility* of early cancer lesions through manipulation of nutrients, hormones, and immune mechanisms. This view clashes with the older, perhaps oversimplified, idea that once a nest of cancer cells is formed the only treatment is physical removal or cytotoxic destruction. It is, to say the very least, a refreshing and hopeful outlook, but obviously we need to learn much more about individual differences in response to the same agent (for example, the Epstein-Barr virus).

It is indeed gratifying to see common threads of knowledge brought together as they have been in this volume from seemingly diverse disciplines in pursuit of a shared goal, namely, a better understanding of cancer and, ultimately, its conquest. It is particularly pleasing to see nutrition science emerge as a unifying force—a meeting ground for scientists involved in a wide variety of investigations. Nutrition has often been regarded as a sort of neglected child. We would prefer to think of it as a slumbering giant whose potential importance is just now being appreciated!

Regrettably, Dr. Cecile Leuchtenberger was not able to attend the symposium because of the illness of her husband and co-investigator, Dr. Rudolf Leuchtenberger. Their observation, made nearly 40 years ago, that folic acid triglutamate can cure breast cancer in mice was probably the first to suggest a growth-*regulating* role for a vitamin, at a time when conventional wisdom emphasized only the growth-*promoting* effects of vitamins and led to the presumption that somehow vitamins were "bad" for patients with cancer. The Leuchtenbergers' work was overshadowed by developments related to the folic acid antagonists, but deserves renewed attention in light of newer knowledge concerning pteroylpolyglutamate metabolism. Their work was presented *in absentia* by Dr. Untae Kim of the Roswell Park Memorial Institute and their contribution is published as a chapter in these proceedings.

Dr. Denis Burkitt spent some 20 years in Uganda as a surgeon at the Makerere University College Medical School beginning in the mid-1950s. During those years he recognized the unique clinical, pathological, and epidemiological features of the lymphoma that now bears his name. Simultaneously, he recognized remarkable differences in the prevalence, in African natives, of certain diseases that are widespread in Western civilizations. His observations on the importance of dietary fiber in the prevention of diverticular disease, cancer of the colon, and other diseases have had a profound influence on nutrition science in the Western world and on the entire field of preventive medicine. Although he would perhaps modestly disagree, his epidemiological studies demonstrating an overlap between the geographic distribution of malaria and African Burkitt's lymphoma may well rank equally in importance with his observations on dietary fiber—because of a possible association with immunological and nutritional defects in malaria. His achievements are all the more inspiring when one realizes that they were based on two of the simplest, yet most powerful, tools of science: an inquiring intellect and deductive reasoning.

Other contributors have shown how various nutrients appear to influence the genesis, progression, and even treatment of cancer. Clues have come from epidemiology, virology, immunology, genetics, biochemistry, and experience with tissue and cell cultures. Animal experiments have encouraged studies in human subjects on the one hand, while suggesting the extreme, yet intriguing, complexities of such studies on the other. As Dr. Burkitt has shown, investigations of the impact of nutrition on carcinogenesis can enhance our ability to understand and prevent a wide variety of *other* disabling and fatal diseases. Since it was not feasible to cover all of the important recent developments, we attempted to select topics and participants for their timeliness, unique features, and relevance to each other.

In summary, we believe that this volume on the subject of nutrition and cancer represents a major advance in scientific inquiry, for it has brought together distinguished leaders from numerous disciplines to discuss in depth nutrition and cancer causation, treatment, and, perhaps most importantly, *prevention*.

As organizers of the meeting and guest editors of the proceedings we again would like to express our appreciation to the Bristol-Myers Company for the financial support that made the meeting possible, and for the spirit of complete academic freedom in which the support was given.

C. E. Butterworth, Jr.
Martha L. Hutchinson

1

Why Isolate Cancer?

Denis Burkitt

Unit of Geographical Pathology
St. Thomas's Hospital Medical School
London, England

I. VIEWING CANCER IN CONTEXT

When using the epidemiological approach in endeavoring to detect factors causative of particular forms of cancer, much can be lost by ignoring other diseases that share similar epidemiological features. In any search for factors in the environment that have the same geographical distribution of some form of cancer and thus may be causally related to it, it would be ridiculous to ignore other diseases exhibiting a similar distribution. The possibility that these might be caused, at least in part, by the same factors that are causative of the cancer could well provide clues to the cause of the latter.

1

Nutritional Factors in the Induction
and Maintenance of Malignancy

Cigarette smoking might have been recognized as a cause of bronchial carcinoma by observing that its distribution geographically and socioeconomically was related to such conditions as chronic bronchitis, emphysema, and nicotine-stained fingers, and then discovering that these conditions were related to smoking, so why not cancer also? Further confirmation of this conclusion would have been provided by recognizing that these nonmalignant disorders and lung cancer tended to occur together in the same patients and thus were interrelated.

With this approach in mind, I wrote a guest editorial in the *Journal of the National Cancer Institute* entitled: "Some Neglected Leads in Cancer Research" (Burkitt, 1971a), and once shocked an audience at the Institute by suggesting that one of the major defects in at least some cancer research was specializing in cancer. In this context it is particularly regrettable that when searching for the causes of large bowel cancer the epidemiological features of polyps have been so neglected. Although it is generally agreed that in Western countries most bowel cancers arise in polyps (Hill *et al.*, 1978), few cancer registries even record the prevalence of polyps, and as a consequence very little is known of their geographical distribution other than their extreme rarity in communities at low risk of developing colorectal cancer and vice versa (Bremner and Ackerman, 1970; Burkitt, 1975a). Might it not be better if research into bowel cancer was temporarily suspended and the cause of polyps sought instead? Their infinitely higher frequency would make investigation easier. This approach is currently being used by Bruce (1983), in intervention studies, determining factors that might reduce their occurrence. Vitamin C, vitamin E, and wheat bran are being added to the diet of three different groups of patients to observe whether they confer any protective effects.

II. DISEASES OF WESTERN CULTURE

There is now a well-recognized list of disorders that are agreed to be characteristic of modern Western culture (Burkitt and Trowell, 1975; Trowell and Burkitt, 1981). These include both benign and malignant diseases, and there is reason to believe that in some instances at least the latter may share some causative factors with the former.

Epidemiological and other evidence suggests that the following nonmalignant Western diseases are diet related: coronary heart disease (I.H.D.), gall stones, appendicitis, diverticular disease of the colon, diabetes, obesity, hiatus hernia, deep vein thrombosis, hemorrhoids, and varicose veins (Burkitt and Trowell, 1975; Trowell and Burkitt, 1981).

The malignant diseases that in like manner have their highest prevalences in economically more developed and affluent societies and their lowest in rural communities in the Third World include colorectal cancer, for which both causative and protective elements in diet have been suggested, and cancer of the breast, endometrium, and prostate, in which dietary factors may also play a causative role. Some explanation is demanded as to why these diseases, whether benign or malignant, tend to be associated with one another in their epidemiological features. Additional diseases characteristic of Western culture, whose causation still remain obscure, include multiple sclerosis, Crohn's disease, ulcerative colitis, and thyrotoxicosis.

III. SIGNIFICANCE OF RELATIONSHIPS

It is a fundamental principle that all the different results of a common cause, or of two or more related causes, tend to cluster together, and thus be interrelated. The frequency of each is maximum where the cause operates maximally and vice versa. This applies to the determinants of disease as well as to other cause and effect relationships (Burkitt, 1969). As mentioned above, the diverse effects of smoking, whether benign or malignant, tend to be associated with one another, whether in individual smokers or in communities of smokers.

When it is observed that two or more diseases tend to be associated in their geographical or cultural distribution, the possibility that they might share a common cause, which need not be a sole cause, must be seriously considered. Examples abound. Diverticular disease of the colon has never been observed to emerge in any community until several decades after appendicitis has emerged and become relatively common. Coronary heart disease has never been known to become a serious problem until several decades after diabetes has become common (Burkitt, 1976a). Postulated reasons for linking these diseases will be outlined below.

The discovery of Burkitt's lymphoma was initially a recognition of relationships. It was the realization that a number of neoplasms, hitherto considered to be different tumors, tended to occur together not only in individual patients but also in their geographical distribution that suggested they were all part of a single tumor process. Subsequently it was the relationship between the geographical distribution of this tumor and various nonmalignant diseases that threw light on the etiology of the condition. The relationships between its distribution and that of various insect-vector diseases initially suggested the possible role of a virus in its causation (Burkitt, 1962), with the resultant discovery of the Epstein-Barr virus, (Epstein *et al.*, 1964), and subsequently its relationship to holoendemic malaria (Kafuko and Burkitt, 1970) disclosed the role of immunodepression in its pathogenesis. Had the study been confined to cancer the clues to causation derived by studying nonmalignant diseases might never have emerged. We must view the problems we tackle initially through a wide angle rather than through a telephoto lens. The approach adopted in the study of Burkitt's lymphoma is surely applicable to other forms of cancer also.

The Western diseases enumerated above share a similar geographical, socioeconomic, and cultural distribution. They are more prevalent in affluent than in poorer communities, and in Africa and Asia they are commoner in urban dwellers and in more educated classes than in rural populations. They all increase in prevalence, although after differing lapses of time, following emigration from low-risk to high-risk situations. Of particular significance is the fact that prevalences are similar in Black and in White Americans today, and that second and subsequent generations of Japanese who have emigrated to Hawaii and California are at comparable risk to members of other ethnic groups in the host country, although these diseases were uncommon in Japan prior to World War II. Moreover there is no evidence that any of these diseases was other than relatively rare even in Western countries prior to the current century. These epidemiological features are shared by the forms of cancer that are common in Western countries, such as tumors of the large bowel, breast, endometrium, and prostate.

Although colorectal cancer has been most clearly related to patterns of eating, diet has also been incriminated in the causation of cancer of the breast (Tannenbaum, 1942) and has been hinted at as a cause of tumors of the prostate (Armstrong and Doll, 1975) and endometrium (Elwood *et al.*, 1977). Just as in the case of Burkitt's lymphoma, relationships between a number of different diseases in their geographical and socioeconomic distribution, and in some instances in individual patients, suggests some common or related causes (Burkitt, 1969).

The question must be asked, what are the changes associated with adoption of Western culture that might play a role in the causation of these diseases?

IV. INCRIMINATION OF DIET

All the nonmalignant Western diseases listed are related either directly or indirectly to the alimentary tract, and this is of course also true of colorectal cancer. There is no doubt that food consumed is the major factor influencing both the content and behavior of the gut, and consequently it is the most likely component of life-style to influence these diseases.

The main contrasts in dietary patterns between Third World countries with minimal prevalences of these diseases and more affluent societies who are at maximum risk are similar in nature to, but less in extent than, the differences between Western diets a century and more ago compared to those of today. Communities at greatest risk consume much more fat and sugar and much less starch and dietary fiber than do populations at minimal risk (Perisse et al., 1969). Similarly, Western diets today contain much more fat and sugar and much less starch and fiber from cereals and tubers than did those of a century and more ago.

Hypotheses have been postulated, backed by considerable evidence, that reduced fiber together with other factors contributes to the cause of I.H.D. (Trowell, 1975), obesity, (Haber et al., 1977), colorectal cancer (Wynder and Reddy, 1975), and possibly breast cancer (Tannenbaum, 1942). Dietary fiber on the other hand is probably protective against dental caries (Adatia, 1975), appendicitis (Burkitt, 1975b), colorectal cancer (Burkitt, 1971a,b; Cummings, 1982; Walker and Burkitt, 1976), and almost certainly against diverticular disease (Painter, 1975). There is now good evidence that fiber is protective against diabetes (Anderson and Ward, 1979), and it is likely to be protective against hiatus hernia (Burkitt, 1981), hemorrhoids (Thomson, 1975), varicose veins (Burkitt, 1976b), and even I.H.D. (Morris et al., 1977; Rydning et al., 1982).

Excessive sugar intake contributes to dental caries (Adatia, 1975) and, because it contributes to excessive energy intake, to obesity.

A high-fat diet is however almost invariably a low-fiber diet and vice versa, so that any causative properties attributed to the former are associated with the protective properties ascribed to the latter. Diets high in fat and low in fiber are epidemiologically associated with high prevalences of Western disease. The converse is also true.

The common causative factors shared by these different diseases could explain relationships between them as referred to above.

V. EVOLUTIONARY ADAPTATION

All biological species tend to wither and perhaps to die when placed in an environment to which they are not adapted. Man is not exempt. Western man has made greater changes in his dietary environment during the past 150–200 years, or 6–8 generations, than he has made during his whole existence on earth. These changes have fundamentally been a fall in starch and fiber consumption and an increased intake of fat, sugar, and salt (Perisse et al., 1969).

VI. WESTERN CANCERS AND WESTERN DIETS

A. Colorectal Cancer

The form of cancer that has been most specifically linked with Western diets is that involving the large bowel. All available evidence points to excessive fat in the diet as a causative factor (Wynder and Reddy, 1975) and adequate fiber as protective (Cummings, 1982; Burkitt, 1971b; Walker and Burkitt, 1976). Until recently, the former hypothesis was considered much the stronger, but during the last few years, the latter has been gaining increased acceptability.

The mechanisms whereby dietary fiber is believed to protect against bowel cancer can be summarized as follows:

1. *Dilution.* Fiber, and cereal fiber in particular, increases fecal bulk and thus dilutes any fecal carcinogens.

2. *Reducing contact time.* By hastening passage of bowel content, particularly through the colon, fiber reduces contact time between fecal carcinogens and the bowel mucosa.

3. *Altering pH.* By reducing fecal pH, fiber probably reduces bacterial degradation of cholesterol and primary bile acids into potential carcinogens. This has certainly been demonstrated in *in vitro* experiments (MacDonald *et al.*, 1978).

4. *Action of butyrate.* Fiber increases butyrate, which has been shown to protect cells from malignant transformation (Hagopian *et al.*, 1977).

5. *Availability of ammonia.* The proliferation of bacteria resulting from increased fiber intake uses up free nitrogen and thus reduces that available for ammonia formation. Ammonia is believed to increase susceptibility of cells to malignant transformation, so its reduction can be considered to be beneficial (Visek, 1972).

B. Breast Cancer

This neoplasm is approximately five times as common in Americans as it is in Africans, but the rates are comparable in Black and White Americans. Like colorectal cancer it is more common in economically developed countries. Epidemiologically high incidence rates are associated with high fat intakes and to some extent with obesity (Armstrong and Doll, 1975). Both high fat intake and deposition of fat in the body increase the development of breast cancer in experimental animals.

Another point that must not be forgotten is that over-nutrition in general has been shown in experimental studies to increase risk of developing a large variety of cancers (Tannenbaum, 1942). The evidence relating diet to cancer of the prostate is less clear.

The enormous possibilities of reducing cancer in Western countries by dietary changes is emphasized by the following quotation: "It is highly likely that the United States will eventually have the option of adopting a diet that reduces the incidence of cancer by approximately one-third, and it is absolutely certain that another third could be prevented by abolishing smoking" (National Research Council, 1982).

VII. RECOMMENDED CHANGES IN DIET

All communities studied that subsist largely on a diet dominated by starch foods retaining their fiber, and with low intakes of fat and sugar are at low risk of developing any of the characteristically Western diseases, and all communities consuming diets rich in fat and sugar and with low levels of starch and fiber appear to be at high risk. Not only does this apply geographically, but there is no evidence that these diseases were other than relatively rare even in Western countries when their diets contained less fat and more starch and fiber than is the case now. It must of course be emphasized that associations do not necessarily imply causative associations, but they enable the erection of hypotheses that can then be tested and either refuted or confirmed. There is much evidence to substantiate a causal relationship between these diseases and dietary factors. Seven Western nations, including the United States, have now published recommended dietary guidelines, all of which advise an increase in starch and fiber and a reduction in fat and sugar consumption.

It would consequently seem reasonable to recommend that both starch and fiber intake be approximately doubled, sugar consumption halved, and fat reduced by about one-third. Halving salt would also be beneficial because of its influence on hypertension.

This in practice would imply the following.

Eating much more bread, perhaps three times the present amount, but brown or preferably wholemeal in place of white.

Eating many more potatoes provided they are neither cooked in nor eaten with fat, and also eating more of other root vegetables and pulses.

Much less "red" meat should be consumed, since over 30% of even lean meat (unless fish or fowl) can be fat. An additional reason for reducing meat consumption is that over 20 units of energy must be fed to animals to produce 1 unit for human consumption, a situation difficult to justify in a starving world.

Fried foods should as far as possible be abandoned.

Fiber-rich breakfast cereals could with advantage be eaten in greater quantities.

The addition of millers bran, about 1 heaping tablespoonful, to the breakfast meal is a good cost-effective way of increasing fiber intake.

VIII. ACTION CONCURRENT WITH INVESTIGATION

There is a widely held opinion that recommendations regarding dietary and other changes in life-style that might prevent disease must await understanding of mechanisms involved and sufficient evidence to turn well-founded hypotheses into proved facts.

The continuing flood of unsubstantiated claims that are made for the therapeutic value of numerous fad diets not unnaturally fosters this caution. Nevertheless, when evidence as substantial as that which supports the dietary changes recommended in Section VII indicates advantages that are most unlikely to be offset by any significant disadvantages, withholding action seems illogical.

There would seem to be much to be gained and nothing to be lost by subscribing to these recommendations. This conviction in no way belittles the importance and urgency of investigations to substantiate or refute these claims and to discover mechanisms whereby individual dietary components or their interaction with one another play a protective or causative role in the pathogenesis of disease.

REFERENCES

Adatia, A. (1975). *In* "Refined Carbohydrate Foods and Disease" (D. P. Burkitt and H. C. Trowell, eds.), pp. 251–277. Academic Press, New York.
Anderson, J. W., and Ward, K. (1979). *Am. J. Clin. Nutr.* **32**, 2312–2321.
Armstrong, B., and Doll, R. (1975). *Int. J. Cancer* **15**, 617–631.
Bremner, C. G., and Ackerman, L. V. (1970). *Cancer* **26**, 991–999.
Bruce, W. R. (1983). *Proc. Int. Cancer Congr., 13th, 1982* (in press).
Burkitt, D. P. (1962). *Br. Med. J.* **2**, 1019–1023.
Burkitt, D. P. (1969). *Lancet* **2**, 1229.
Burkitt, D. P. (1971a). *JNCI, J. Natl. Cancer Inst.* **47**, 913–919.
Burkitt, D. P. (1971b). *Cancer* **28**, 3–13.
Burkitt, D. P. (1975a). *In* "Refined Carbohydrate Foods and Disease" (D. P. Burkitt and H. C. Trowell, eds.), pp. 87–97. Academic Press, New York.
Burkitt, D. P. (1975b). *In* "Refined Carbohydrate Foods and Disease" (D. P. Burkitt and H. C. Trowell, eds.), pp. 87–97. Academic Press, New York.
Burkitt, D. P. (1976a). *Can. Fam. Phys.* **22**, 63–71.
Burkitt, D. P. (1976b). *Arch. Surg. (Chicago)* **111**, 1327–1332.
Burkitt, D. P. (1981). *Am. J. Clin. Nutr.* **34**, 428–431.
Burkitt, D. P., and Trowell, H. C. (1975). "Refined Carbohydrate Foods and Disease." Academic Press, New York.

Cummings, J. (1982). *In* "Nutrition and Health" (M. R. Turner, ed.), pp. 35–48. M. T. P. Press Ltd., Lancaster, England.

Elwood, J. M., Cole, P., Rothman, K. J., and Kaplan, S. D. (1977). *JNCI, J. Natl. Cancer Inst.* **59,** 1055–1060.

Epstein, M. A., Achong, B. G., and Barr, Y. M. (1964). *Lancet* **1,** 702–703.

Haber, G. B., Heaton, K. W., Murphy, D., and Burrows, L. F. (1977). *Lancet* **2,** 679–682.

Hagopian, H. K., Riggs, M. G., and Swartz, L. A. (1977). *Cell* **12,** 855–860.

Hill, M. J., Morson, B. C., and Bussey, H. J. R. (1978). *Lancet* **1,** 245–247.

Kafuko, G. W., and Burkitt, D. P. (1970). *Int. J. Cancer* **6,** 1–9.

MacDonald, I. A., Webb, G. R., and Maloney, D. E. (1978). *Am. J. Clin. Nutr.* **31,** S233–238.

Morris, J. N., Marr, J. W., and Clayton, D. G. (1977). *Br. Med. J.* **2,** 1307–1314.

National Research Council (1982). "Diet, Nutrition and Cancer," Nat. Acad. Press, Washington, D.C.

Painter, N. S. (1975). "Diverticular Disease of the Colon." Heinemann, London.

Perisse, J., Sizaret, F., and Françoise, P. (1969). *FAO Nutr. Newsl.* **7,** 1–9.

Rydning, A., Berstad, A., Aadland, F., and Odegaard, B. (1982). *Lancet* **2,** 736–738.

Tannenbaum, A. (1942). *Cancer Res.* **2,** 468–475.

Thomson, W. H. F. (1975). *Br. J. Surg.* **62,** 542–552.

Trowell, H. C. (1975). *In* "Refined Carbohydrate Foods and Disease" (D. P. Burkitt and H. C. Trowell, eds.), pp. 195–226. Academic Press, New York.

Trowell, H. C., and Burkitt, D. P. (1981). "Western Diseases, Their Emergency and Prevention." Harvard Univ. Press, Boston, Massachusetts.

Visek, W. J. (1972). *Fed. Proc., Fed. Am. Soc. Exp. Biol.* **31,** 1178–1193.

Walker, A. R. P., and Burkitt, D. P. (1976). *Am. J. Dig. Dis.* **21,** 910–917.

Wynder, E. L., and Reddy, B. S. (1975). *JNCI, J. Natl. Cancer Inst.* **54,** 7–10.

2

Nutritional Considerations in the Epidemiology of Lymphoma

David T. Purtilo

Department of Pathology and Laboratory Medicine
University of Nebraska Medical Center
Omaha, Nebraska

I. INTRODUCTION

Differences in the geographic distribution of subtypes of malignant lymphoma (ML) offer clues to etiologic factors in lymphomagenesis. Comparisons in the frequency and sub-

11

Nutrition Factors in the Induction
and Maintenance of Malignancy

types of ML occurring in the United States, tropical Africa, and Japan suggest that ecogenetic factors (i.e., genetic and environmental) are determinants of lymphomagenesis. Table I summarizes a few risk factors and etiologic agents of lymphoma. No single factor or agent is capable of inducing ML. Exposure to certain agents impairs immune regulation, whereas other agents promote lymphoid proliferation. The ultimate step in lymphomagenesis may induce specific chromosomal damage and rearrangement. In this chapter ML is divided into Hodgkin's disease (HD) and non-Hodgkin's lymphoma (NHL).

One working model of lymphomagenesis considers that disregulated T cell immunity can lead to a hyperplastic proliferation of the lymphoid cells. For example, multiple factors can drive B cell proliferation (Fig. 1). A specific cytogenetic error is proposed to occur in one proliferating cell.

TABLE I

Risk and Postulated Etiologic Factors in Lymphomagenesis

Genetic
  Inherited immune deficiency, i.e., X-linked lymphoproliferative syndrome
  Inherited chromosomal breakage, i.e., ataxia telangiectasia
  Inherited immune regulatory defects, i.e., systematic lupus erythematosus
Inherited familial lymphoma, i.e., HD, NHL, all subtypes
Male predisposition is greater than female
Viruses
  Epstein-Barr virus, i.e., Burkitt's lymphoma, opportunistic ML
  Retrovirus human T cell leukemia virus, i.e., acute adult T cell leukemia
  Rubeola as cofactor in Burkitt's lymphoma
Immune deficiency
  Inherited, i.e., Wiskott-Aldrich syndrome
  Acquired, i.e., renal, cardia, thymic, bone marrow transplantation
Physical and chemical agents
  Radiation
  Benzene
  Asbestos
  Nitrates
  Dilantin
  Penicillin, i.e., angioimmunoblastic lymphadenopathy
Nutrition
  Bovine protein consumption in excess?
  Protein-calorie malnutrition, cofactor in BL?
Plant mitogen exposure
  Jackbean
Other
  Malaria
  Filaria
  Toxins

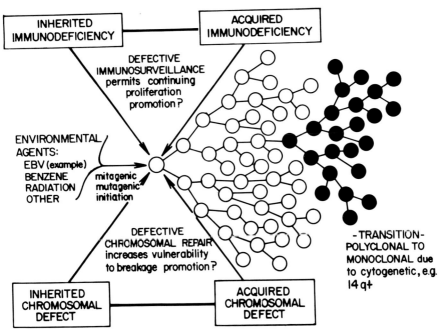

Fig. 1. Hypothesis regarding etiologic factors in lymphomagenesis. Both inherited and acquired immune deficiency and chromosomal breakage are important predisposing conditions. A specific cytogenetic change (i.e., 14q+) may convert a polyclonal B cell proliferation to a monoclonal malignancy.

This genetic change endows a cell with the ability to grow as a malignant clone. The altered cell has survival advantages that allow it to escape from immunoregulatory and other control mechanisms (Purtilo, 1981). This hypothesis has been developed by studying Burkitt's lymphoma in tropical Africa (Klein, 1979). More recently, Yunis *et al.* (1982) have described specific chromosomal alterations in other types of NHL.

II. TROPICAL AFRICA

The epidemiologic studies on lymphoma carried out by Burkitt (1958) serve as a model for studying lymphomagenesis. He had attributed the geographic clustering of Burkitt's lymphoma (BL) to a transmissible agent, possibly harbored by mosquitoes that preferred warm and moist habitats. Moreover, he noted holoendemic malaria overlapped the geographic distribution of BL. Epstein's studies led to the identification of a unique herpesvirus, Epstein-Barr virus (EBV) (Epstein *et al.*, 1964). Subsequent studies by G. Henle *et al.* (1968) revealed that this virus is the etiologic agent of infectious mononucleosis (IM). Nasopharyngeal carcinoma (Zur Hausen *et al.*, 1970) and a variety of lymphoproliferative diseases in immune compromised individuals have been associated with EBV (Purtilo, 1975; Purtilo and Klein, 1981).

Klein (1979) has postulated that three steps occur sequentially in Burkitt lymphomagenesis: (1) initiation of polyclonal B cell proliferation by EBV; (2) expansion of B cell proliferation under the mitogenic influence of malarial antigens; and (3) a specific cytogenetic alteration involving reciprocal translocations of material between the long arms of chromosomes 8 and 14, 14q+ (Fig. 2). Presumably, this specific cytogenetic translocation endows one cell with the capacity to outstrip host defenses. Thus a monoclonal tumor is established. Recently, Rowley (1982) has summarized the work from several laboratories indicating that karyotyped BL cells show specific chromosomal rearrangements involving translocations of materials at the breakpoint of immunoglobulin gene loci on chromosomes 14 (heavy chain), 22 (lambda), and 2 (kappa). The

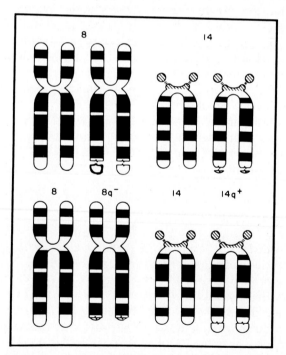

Fig. 2. Schematic of reciprocal translocation between chromosomes 8 and 14, i.e., t(8;14) resulting in 14q+. (From Merz, 1982. Copyright 1982, American Medical Association.)

specific translocation determines the immunoglobulin phenotype on the surface of the BL cells (Lenoir et al., 1982). The reapproximation of the genetic loci for immunoglobulin synthesis (on 14, 2 or 2) adjacent to an oncogene at the breakpoint on chromosome 8 is thought to promote oncogene expression; uncontrolled proliferation commences (Rowley, 1982).

III. IMMUNODEFICIENCY PREDISPOSES TO LYMPHOMAGENESIS

Immunoincompetence has not been sufficiently emphasized as a predisposing factor to Burkitt's lymphomagenesis. In tropical Africa several factors could act synergistically to produce immune deficiency to EBV: (1) infection occurs during early life (de-Thé, 1977); (2) males are predominantly involved (Purtilo, 1977); (3) the African child often shows borderline malnutrition (Purtilo, 1980), often the major source of calories is from cassava which may contain cyanide (Cock, 1982) or moldy maise containing aflatoxin; (4) chromosomal aberrations have been reported in lymphoid cells in children with protein–calorie malnutrition (Upadhyaya et al., 1975); (5) infection by measles (rubeola) can be chronic in malnourished children (Dossetor, 1976); and (6) malaria is immunosuppressive (Taylor and Siddiqui, 1982). All of these conditions can impair T cell function and could depress immune surveillance against EBV-infected B cells. Smoldering EBV infections have been detected in prospective studies in the West Nile region; BL evolves in 1/10,000 children at risk per year after approximately 2.5 years of increasing viral burden (de-Thé et al., 1978). In vitro studies may provide useful information regarding the influence of nutrition on activation of EBV in B cells.

IV. MODULATION OF EBV ACTIVITY IN VITRO

Normally, in vitro EBV pursues one of two alternate pathways: (1) The productive cycle leads to death of the cell following lysis. The initial transforming protein encoded by the virus is termed EB nuclear associated antigen (EBNA). It is seen in both the productive and nonproductive or proliferative B cells (Fig. 3). (2) In the productive pathway, viral synthesis produces early antigen (EA), and the viral capsid antigen (VCA) is formed as viral particles are assembled. Tumor-promoting chemicals can induce the viral productive cycle (Yamamoto et al., 1979). Alternatively, various vitamins including retinoic acid (Roubal et al., 1980) inhibit expression of EA in vitro.

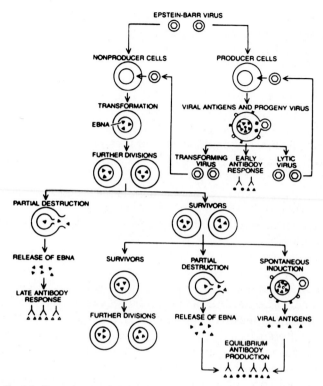

Fig. 3. Epstein-Barr virus molecular expressions in human B cells. Productive or lytic infection lead to cellular death, whereas nonproductive infection can lead to proliferation of transformed B cells. Both pathways begin when EBV infects B cells producing EB nuclear-associated antigen (EBNA). Productive infections proceed to elaborate early antigen (EA) and viral capsid antigen (VCA). (From W. Henle *et al.*, 1979, courtesy of *Scientific American.*)

Ito (1982) has proposed that various natural toxic plant substances, liberated in the oral cavity of African children, are responsible for inducing the viral cycle and thereby promote the development of BL in the jaws of African children. However attractive this model might appear, induction of the lytic cycle would favor death of the B cell and not lymphoproliferation. Malnutrition and the attendant immune deficiency might predispose to opportunistic infections and ML.

V. MALNUTRITION AND IMMUNE COMPETENCE

Good *et al.* (1982) have noted that nearly every aspect of the body's defense can be damaged by inadequate nutrition: antibody production, phagocytic function, inflammatory responses, complement function, and secretory and mucosal immunity. Thymus-based immune functions can particularly be depressed in individuals with protein–calorie malnutrition (PCM). Thymolymphatic atrophy and opportunistic infections are well known in children with profound PCM (Smythe *et al.*, 1971; Purtilo and Connor, 1975).

Objective measurements of the impact of malnutrition on immune function have been described recently by Chandra (1981). T cells numbered only 26% of lymphoid cells from malnourished children compared to 67% in controls. The T4 (helper/inducer) subpopulations numbered 15% compared to 41% for controls, and T8 (suppressor/lytic) subpopulations numbered 17.6% compared to 25% in normal controls. Nutritional therapy was capable of reversing the abnormal T cell subpopulations within 4 to 8 weeks. Purtilo *et al.* (1976) have demonstrated hyperimmunoglobulinemia of parasitized children with PCM. Information is almost nonexistent regarding the role of undernutrition on lymphomagenesis. However, addressed later is the association of overconsumption and a high incidence of ML (see Section VI,C and Fig. 4).

Correa and O'Connor (1973) found five gross differences in the distribution of lymphomas worldwide that might, in part, be attributable to nutritional differences: (1) tropical countries with epidemic proportions of Burkitt's lymphoma; (2) tropical countries where Burkitt's lymphoma was not excessive, with high proportions of Hodgkin's disease (HD) in children and low proportions in young adults; (3) tropical and subtropical countries with features of the second group but with additional high proportions of HD in young adults and high frequencies of the nodular sclerosis subtype; (4) affluent societies with a low incidence of HD in children, a predominance of nodular sclerosis, and frequent multiple myeloma; and (5) Oriental countries with a low frequency of HD and a high frequency of so-called "reticulum cell sarcoma" (tumors now regarded to be of lymphocyte derivation). Provocative differences in the epidemiology of malignant lymphoma in Japan and the United States prevail.

VI. LYMPHOPROLIFERATIVE DISORDERS IN JAPAN

A. Malignant Lymphoma in Japan

Meetings held during March 1981, in Honolulu, and in September 1982, in Seattle, concerned the differences in lymphocytic diseases in the United States and Japan (Miller *et al.*, 1981). In general, there is a reciprocal relationship between the frequencies of autoimmune disorders and malignant lymphoproliferative disorders in the two countries. Malignant lymphoma is rather uncommon, and autoimmune disorders are common in Japan. Binational differences between Japan and the United States with regard to lymphocytic diseases are noteworthy.

B. Deficiency of Lymphoproliferative Diseases in Japan

1. There is an absence of the early age peak of HD at 25–29 years (i.e., "Grand Tetons") age peaks in the United States.
2. Chronic lymphocytic leukemia is rare in Japan, versus 30% of all leukemias in American adults.
3. Follicular (non-Hodgkin's) lymphoma is almost absent in Japan.
4. Clinically apparent IM is rare. Silent EBV infection occurs in Japanese during infancy before the immune system has fully matured.

C. Excesses of Lymphoproliferative Diseases in Japan

1. Adult T cell leukemia clusters in eastern Kyushu and Okinawa, whereas this cancer is very rare in Western countries.
2. Kawasaki's disease (mucocutaneous lymph node syndrome) initially became epidemic in Japan and then appeared in other countries.
3. Subacute necrotizing lymphadenitis clusters in Hokkaido. About 70% of the patients are women 20 to 35 years of age.
4. Ill-defined lymphoproliferative/autoimmune disorders including Takatsuki's, Kimura's disease, Takayasu's, Hashimoto's thyroiditis, and systemic lupus erythematosus occur more commonly in Japan than in the United States (Miller et al., 1981).

Differences in socioeconomic, genetic, and cultural practices may account for the distribution of these disorders. A migrant effect is noted when Japanese people move to the United States and presumably adopt Western diets (Mason and Fraumeni, 1974). An increased frequency of lymphomas is found in migrants moving to the United States.

Diet is a determinant of the frequency and subtypes of malignant lymphoma. The consumption of animal protein, particularly bovine, has been suggested as a determinant of lymphomagenesis (Cunningham, 1976). The relationship between bovine protein consumption and the incidence of lymphoma deaths is shown in Fig. 4. Incidence of mortality from NHL and HD in the mid-1960s in the United States was 3.6 and 1.76 per 10^5, respectively. Cunningham's (1976) comparative study of 15 nations showed the United States to have the highest frequency of ML deaths and nearly the highest daily bovine protein consumption. Ap-

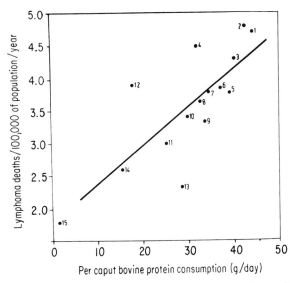

Fig. 4. Comparison of bovine protein consumption with incidence of non-Hodgkin's lymphoma. (From Cunningham, 1976, courtesy of the *Lancet*.)

proximately 25-fold more bovine protein is consumed in the United States compared to Japan. In experimental rats fed too much protein (Ross and Bras, 1965), a high frequency of lymphomas developed. Similarly, the same investigators found too little protein in diet produced lymphomas in the animals (Ross and Bras, 1973).

Armstrong and Doll (1975) have found impressive correlations with consumption of meat and colonic cancer and fat consumption with cancers of the breast and corpus uteri. These malignancies are less common in Japan than in the United States. Perhaps hyperlipidemia impairs immune response: Waddell *et al.* (1976) have depressed lymphocyte proliferation by hyperlipidemic plasma.

Recently, groups of American leukemia researchers led by Robert Gallo (Poiesz *et al.*, 1981) and Japanese investigators led by Yorio Hinuma *et al.* (1981) have identified a virus that may be responsible for adult T cell leukemia (ATL), which geographically clusters in southeast Japan. The retrovirus is termed human T cell leukemia virus (HTLV). In general, the Japanese experience more T cell lymphoproliferative malignancies than Americans. Tajima *et al.* (1981) have hypothesized that the limitation of HTLV to coastal regions in Kyushu is related to geographic isolation of the virus, malnutrition, and repeated exposure to filarial antigens. They also have noted familial aggregation of cases.

Curiously, along the Mediterranean coastal area of North Africa, αchain lymphoma can be identified in the intestine. This has been postulated to be due to chronic intestinal infestation with microbes (Ramot and Magrath, 1982). Nutrition is probably also important in the intestinal lymphomagenesis. For example, celiac disease is associated with a nearly 100-fold increased frequency of malignant lymphoma (Brandt *et al.*, 1978). These individuals have a hypersensitivity response to gluten. Hence, intestinal mucosa becomes damaged. Recently, we have identified, in patients with celiac disease and malignant lymphoma of the small intestine, abnormally elevated EBV-specific antibody titers and dysgammaglobulinemia (D. T. Purtilo, unpublished). These individuals are known to inherit a specific HLA DR3 haplotype which may predispose to abnormal immune responses to gluten (Mackintosh and Asquith, 1978).

While the incidence of malignant lymphoma, especially Burkitt's lymphoma, appears to be declining in some areas of tropical Africa, where there is malarial eradication, the incidence of ML in the United States appears to be increasing (Cantor and Fraumeni, 1980).

VII. MALIGNANT LYMPHOMA IN THE UNITED STATES

Many epidemiologic characteristics of the two large subgroups of ML, HD and NHL, occur in parallel in the United States. However, given that studies tend to consider only one group at a time, HD and NHL will be discussed separately here. The patterns of NHL mortality during the period of 1950 to 1975 in the United States show upward trends. The southern United States has the lowest incidence of NHL. Elevated incidence occurs in coastal California and in certain areas in the midwest. These differences in incidence are partly related to socioeconomic status; high incidence of NHL is related to high socioeconomic attainment. In countries where food packing and processing is a major occupation (i.e., sugar refining and canning of fruits, vegetables, and seafoods) incidence is high. Also highly correlated are fuel use and consumption of sugar, total fat, and eggs (Armstrong and Doll, 1975). Persons working in printing, publishing, and petrochemical industries, including rubber products and fabricated metal products, show less association with NHL (Cantor and Fraumeni, 1980).

The incidence of HD is correlated with socioeconomic class: recently Guttensohn (1982) showed Jewish families to be at highest risk. Both IM and HD occur predominantly in middle and upper class families showing high educational accomplishment.

Purtilo and Sakamoto (1982) have proposed that social class, age at

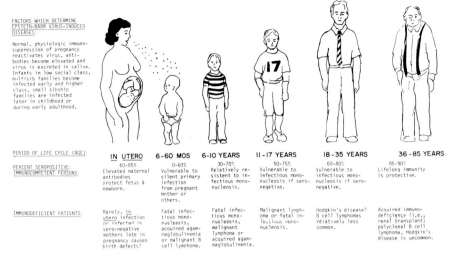

FACTORS WHICH DETERMINE
EPSTEIN-BARR VIRUS-INDUCED
DISEASES:

Normal, physiologic immunosuppression of pregnancy
reactivates virus, anti-
bodies become elevated and
virus is excreted in saliva.
Infants in low social class,
multisib families become
infected early and higher
class, small sibship
families are infected
later in childhood or
during early adulthood.

PERIOD OF LIFE CYCLE (AGE):	IN UTERO	6-60 MOS	6-10 YEARS	11-17 YEARS	18-35 YEARS	36-85 YEARS
PERCENT SEROPOSITIVE; IMMUNOCOMPETENT PERSONS:	60-85% Elevated maternal antibodies protect fetus & newborn.	0-60% Vulnerable to silent primary infection from pregnant mother or others.	30-70% Relatively re-sistent to in-fectious mono-nucleosis.	50-75% Vulnerable to infectious mono-nucleosis if sero-negative.	60-80% Vulnerable to infectious mono-nucleosis if sero-negative.	85-90% Lifelong immunity is protective.
IMMUNODEFICIENT PATIENTS:	Rarely, in utero infection or infected in sero-negative mothers late in pregnancy causes birth defects?	Fatal infec-tious mono-nucleosis, acquired agam-maglobulinemia or malignant B cell lymphoma.	Fatal infec-tious mono-nucleosis, malignant lymphoma or acquired agam-maglobulinemia.	Malignant lymph-oma or fatal in-fectious mono-nucleosis.	Hodgkin's disease? B cell lymphomas relatively less common.	Acquired immuno-deficiency (i.e., renal transplant) polyclonal B cell lymphoma, Hodgkin's disease is uncommon.

Fig. 5. Various outcomes of Epstein-Barr virus are determined by socioeconomics and the immunocompetence of individuals at various times in the life cycle. (From Purtilo and Sakamoto, 1982, courtesy of *Medical Hypotheses*.)

time of infection, and immune competence are determinants of clinical outcomes of EBV infections (Fig. 5). Upper socioeconomic individuals tend to be shielded from infections by viruses; however, when they occur the illness is often more severe.

Hodgkin's disease has been postulated to result from a slow viral infection or graft-versus-host-like disease (DeVita, 1973). Purtilo has postulated that the bimodal distribution of HD is due to genetic or environmental factors. The early peak is possibly predominantly due to inherited immune deficiency and viral infection. Bjorkholm (1978) has identified immune deficiency in patients and families with HD. Environmental factors may be responsible for the late peak (Olsson and Brandt, 1979; Purtilo, 1981). A high frequency of HD is found in elderly individuals employed in industries where exposure to petrochemicals occurs (Olsson and Brandt, 1979). If my hypothesis (Purtilo, 1981) is correct, then the lack of the early peak of HD in Japan would be due to absence of genetic factors responsible for predisposition to the malignancy at an early age. Japanese also seem to be very resistant to chronic lymphocytic leukemia (Miller *et al.*, 1981).

The aggregation of HD and certain leukemias in agricultural communities in the Midwest may be due to exposure to substances related to farming. The modern farmer can be exposed to literally tons of chemicals each year. Herbicides, pesticides, fertilizers, and insecticides are agents that could damage the immune system. In addition, the plant lectins, commonly employed in the laboratory to assess lymphocyte proliferative responses, may be mitogenic in the environment of the rural person. For example, HD clustered in a town of 1250 people in Michigan. A very large elevator storing navy beans produced a cloud of bean dust, during the harvest season, covering the houses with dust. The navy beans contain glycoprotein similar to phytohemagglutinin. These observations provoked formulation of a testable hypothesis. Plouffe *et al.* (1979) stimulated lymphocytes with extracts of navy bean. dust. The residents from the town showed increased levels of transformation as compared to nonresident controls who were not exposed to the bean dust.

Both experiments of nature and of man that impair cellular immunity are frequently associated with ML. We have identified EBV as an etiologic agent of NHL in individuals with X-linked lymphoproliferative syndrome (XLP) and renal transplant recipients (RTR) (Purtilo and Klein, 1981). More difficult to establish is the exact role of nutritional factors in lymphomagenesis. Thus, investigators have turned to experimental animal models to determine the impact of over- or under-nutrition on lymphomagenesis.

VIII. MALNUTRITION IN MURINE MODELS OF LYMPHOMAGENESIS

Good *et al.* (1982) have described enhancement of thymus-dependent immunity of underfed mice. Certain strains of short-lived mice prone to autoimmunity and lymphoproliferative disorders may show dramatic inhibition of disease by dietary restriction. In contrast, normal *ad libitum* diet may accelerate or exacerbate genetically determined diseases involving the immune system. Total calorie intake, protein, fat, and zinc may be key determinants of thymic immunity. For example, zinc deficiency can have a profound and lasting effect on the immunity in mice. Deprivation of zinc in pregnant mice induced immunodeficiency (Fig. 6), which persisted for 3 generations (Beach *et al.*, 1982).

Jose and associates (1970) demonstrated that moderately protein-deprived Australian aboriginal children showed impaired antibody production despite paradoxical enhancement of proliferative responses of lymphocytes to certain T cell mitogens. This paradox has been described in studies of animal models of PCM (Fernandes *et al.*, 1976). While B cell functions were impaired proportionally to the degree of dietary restriction, T cell functions were unchanged or even enhanced in mice,

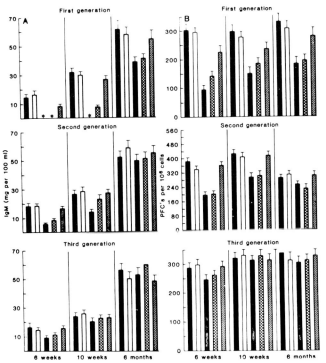

Fig. 6. (A) Concentrations of IgM in serum in F_1, F_2, and F_3 offspring of mice fed a diet moderately deficient in zinc during the last two-thirds of pregnancy and in controls, as determined by radial immunodiffusion. Solid bars represent control offspring of dams fed the 100 ppm zinc diet *ad libitum;* open bars, offspring of pair-fed controls; shaded bars, non-cross-fostered offspring of dams given the zinc-deficient diet; cross-hatched bars, offspring of zinc-deprived dams, cross-fostered to dams fed the 100 ppm zinc throughout pregnancy; and hatched bars, offspring of control dams fed *ad libitum,* cross-fostered to dams given the zinc-deficient diet. Asterisks indicate no IgM detectable. (B) Plaque-forming cell response to sheep erythrocytes in the F_1, F_2, and F_3 offspring. Response was determined 4 days after inoculation with 2×10^8 sheep red cells. (From Beach *et al.,* 1982, copyright 1982 by the American Association for the Advancement of Science.)

rats, guinea pigs, and in a few monkeys. Tumor immunity was also enhanced in nutritionally deprived animals. Mice and rats immunized with syngeneic, allogeneic, or xenogeneic tumors responded with normal or heightened killer T cell activity even when protein was reduced from 28 to 5% of the caloric content of the diet. Surprisingly, the cell-mediated tumor killing was preserved or even increased in deprived mice.

In contrast, dietary excess can lead to a rapid decline in thymus activities in murine strains genetically apt to develop autoimmunity and

lymphoproliferative diseases (Walford *et al.*, 1974). For example, restriction of total food intake or the fat component in hybrid (NXB×
NZW)F_1 mice inhibited the involution of thymic and T cell immunological function. Thus circulating immune complexes, anti-DNA antibodies,
and viral glycoproteins were reduced. In addition, mice of the MLR/lpr
showed inhibition of development of the autoimmune and lymphoproliferative disorders on diets with restricted total calories (Good *et al.*,
1982).

IX. HORMONAL AND ANTIGENIC STIMULI

Two additional features must be mentioned regarding lymphomagenesis: hormonal and chronic antigenic stimuli. Females show more
frequent autoimmune disorders and fewer malignant lymphomas than
do males (Purtilo and Sullivan, 1979). Studies of the NZB/NZW mouse
have demonstrated a possible reason for the marked female predominance of autoimmune and lymphoproliferative diseases (Talal, 1976).
Castration of the males at an early age leads to a high frequency of the
autoimmune-lymphoproliferative diseases. The implication is that es-
trogens or feminizing hormones promote autoimmune disorders.

A paradox of the immune surveillance hypothesis has been the failure
of the athymic nude mouse to exhibit a high frequency of malignancies.
However, nude athymic mice (Baird *et al.*, 1982) bearing tumor xeno-
grafts or carrying pinworms show stimulation of the lymphoid system.
Within a few days, the mice produce large amounts of murine leukemia
virus antigen, and lymphoma develops in approximately 1 month.

Difficulties prevail in the interpretation of the results of studies of the
experimental murine models of lymphomagenesis. Chronic antigenic
stimulation from allografted organs and/or parasites in the intestinal
tract or in blood (i.e., malaria, microfilaria) may promote viral on-
cogenesis, i.e., EBV induction of BL in Africa, and HTLV induction of
ATL in southern Japan.

X. SUMMARY AND CONCLUSIONS

Most malignant lymphoproliferative disorders arise from multiple factors impinging on the immune system. Immune dysregulation, hyperplasia of a cell type, and cytogenetic alteration could potentially spawn a
malignant clone of cells. Inherited (i.e., XLP) or acquired immunodeficiency (i.e., renal transplant recipients) to EBV predisposes to oppor-

tunistic ML carrying EBV. Comparative epidemiologic studies of tropical Africans, Japanese, and North Americans reveal striking contrast in the subtypes and frequencies of malignant lymphoproliferative disorders. Prevailing socioeconomic and cultural conditions probably determine the time of exposure to viruses and also the type of viruses the individuals encounter. For example, EBV tends to infect the African child early in life, whereas in western countries, exposure to this virus during adolescence or early adulthood often leads to IM. Human T cell leukemia virus is apparently restricted geographically, primarily to southern Japan, and thus adult T cell leukemia is unusually frequent there. The African child may be predisposed to developing BL due to relative immune deficiency associated with malnutrition, malaria, chronic measles infection, and the relative immune deficiency that males possess. *In vitro*, EBV can be activated to pass through its viral cycle with tumor-promoting agents or is inhibited in expression of early antigen by ascorbic and retinoic acids. Malignant lymphoma in the United States may be associated with excessive intake of protein, fat, and total calories. Murine models of lymphomagenesis suggest that restriction of caloric intake or fats can delay the development of autoimmune and lymphoproliferative disorders. Both genetic and environmental factors are determinants of lymphomagenesis in humans. Recognition of the environmental factors predisposing to lymphoma may allow prevention of ML.

ACKNOWLEDGMENTS

This work was supported in part by Grant CA30196-01 from the National Cancer Institute, the American Cancer Society Grant RD161, the Nebraska Cigarette Tax Grant LB506, and a grant from the Lymphoproliferative Research Fund.

REFERENCES

Armstrong, B., and Doll, R. (1975). *Int. J. Cancer* **15**, 617–631.
Baird, S. M., Beattie, G. M., Lannom, R. A., Lipsick, J. S., Jensen, F. C., and Kaplan, N. O. (1982). *Cancer Res.* **42**, 198–206.
Beach, R. S., Gershwin, M. A., and Hurley, L. S. (1982). *Science* **218**, 469–471.
Bjorkholm, M. (1978). *Scand. J. Haematol.* **33**, 1–74.
Brandt, L., Hagender, B., Norden, A., and Stenstam, M. (1978). *Acta Med. Scand.* **204**, 467–470.
Burkitt, D. P. (1958). *Br. J. Surg.* **46**, 218–223.
Cantor, K. P., and Fraumeni, J. F. (1980). *Cancer Res.* **40**, 2645–2652.
Chandra, R. K. (1982). *Nutr. Rev.* **39**, 225–231.
Cock, J. H. (1982). *Science* **218**, 755–762.

Correa, P., and O'Connor, G. T. (1973). *JNCI, J. Natl. Cancer Inst.* **50,** 1609–1617.

Cunningham, A. S. (1976). *Lancet* **2,** 1184–1186.

de-Thé, G. (1977). *Lancet* **1,** 335–338.

de-Thé, G., Geser, A., Day, N. E., Tukei, P. M., Williams, E. H., Beri, D. P., Smith, P. G., Dean, A. G., Bornkamm, G. W., Feorino, P., and Henle, W. (1978). *Nature (London)* **274,** 756–761.

DeVita, V. T. (1973). *N. Engl. J. Med.* **289,** 801–802.

Dosseter, J. F. (1976). *Brit. Med. J.* **2,** 1231.

Epstein, M. A., Achong, B. G., and Barr, M. (1964). *Lancet* **1,** 702–703.

Fernandes, G., Yunis, E. J., and Good, R. A. (1976). *Proc. Natl. Acad. Sci. U.S.A.* **78,** 1279–1283.

Good, R. A., West, A., Day, N. K., Dong, Z., and Fernandes, G. (1982). *Cancer Res.* **42,** 737s–746s.

Guttensohn, N. M. (1982). *Cancer Treat. Rep.* **66,** 689–695.

Henle, G., Henle, W., and Diehl, V. (1968). *Proc. Natl. Acad. Sci. U.S.A.* **59,** 94–101.

Henle, W., Henle, G., and Lennette, E. T. (1979). *Sci. Am.* **241** (July), 48–59.

Hinuma, Y., Nagata, K., Hanaoka, M., Nakai, M., Matsumoto, T., Kinoshita, K., Shirakawa, S., and Miyoshi, I. (1981). *Proc. Natl. Acad. Sci. U.S.A.* **78,** 6476–6480.

Ito, Y. (1982). *Adv. Comp. Leuk. Res., Proc. Int. Symp., 10th, 1981* pp. 559–560.

Jose, D. G., Welch, J. S., and Deherty, R. L. (1970). *Aust. Paediatr. J.* **6,** 192–202.

Klein, G. (1979). *Proc. Natl. Acad. Sci. U.S.A.* **76,** 2442–2446.

Lenoir, G. M., Preud'homme, J. L., Bernheim, A., and Berger, R. (1982). *Nature (London)* **298,** 474–476.

Mackintosh, P., and Asquith, P. (1978). *Br. Med. J.* **34,** 291.

Mason, T., and Fraumeni, J. F. (1974). *Lancet* **1,** 215.

Merz, B. (1982). *Med. News* **248,** 2424–2426.

Miller, R. W., Gilman, P. A., and Sugano, H. (1981). *JNCI, J. Natl. Cancer Inst.* **67,** 739–740.

Olsson, H., and Brandt, L. (1979). *Br. Med. J.* **2,** 580–581.

Plouffe, J. F., Silva, J., Schwartz, R. S., Callen, J. P., Kane, P., Murphy, L. A., Goldstein, I. J., and Fekety, R. (1979). *Clin. Exp. Immunol.* **35,** 163–170.

Poiesz, B. J., Ruscetti, F. W., Reitz, M. S., Kalyanaraman, V. S., and Gallo, R. C. (1981). *Nature (London)* **294,** 268.

Purtilo, D. T. (1975). *Lancet* **1,** 935–950.

Purtilo, D. T. (1977). *Semin. Oncol.* **4,** 335–343.

Purtilo, D. T. (1980). *Lancet* **1,** 300–303.

Purtilo, D. T. (1981). *Cancer Genet. Cytogenet.* **4,** 251–268.

Purtilo, D. T., and Connor, D. H. (1975). *Arch. Dis. Child.* **50,** 149–152.

Purtilo, D. T., and Klein, G. (1981). *Cancer Res.* **41,** 4209.

Purtilo, D. T., and Sakamoto, K. (1982). *Med. Hypotheses* **8,** 401–408.

Purtilo, D. T., and Sullivan, J. L. (1979). *Am. J. Dis. Child.* **133,** 1251–1253.

Purtilo, D. T., Riggs, R. S., Evans, R., and Neafie, R. C. (1976). *Am. J. Trop. Med. Hyg.* **25,** 229–232.

Ramot, B., and Magrath, I. (1982). *Br. J. Haematol.* **52,** 183–189.

Ross, M. H., and Bras, G. (1965). *J. Nutr.* **87,** 245–260.

Ross, M. H., and Bras, G. (1973). *J. Nutr.* **103,** 944–963.

Roubal, J., Luka, J., and Klein, G. (1980). *Cancer Lett.* **8,** 209–212.

Rowley, J. D. (1982). *Science* **216,** 749–750.

Smythe, P. M., Brereton-Stiles, G. G., Grace, H. J., Mafoyane, A., Schonland, M., Coovadia, H. M., Leoning, W. E. K., Parent, M. A., and Vos, G. H. (1971). *Lancet* **2,** 939–943.

Tajima, K., Tominaja, S., Shimiza, H., and Suchi, F. (1981). *Gann* **73,** 684–691.

Talal, N. (1976). *Transplant. Rev.* **31**, 240–263.

Taylor, D. W., and Siddiqui, W. A. (1982). *Annu. Rev. Med.* **33**, 69–96.

Upadhyaya, K. C., Verma, I. C., and Ghai, O. P. (1975). *Lancet* **2**, 704.

Waddell, C. C., Taunton, O. D., and Twomey, J. J. (1976). *J. Clin. Invest.* **58**, 950–954.

Walford, R. L., Liu, R. K., Gerbase-Delima, M., Mathies, M., and Smith, G. S. (1974). *Mech. Ageing Dev.* **2**, 447–454.

Yamamoto, N., Bister, K., and Zur Hausen, H. (1979). *Nature (London)* **278**, 553–554.

Yunis, J., Oken, M. M., Kaplen, M. E., Ensrud, K. M., Howe, R. R., and Theologides, A. (1982). *N. Engl. J. Med.* **307**, 1231.

Zur Hausen, H., Schulte-Holthausen, H., Klein, G., Henle, W., Clifford, P., and Santesson, L. (1970). *Nature (London)* **228**, 1056–1058.

3

Viral-Induced Changes in Metabolic Function and Nutritional Requirements of Cultured Human Cells

Fred Rapp

Department of Microbiology
The Milton S. Hershey Medical Center
The Pennsylvania State University
Hershey, Pennsylvania

Nutritional Factors in the Induction
and Maintenance of Malignancy

I. INTRODUCTION

The use of cell culture systems has dramatically influenced the development of the field of virology. Specifically, the ability to grow cells in culture has allowed the scientist to study in more detail the properties of viruses, of cells and of host-cell interactions. This chapter will focus on changes in the nutritional requirements and metabolic function of cultured human cells that are induced by virus infections.

Alexis Carrel (1928) said it all:

> It is certain that the modern methods, by which pure strains of given cell types are cultivated in flasks in a medium of known composition and maintained in a condition of measurable activity for long periods of time, will help to ascertain the nature and fundamental properties of viruses. A virus may be a very minute organism, or it may be a chemical substance manufactured by the cells themselves. In either case, its multiplication depends upon the activity of a living tissue. Since pure strains of cells are caused to live *in vitro* under such simple conditions that the effects of viruses on cell morphology and reactivity and the relation of the nature and metabolic condition of cells to the viruses may be analyzed, new discoveries will certainly be made.

Stated in 1928, it has taken a considerable period of time to achieve that goal, and the end of the road is not yet in sight.

II. USE OF CULTURED CELLS IN VIRUS RESEARCH

A. Historical Background

The early demonstration by Harrison (1907) that fragments of tissue could be maintained *in vitro* encouraged other scientists to experiment with tissue culture for the growth and study of viruses. As early as 1913, vaccinia virus was grown in rabbit and guinea pig cornea fragments (Steinhardt *et al.*, 1913). However, progress was very slow, since it was difficult to observe the effects of viruses in tissue and also because little was known about the nutritional requirements that were necessary to maintain the tissues and cells in culture. The use of cultured cells in virus research became indispensable after Enders and his colleagues observed in 1950 that polioviruses could be propagated successfully in cultures of human tissue of nonneural origin (Robbins *et al.*, 1950). Until that time, nervous tissue was thought to be the virus's primary target in the body. Thus, the long-held belief of virologists that viruses could be cultivated in the laboratory only in fragments of target tissue taken from the host was finally and firmly disproved.

For the past 35 years, tissue and cell cultures have been widely used in virology. Cells are most often grown as monolayers in bottles, tubes, or Petri dishes or in suspension. Different types of media have been developed to properly support the growth of cells.

Formerly, media used routinely for propagation of cells consisted of a balanced salt solution that was enriched with combinations of serum and embryo tissue extracts. However, the use of these complex solutions did not pinpoint the specific ingredients required for growth. This problem became less complex following the finding of Eagle (1955) that mouse L cells and human HeLa cells could be propagated in a medium containing a random mixture of amino acids, vitamins, carbohydrates, salts, and supplemented with serum. The deletion of just one of these components resulted in the early death of the culture, and more importantly, facilitated the determination of nutrients required for the growth and multiplication of mammalian cells in culture.

Media used most often by virologists include medium 199 (Morgan *et al.*, 1950) (Table I) and Eagle minimum essential medium (Eagle, 1959) (Table II). These fully synthetic media are usually fortified with serum and sometimes with various embryonic or yeast extracts or tryptose phosphate broth. Medium 199 contains many components because it was thought that as many nutritional factors as possible should be included in the media, although several components had no apparent effect. The rationale behind the development of synthetic medium was

TABLE I

Medium 199[a]

L-Arginine	DL-Glutamic acid	Uracil	*p*-Aminobenzoic acid
L-Histidine	DL-Aspartic acid	Thiamine	Vitamin A
L-Lysine	DL-Alanine	Riboflavin	Calciferol
L-Tyrosine	L-Proline	Pyridoxine	Menadione
DL-Tryptophan	L-Hydroxyproline	Pyridoxal	Desoxyribose
DL-Phenylalanine	Glycine	Niacin	Ascorbic acid
L-Cystine	Cysteine	Niacinamide	Glutathione
D-Methionine	Adenine	Pantothenate	Oleic acid
DL-Serine	Guanine	Biotin	Cholesterol
DL-Threonine	Xanthine	Folic acid	Sodium acetate
DL-Leucine	Hypoxanthine	Choline	L-Glutamine
DL-Isoleucine	Thymine	Inositol	Adenosine
DL-Valine	Adenylic acid	Ribose	triphosphate
Ferric nitrate			
α-Tocopherol phosphate			

[a] Morgan *et al.* (1950).

TABLE II

Eagle Minimum Essential Medium[a]

L-Amino-acids	Salts	Serum protein	Vitamins	Carbohydrate
Arginine	$CaCl_2$	Whole or	Choline	Glucose
Cystine	KCl	dialyzed serum	Folic acid	
Glutamine	$MgCl_2 \cdot 6H_2O$		Inositol	
Histidine	$NaHCO_3$		Nicotinamide	
Isoleucine	NaCl		Pantothenate	
Leucine	$NaH_2PO_4 \cdot 2H_2O$		Pyridoxal	
Lysine			Riboflavin	
Methionine			Thiamine	
Phenylalanine				
Threonine				
Tryptophan				
Tryosine				
Valine				

[a] Eagle (1959).

to synthesize an artificial medium in which the maintenance and multiplication of cell life was adequate. Synthetic media were designed to support the long-term growth of cells.

Serum supplementation was always required in the formulation of cell culture media in order to maintain long-term culture of cells. Studies conducted by Sato and his colleagues (Barnes and Sato, 1980a,b) investigated the hormone and growth factor requirements of many cell lines. These investigators have identified those substances that can be substituted for the growth-promoting activity of serum (Table III). These substances include peptides such as insulin and epidermal growth factor; steroids, such as hydrocortisone, testosterone, and progesterone; prostaglandins; and trace elements, such as cadmium and selenium. Most cell lines share a requirement for insulin and transferrin; however, individual cell lines may require specific components to support their growth. Sato and his group of researchers developed defined serum-free media that (1) promote growth comparable to that in serum-containing media, and (2) allow cells to maintain their differentiated characteristics (Bottenstein *et al.*, 1979; Barnes and Sato, 1980a). Recently, Sato and his colleagues have developed a serum-free medium that is supplemented with growth factors and supports the growth of lymphocyte hybridomas (Murakami *et al.*, 1982). They identified ethanolamine and phosphoethanolamine as necessary growth-promoting agents and found that they are required compounds for the growth of all hybridoma lines tested to date.

There are several advantages to using serum-free cell culture. They include (1) less expense, (2) better support for the survival and proliferation of certain cell types than serum-containing medium, (3) ability to select for a specific cell type in a mixture of cell types by manipulating the composition of the medium, (4) facilitation of studies on the interaction of hormones with cells, (5) ability to use new approaches for cell selection and somatic cell genetics, (6) ability to study nutrition and secretion at the cellular and molecular level, and (7) facilitation of new approaches in the recognition and treatment of proliferation and differentiation disorders (Barnes and Sato, 1980b).

A new development in the culture of human hematopoietic cells is the growth of human T lymphoblasts. Growth of these cells became possible by the addition of T cell growth factor (Morgan *et al.*, 1976; Ruscetti *et al.*, 1977), and several normal T cell lines and T cell lines derived from

TABLE III

Serum-Free Supplements to Medium[a]

Hormones and growth factors	Binding proteins
Insulin	Transferrin
Glucagon	Fatty acid-free BSA
Epidermal growth factor	Attachment and spreading factors
Nerve growth factor	Cold-insoluble globulin
Gimmel factor	Serum spreading factor
Fibroblast growth factor	Fetuin
Follicle-stimulating hormone	Collagen gel
Growth hormone	Polylysine coat
Luteinizing hormone	Low molecular weight nutrient factors
Thyrotropin-releasing hormone	H_2SeO_3
Luteinizing-hormone releasing	$CdSO_4$
hormone	Putrescine
Prostaglandin E_1	Ascorbic acid
Prostaglandin $F_{2\alpha}$	α-Tocopherol
Triiodothyronine	Retinol
Parathyroid hormone	Linoleic acid
Somatomedin C	
Hydrocortisone	
Progesterone	
Estradiol	
Testosterone	

[a] Bottenstein *et al.*, 1979; Barnes and Sato, 1980a.

patients with T cell malignancies have been established (Ruscetti *et al.*, 1977; Poiesz *et al.*, 1980a,b). This led to the isolation of the first human retroviruses (Poiesz *et al.*, 1980b, 1981; Yoshida *et al.*, 1982) and has enabled investigations into the distribution of these viruses and virus antibodies in the human population.

The availability of antibiotics to reduce bacterial contamination of cell cultures greatly advanced the progress of research. Also, of major significance, was the use of the enzyme, trypsin, to disperse cells. This method, originally described by Rous and Jones (1916) and adapted by Dulbecco (1952) for virological studies, facilitated the widespread use of cell culture in virology.

Virus research has flourished with the availability of cell and tissue culture systems. The use of quantitative techniques has enabled virologists to study the properties of viruses and their interactions with cells in greater detail. Many other fields have been affected positively by advances made in virology through the use of cell culture systems. Perhaps, the area on which it has made the most impact is infectious diseases: the development of vaccines and antiviral agents has significantly aided the control of virus-caused diseases throughout the world.

B. Isolation and Identification of Viruses

Cell culture systems are essential for detecting viruses because viruses can only be isolated from blood, urine, stool, throat swabs, lesions, autopsy material, and biopsies after inoculation of the material into cell monolayers or cell suspensions. The cell used for the culture is one that is sensitive to the virus being sought (Table IV). Usually, cultures are checked daily for the development of cytopathic effects and passaged into fresh cells. Serologic techniques are then used to identify the virus. When cytopathic effects do not occur, virus replication can often be detected by adding strains to the culture to reveal the presence of intranuclear or intracytoplasmic inclusions. Electron microscopy, hemadsorption, metabolic effects, and newer, more sophisticated molecular techniques also can be employed to detect the presence of a virus and to identify it. If virus is not detected early, prolonged passage may permit a gradual accumulation of the virus in culture until cytopathic effects can be observed.

The identification of a virus presents more difficulties than its isolation. Clues to virus identification are present in the cytopathic changes produced by many viruses (Syverton, 1957; Rapp and Melnick, 1966); the speed of cell changes and the type of change are often key factors in identification. However, certain viruses cause cytopathic effects in some

TABLE IV

Properties of Viruses in Cultured Human Cells[a]

Viruses	Sensitivity to human cells	Cytopathic effect	Morphologic transformation
DNA viruses			
Adenovirus	+	+	+
Herpes simplex	+	+	+
Pseudorabies	+	+	
Vaccinia	+	+	
Cytomegalo	+	+	+
Varicella	+	+	
Papovaviruses	+	+	+
RNA viruses			
Coxsackie	+	+	
Reovirus	+	+	
Influenza	+	+	
Newcastle	+	+	
Polio	+	+	
Rabies	+	±	
Vesicular stomatitis	+	+	
Measles	+	+	
Rous sarcoma	+	+	+

[a] Adapted from Bang (1966).

cells but not in others (Table V). One of the most impressive changes occurs when virus replication results in cell lysis (Reissig *et al.*, 1956). Specific types of cellular changes are characteristic of infection with certain viruses (Boyer *et al.*, 1957). For example, several viruses cause the formation of multinucleated giant cells in culture, including pox (Per-

TABLE V

Effect of Virus Infection on Host Cells

Effect on cells	Virus(es)
Death	Most viruses
Proliferation	Poxvirus, papovavirus, papillomavirus
Fusion resulting in multinucleate hydrid cells	Respiratory syncytial virus, measles virus, Sendai virus, herpesvirus
Transformation to malignancy	Polyomavirus, papovavirus, herpesvirus, adenovirus, retrovirus
No visible change for weeks	Rubella virus, some adenoviruses

eira, 1961), herpes B (Reissig and Melnick, 1955), herpes simplex (Hoggan and Roizman, 1959), varicella-zoster (Weller *et al.*, 1958), measles (Enders and Peebles, 1954; Seligman and Rapp, 1959), mumps (Henle *et al.*, 1954), parainfluenza (Marston, 1958), respiratory syncytial (Chanock and Finberg, 1957) and simian orphan viruses (Rustigian *et al.*, 1955). Simian virus 40 (SV40) produces cytoplasmic vacuolation in monkey cells (Sweet and Hilleman, 1960), although vacuolation is usually not observed in rhesus, baboon, or human cells. It is very important to realize that changes in cells due to virus infection may be helpful in determining the identity of the virus but are not pathognomonic.

III. NUTRITION OF CULTURED HUMAN CELLS

Carrel (1912) was the first to expound on the importance of considering the cell system and medium as a whole, each interacting with the other at all times. Lewis and Lewis (1912) worked diligently on the problem of totally defined environment for cell cultures and looked forward to the time when cell culture systems could be reproduced from

TABLE VI

Commonly Used Defined Media

Medium	Use	Reference
Medium 199	Primary chick embryo cells	Morgan *et al.* (1950)
Medium M150	Primary chick embryo cells	Morgan *et al.* (1955)
Basal medium	Human and mouse cell lines	Eagle (1955)
McCoy's 5A	Rat tumor cells	McCoy *et al.* (1959)
Minimum essential medium	Mammalian cell lines	Parker (1961)
CMRL 1066	Mouse cell lines	Parker (1961)
L-15	Human and mouse cell lines	Leibovitz (1963)
F-10	Diploid human and hamster cells	Ham (1963)
Nagle suspension medium	Mammalian cells in suspension	Nagle *et al.* (1963)
F-12	Diploid and established hamster and mouse cells	Ham (1965)
CMRL 1415	Primary mouse embryo cells	Healy and Parker (1966)
RPMI 1640	Human normal and leukemic cells, hamster tumor cells	Moore *et al.* (1967)
Nagle autoclavable	Mammalian cell lines in suspension	Nagle (1968)
7C's	Rat tumor cells	Ling *et al.* (1968)

TABLE VII

Nutritional Requirements of a Cell[a]

Essential amino acids	Vitamins	Salts	Other
Glycine	Thiamine hydro-	Sodium chloride	Dextrose
L-Lysine HCl	chloride	Potassium chloride	Buffer, pH 7.2
L-Methionine	Calcium panto-	Calcium nitrate	Phenol red
L-Threonine	thenate	Magnesium chlo-	Sodium hydroxide
DL-Valine	Riboflavin	ride	Hypoxanthine
L-Arginine HCl	Pyridoxine hydro-	Sodium phosphate	Glutamine
L-Histidine HCl	chloride	Potassium phos-	
L-Proline	Folic acid	phate	
DL-Isoleucine	Biotin	Sodium bicarbonate	
β-Phenyl-L-alanine			
L-Leucine			
L-Tryptophan			
L-Glutamic acid			
L-Aspartic acid			
L-Cystine			
L-Tyrosine			

[a] Waymouth (1955).

laboratory to laboratory. The development of chemically defined media (Table VI) immensely aided the progress of virus research; however, it is critical to remember that although conditions are now standardized, they are nonetheless artificial and that no "normal" condition of cells in culture exists.

The nutrition of a cell refers to the nutrients that are essential for its growth (Waymouth, 1957). Metabolism, a chemical and physical process that occurs continuously within a cell, involves the buildup and breakdown of nutrients used by the cell (Lwoff, 1957; Waymouth, 1957). What are the nutritional requirements of a cell (Table VII)? This question is difficult to answer because considerations have to include whether the needs of the cell population are for indefinite survival, for active proliferation, or for a specific function such as the production of a characteristic secretion. A clear statement on the role of nutrition in cell culture was made by Knight (1945). He said,

> . . . a given substance, required as a component of one of the essential metabolic processes, might appear in three different roles . . . (1) as an "essential nutrient," when its rate of synthesis by the cell was so slow as to be unsignificant; (2) as a growth stimulant, when its rate of synthesis was somewhat

faster but still slow enough to be a limiting factor; or (3) as a substance not required at all for nutrition, because the cell could synthesize it so fast that it was not a limiting factor in growth. It is the metabolic process which is the essential thing.

IV.   METABOLISM OF VIRUS-INFECTED CELLS

When a virus infects a cell, dramatic changes usually occur in the metabolism of the cell. These viral-induced changes often reorient the cell's metabolic machinery toward the production of viral components. Sometimes a virus can induce cells to produce the enzymes it needs for multiplication.

In cultured cells, the study of metabolism is usually limited to the processes involved in energy transfer or in the synthesis of various substances. The metabolic effects of viral infections, however, can range from relatively minor changes in physiological activity to cell death and from a striking increase in the number of normal cells to the transformation of normal cells into malignant ones.

When an animal virus infects a cell *in vivo* or *in vitro,* several changes in the physiology of the cell can result. These changes may be manifested by (1) accelerating functions, such as DNA replication and cell division; (2) discontinuing the biosynthesis of the cell's products with resultant cell death; (3) heritably changing the biochemical properties of the cell and its potential for growth; or (4) exhibiting no effect on cellular functions or biosynthetic capacity at all. Which form the cell's response will take depends on the interaction(s) between viral gene products and the genetic and biosynthetic capabilities of the cell. The mechanisms that control the cell's response to virus infection are not yet understood.

V.   EFFECTS OF METABOLIC CHANGES ON CELL GROWTH

A.   Acceleration of Cellular Functions

A fine example of virus infection responsible for the stimulation of specific cellular functions is the ability of simian virus 40 (SV40) and polyoma virus to stimulate the synthesis of several cellular enzymes used in the biosynthesis of deoxypyrimidines and DNA replication. Although SV40 stimulates the specific activities of many cellular enzymes, there are other cellular enzymes, such as dAMP kinase, that are not stimulated; thus the process is a selective one. Evidence suggests that

RNA and protein synthesis are required for the increase in the specific activity of the cellular enzymes after virus infection. Similar results have been obtained following adenovirus infection, and Rous sarcoma virus, a retrovirus, can selectively stimulate the transcription of certain fetal genes but not the same type of adult genes.

B. Cessation in Biosynthesis of Cell Products

Infection with viruses (e.g., adenoviruses, herpesviruses, poxviruses, picornaviruses, diplornaviruses, togaviruses, and rhabdoviruses) can result in the inhibition and ultimately the cessation of cellular biosynthetic processes. Apparently, virus functions are required for the cessation of cellular DNA, RNA, and/or protein synthesis. In some cases, virus proteins are directly involved in the cessation of cellular functions, although under other circumstances, a virus gene product must be synthesized in order to affect the host.

C. Heritable Changes in Biochemical and Growth Properties

Certain DNA-containing viruses (papovaviruses, adenoviruses, herpesviruses, poxviruses) and the RNA-containing retroviruses have all been shown to transform cells in culture and to produce tumors in appropriate animal hosts. How these cells are transformed is still unclear, but the biochemical changes in these virally altered cells are profound. The enhanced growth potential of virus-transformed cells is another interesting dimension to be considered.

D. No Changes in Cellular Function

Some viruses (myxoviruses and retroviruses) infect cells but do not destroy them. A myxovirus infection can produce an alteration in the host cell, but cell death does not result. Sarcoma viruses are particularly intriguing because they can produce biochemical and morphological changes in the host cell and bestow new growth potential without affecting the viability of the cell. It is still not clear how such dramatic changes can take place in the host with so little trauma to the host cell.

What actually happens when a virus infects a cell? First, there are mechanisms that will either inhibit or stimulate necessary host cell functions. Then, the activity of certain enzymes will often increase. This can result from virus-coded enzymes and also by increases in the synthesis of cellular enzymes. The presence of virus in the cell may also explain why a greater portion of cell DNA is expressed early in the infection, as compared to uninfected cells. There are also major immunological changes in virus-infected cells: specifically, new antigenic determinants are present on the cell surface and cells become more agglutinable by concanavalin A.

Some viruses are capable of stimulating the synthesis of several enzymes the cell uses to replicate DNA, whereas other viruses inhibit this synthesis to a pronounced degree. Still others have no observable effects whatsoever. However, most DNA-containing viruses (and some retroviruses) can transform cells in culture and produce tumors in an appropriate host animal. These virus-transformed cells not only undergo many biochemical and immunological changes but acquire new dimensions of growth manifested by changes in cell morphology and immortality.

VI.   MALIGNANT TRANSFORMATION OF CELLS IN CULTURE

Many viruses have been used to transform a variety of animal cells *in vitro*. Cells derived from rodent and avian species have been used most often, but human and monkey cells have also been employed. For virus transformation to occur, it is necessary that the cell be nonpermissive for virus replication or that the virus be rendered unable to cause cytopathology, if virus multiplication causes cell destruction. The problem of cytopathology is greater for DNA-containing oncogenic viruses than for RNA-containing oncogenic viruses (Rapp, 1973).

Virus-transformed cells develop properties (Table VIII) that are more typical of cultured tumor cells than of cultured normal cells. As a result, cells transformed by viruses in culture systems are now used to study the process of tumor initiation. The properties of virus-transformed cells include change in cell morphology, loss of contact inhibition, alteration in growth rate, greater ability to survive extended culture *in vitro*, ability to grow in soft agar, reduction in serum requirements, alteration in surface properties, development of karyotypic abnormalities, ability to form tumors in receptive animals, presence of virus-specific functions, and increased resistance to superinfection by the transforming virus (Rapp and Westmoreland, 1976).

There are several biological properties characteristic of transformed cells in culture; none is a necessary or sufficient criterion for transformation, and many are secondary to the transforming event. Nevertheless, much effort has been expended on comparing the properties of cells transformed by DNA viruses with those of cells transformed in other

TABLE VIII

Properties of Virus-Transformed Cells

Change in morphology
Loss of contact inhibition
Alteration in growth rate
Enhanced ability to survive extended culture *in vitro*
Ability to grow in soft agar
Reduction in serum requirements
Alteration in surface properties
Development of karyotypic abnormalities
Presence of virus-specific functions
Increased resistance of the cell to superinfection
Ability to form tumors in susceptible hosts

---

ways, and trying to determine whether any of the observed similarities and differences are significant.

Transformed cells frequently have an abnormal morphology that may be determined, at least in part, by the transforming virus. For example, hamster and mouse cells transformed by polyoma virus tend to be spindle shaped and form swirls in culture, whereas cells transformed by SV40 frequently have a more epithelioid appearance. Colonies of cells that have been doubly transformed by SV40 and polyoma virus, and that have tumor (T) antigen and transplantation-specific tumor antigen (TSTA) specified by both viruses, have morphological features characteristic of both types of virus transformation. Similarly, cells transformed by PARA (SV40)–adenovirus hybrids often appear intermediate in appearance between the larger epithelioid morphology characteristic of SV40 transformation, and the small, rounded, densely packed epithelioid cell with little cytoplasm that is typical of adenovirus transformation. The morphology of transformed cells can revert to a more normal appearance under certain environmental conditions [such as growth at elevated temperature in the case of cells transformed by temperature-sensitive (ts) mutants or negative selection using fluorodeoxyuridine, colchicine, low serum, or concanavalin A] and may be a function of intracellular levels of cyclic AMP.

The observation that Epstein-Barr virus (EBV)-lymphoid cells hybridized to other human cells form multilayered foci in culture is dramatic because the ability to pile up into dense colonies is a characteristic feature of the growth of transformed cells and one that has frequently been exploited in the isolation of transformed cells. The failure of normal cells to pile up is frequently ascribed to contact inhibition, since it was at one time believed that when two cells came in contact, there was mutual inhibition of division and movement. At one time, transformed cells were defined as being less sensitive to contact inhibition, and therefore able to grow to high saturation densities. It is now clear that the situation is far more complex. Although cell contact is important, especially in inhibition of movement, factors in the medium (such as pH and serum concentration) are probably of much greater significance in determining cell division. Transformed cells generally have less stringent requirements for growth factors in the medium and, as a result, are less susceptible to starvation in dense culture. Although the insensitivity of transformed cells to controls that regulate normal cell multiplication is probably their most significant property in terms of malignancy, little is known of the signals involved in normal growth regulation, and still less is known about the lesion(s) permitting transformed cells to become unresponsive to them. Recently, the role of cyclic AMP and other nucleotides in growth control has received considerable attention. However, the means by which intracellular levels of cyclic AMP (which do correlate with cell division and other biological properties such as differentiation) are regulated are themselves largely obscure. Normal epithelioid and fibroblastoid cells cannot grow in liquid suspension and do not form colonies in soft agar as do cells transformed by polyoma, SV40, adenovirus, and herpes simplex virus (HSV) types 1 and 2 (HSV-1 and HSV-2, respectively).

Another property frequently utilized in the isolation of virus-transformed cells is their capacity for growth in continuous culture. Although it was earlier believed that cultures of normal cells could potentially replicate indefinitely, this is no longer held to be true, and only a rare "spontaneous" transformant is thought to have the ability to grow indefinitely *in vitro*. For a cell line to be defined as "transformed," it is usual to demonstrate survival in culture beyond the level at which control cultures have senesced. The property of prolonged life *in vitro* has been particularly useful in the isolation of HSV-transformed cells in which there is no known transformation-associated marker, i.e., the T antigen commonly observed in papovavirus and adenovirus systems.

Virus-induced changes in the cell membrane are potentially significant if the cell survives infection and divides, passing virus-specified membrane changes on to subsequent generations of cells. Cell behavior is governed by stimuli from the environment transmitted via the plasma membrane; thus, any alteration in the membrane may prevent the cell from responding appropriately to such stimuli. Malignant transformation is often regarded as a consequence of a breakdown in the cell's ability to respond to its environment; hence, there have been many investigations into possible differences between the membrane of normal and transformed cells.

A decrease in cell glycosyltransferase activity after transformation, leading to a simplification of membrane glycolipids has been detected in polyoma virus- and SV40-transformed cells. Cells transformed by SV40 or polyoma virus also apparently have shortened glycoprotein carbohydrate chains. Similarly, a block in the biosynthesis of complex glycolipids has been reported in malignant, but not nonmalignant, HSV-2-transformed hamster cells. An increase in the production of exogenous sialidase has been described for oncogenic HSV-2-transformed cells, and this may be responsible for a breakdown of membrane gangliosides in these cells.

It seems most likely that many of the observed differences between normal and transformed cells are consequences of the abnormal growth properties of the latter. Alterations observed in the pattern and synthesis of gangliosides in papovavirus transformed cells were not observed in spontaneously transformed or lytically infected cells, and their significance is not clear. Emmelot (1973) proposed that the configuration of membrane components is of greater importance than membrane composition in determining growth patterns. Some support for configurational changes in the membrane of transformed cells has been provided by the work of Nicolson (1971, 1974), who proposed that the increased agglutinability and sensitivity to toxic effects of plant lectins, such as concanavalin A, are not due to an increase in the number of lectin-binding sites on these cells, but rather to the clustering of existing sites into localized patches to which lectins can bind more easily. In malignant transformation, such clustering may result from chemical changes within the membrane, or from the insertion of virus-induced products that act as a nucleus for the aggregation of lectin-binding sites. Most of the studies on plant lectin binding by transformed cells have involved papovavirus-transformed cells or, more rarely, retrovirus-transformed or spontaneously transformed cells; concanavalin A agglutination by adenovirus-transformed cells also has been described. Plant lectin binding by HSV-transformed cells has not been studied in depth, but experiments in this laboratory have suggested that many HSV-transformed lines do not have a high concanavalin A binding capacity.

Deviations from a normal diploid karyotype are rare in cultures of primary cells or cells at low passage levels. In contrast, transformed cells frequently have a variable degree of aneuploidy and marker chromosomes. Many viruses, including members of the papovavirus, adenovirus, and herpesvirus groups, cause severe chromosomal damage during the course of lytic infection. These lesions do not seem to be related to those observed in transformed or tumor cells in any specific way; indeed, much of the chromosome damage in virus infections appears to be random. Exceptions to this include adenovirus 12-induced breaks on human chromosomes 1 and 17, SV40 lesions on acrocentric chromosomes, and HSV-induced breaks on at least four human autosomes. The best studied of these effects is the break in chromosome 17 in adenovirus 12-infected human cells. The human gene for thymidine kinase (TK) is known to be carried on this chromosome and, moreover, adenovirus 12 induces human TK early in infection.

Chromosome abnormalities are detected in SV40-transformed cells after they have developed abnormal growth properties but before the establishment of transformed cell morphology. Although the observed abnormalities do not appear entirely random, no typical karyotype for SV40-transformed cells can be described, and the extent to which chromosome damage occurs depends on the host cell. Polyoma virus transformation of hamster cells leads to a similar sequence of events with chromosome abnormalities increasing with the age of the transformed culture.

Chromosome analysis of hamster cells transformed by HSV and cytomegalovirus (CMV) demonstrates that those cells have an abnormal but stable karyotype. It is almost certain that the karyotypic abnormalities in transformed cells are secondary phenomena due to cell selection during prolonged culture. It can be anticipated that any chromosome aberration resulting from virus integration or virus-controlled gene expression, which might play a role in initiation of transformation, will be far more subtle and is probably masked by subsequent extensive karyotypic changes as the transformed clone becomes established.

The phenomenon of cell transformation assumes much greater significance when the relationship between transformation and malignancy is considered. However, this relationship is not precisely defined because the situation within an intact animal is far more complex than that in cell culture. Nevertheless, it is clear that the transformed cell and the tumor cell are both released from normal growth controls. When cultured *in vitro*, tumor cells have many properties in common with transformed cells, while transformed cells frequently grow as tumors when transplanted to susceptible hosts. Agents known to be oncogenic, whether viral or chemical, are frequently able to transform cells to malignancy *in vitro*. For this reason, demonstration of the ability of a virus to transform cells, particularly if the transformed cells can be shown to be oncogenic, provides at least circumstantial evidence that the virus has the potential to induce tumors under natural conditions.

Cells transformed by SV40, polyoma virus, or adenovirus rarely contain virus capsid antigens. This is not unexpected since virion antigens are produced late after virus DNA synthesis, and all evidence indicates that virus DNA synthesis and late protein production are incompatible with cell survival, and hence transformation. Those herpesviruses whose biological cycle has been studied do not show a marked shift from early pre-DNA synthesis–transcription to late post-DNA synthesis–transcription. Almost the entire genome seems to be transcribed and translated early in infection, and empty virus nucleocapsids can be made in the absence of DNA synthesis. Control of transcription appears to be a quantitative rather than a qualitative sequence of events. Thus, it is conceivable that virus structural proteins may be produced in transformed cells that do not synthesize virus DNA or infectious progeny. There is as yet no evidence as to the nature of the virus-specific cytoplasmic antigens observed in HSV-transformed cells. Further evidence that HSV-transformed cells can express virion antigens is provided by the observation that animals bearing tumors induced by these cells develop specific neutralizing antibodies to the transforming virus. Animals bearing tumors induced by non-virus-producing SV40-transformed cells develop antibodies to SV40 T antigen but do not produce virus-neutralizing antibody. The production of neutralizing antibody by animals bearing HSV tumors may be due to recognition by the host of virus-specific membrane antigens on some HSV-transformed lines.

Virus-specific TK has been demonstrated in mouse L cells biochemically transformed from TK negative (TK^-) to TK positive (TK^+) by HSV. The enzyme is believed to be virus specific because its kinetics of heat inactivation are similar to those of the enzyme from virus-infected cells, and the electrophoretic mobility resembles that of the virus enzyme. The regulation of its expression, unlike that of the cell enzyme, does not appear to be coordinated with the cell cycle and is inducible by superinfection of cells with TK^- HSV-1. The presence of at least one other HSV-specific antigen in the biochemically transformed TK^+ cells has been demonstrated by immunodiffusion.

The origin of TK expressed in rat cells transformed by HSV is more equivocal. Initially, the enzyme appeared to be virus specific. However, the cells lost the virus TK on passage, and a TK with the properties of a normal cellular enzyme reappeared. It has been suggested that derepression of host TK was facilitated by the initial presence of the virus enzyme. This probably enabled the functionally TK^- cell to survive a few generations in HAT medium, during which time the normal cell TK could be switched-on.

L(TK^+) cells, which are biochemically transformed by HSV, maintain the expression of virus-specific TK. In these cells the host gene for TK has been lost and, thus, is not available for derepression. The rat cells transformed by HSV persistently carry what appear to be virus type-specific proteins, and it may be that the virus TK gene is not lost but that its expression is suppressed. Under different selective conditions, HSV-infected L(TK^+) cells can suppress or lose the virus gene for TK.

Retroviruses have been implicated in the malignant diseases of several animal species for more than 70 years, and are primarily of the type C group (Bishop, 1982). The first breakthrough associating a retrovirus with the initiation of cancer occurred in 1951, when Gross (1951) demonstrated that newborn mice with a low incidence of leukemia developed the disease after inoculation with cell-free extracts from mice that developed leukemia early in life and at a high frequency. Earlier attempts to transmit leukemia in mice with filtered extracts had failed because the recipient animals had been adult mice. Similar studies with cell-free extracts have since demonstrated that cat leukemia, bovine leukemia, and lymphosarcomas of northern pike and gibbon apes are also transmissible. Type C virus particles can be detected in these tumor cells.

Retroviruses associated with the etiology of cancer differ from DNA viruses in two major ways. Retroviruses have considerably less genetic information in the virus genome (Bishop, 1978), and this small genome has enabled investigators to learn much about its structure and function. Second, retroviruses can replicate without causing cell injury or death. Thus, in contrast to DNA viruses that require restriction of virus replication for transformation to occur, some retroviruses replicate and transform simultaneously. The retrovirus genome contains at most four different genes and a "common" (C) region. The *gag* gene codes for a precursor, which is cleaved to yield four internal structural proteins of the virion. The *pol* gene codes for virion reverse transcriptase, the *env* gene for virion envelope glycoproteins, and the *onc* (or *src*) gene for the transformation-related protein. One current theory is that the *src* gene was added to the virus genome during evolution as a result of recombination with host cell information. Similar host cell sequences are designated *sarc*. The C region is found in most retroviruses, but is not identified as a fifth gene because no mRNA or gene product for the C region has been detected.

The avian sarcoma viruses, Rous sarcoma (RSV), and B77 are the only retroviruses that possess and express all four genes. They are not defective for replication and can transform cultured fibroblasts and other cells. Through the use of mutants defective in the transforming (*src*) gene, the product of the gene has been isolated and characterized. The *src* protein is a phosphorylated protein with a molecular weight of 60,000 and protein kinase activity (Brugge and Erikson, 1977; Collett and Erikson, 1978).

The amount of phosphorylated tyrosine within cells increases tenfold as a result of transformation by *src* (Hunter and Sefton, 1980). pp60[src] is unusual in that most protein kinases phosphorylate the amino acids serine and threonine. Since the function of pp60^{src} became known, it has been demonstrated that phosphorylation of tyrosine may have a role in the regulation of normal cell growth. The finding that pp60^{src} protein kinase activity is temperature sensitive when isolated from virions of a ts transformation mutant of RSV suggests that phosphotransferase plays a role in transformation by this virus (Sefton *et al.*, 1980). A single protein kinase could generate the cellular changes associated with transformation either by interacting directly with a single primary target that subsequently induces multiple changes or by acting on several different primary targets.

The significance of phosphotransferase activities became even more apparent with the finding that other retroviruses possess proteins with this enzymatic activity. Not only are these proteins similar in enzymatic activity, but they also are similar in their compartmentalization within the cells, a factor that may be highly significant in determining their function. The bulk of pp60^{src} accumulates as the inner surface of the plasma membrane during transformation by avian sarcoma virus. Location at the cell surface would be important if the protein kinases interact with the cytoskeleton or with receptors for cell growth factors or if they affect the ability of cells to adhere to surfaces. Any or all of these cellular elements participate in the conversion of the normal cell to the cancer cell. A protein extremely similar in size and chemical structure has been found in significantly reduced quantities in normal chicken, rodent, amphibian, fish, and human cells. This protein, denoted pp60^{sarc}, also catalyzes the phosphorylation of tyrosine. Detection of pp60^{sarc} in normal cells further suggests that proteins of this nature are significant in differentiation and growth control.

In contrast to the avian sarcoma viruses, all mammalian sarcoma viruses are defective for replication. This group includes Moloney, Kirsten, and Harvey murine sarcoma viruses and feline sarcoma virus. The mammalian sarcoma viruses rapidly cause a variety of sarcomas *in vivo* and can transform cells *in vitro* even though they do not possess the *src* gene or any sequences related to the *src* gene. All known sarcoma viruses of feline origin have been isolated from naturally occurring sarcomas in outbred cats.

VII. FUTURE EXPECTATIONS

The characterization of virus genes involved in changing the normal cell to a malignant phenotype was preceded by observations that enabled investigators to transfer DNA from viruses to cells and subsequently from cell to cell. This has most recently resulted in the transfer of DNA from tumor cells growing in culture to cells that are not yet changed to a malignant phenotype (Cooper *et al.*, 1980; Perucho *et al.*, 1981; Shih *et al.*, 1981; Shilo and Weinberg, 1981). The cell that has been most useful is the NIH 3T3 cell, although it is reasonably certain that in the future other cells will be found that can be utilized for experiments of this type. DNAs from human and experimental tumor cells yield foci of NIH 3T3 cells that have been "transfected" with the tumor cell DNA. While objections have been raised that the 3T3 cells are not normal and are already committed to growth in culture, they nevertheless offer an experimental system to test the DNA from a variety of tumor cell lines for ability to further enhance the growth of the 3T3 cells (i.e., ability to grow as foci in soft agar). Experiments of this type have yielded so-called "oncogenes" from a number of tumor cell lines established from a variety of human tumors. Since the homologs of these genes also appear to be in normal human cells and since expression of the genes introduced into the NIH 3T3 cells does not appear to increase (as it does when the *src* gene of the avian or mouse viruses is used), the reasons for such a change in cell phenotype seem mysterious. However, recent papers (Reddy *et al.*, 1982; Tabin *et al.*, 1982) have reported a genetic change in the oncogene isolated from cell lines from human bladder carcinomas represented by a single point mutation. This change, which affects a protein of molecular weight 21,000 (p21), involves a single amino acid substitution resulting in incorporation of valine instead of glycine at the twelfth position. Thus, incorporation of a single amino acid appears to render this gene "transforming," while the normal homolog in the cell appears to have other normal functions.

It may be surmised that other genes will be found that will yield information concerning how the metabolism of a cell and its nutritional requirements can be altered by small changes in the DNA and reflected in either gene regulation or specific gene products. These are likely to be minor, but in an era of molecular biology and genetic engineering, they should be amenable to exploration. Further results only await the ingenuity of scientific investigators in developing additional test systems to enable monitoring for such changes.

REFERENCES

Bang, F. B. (1966). *In* "Cells and Tissues in Culture" (E. N. Willmer, ed.), Vol. 3, pp. 151–261. Academic Press, New York.
Barnes, D., and Sato, G. (1980a). *Anal. Biochem.* **102,** 255–270.
Barnes, D., and Sato, G. (1980b). *Cell* **22,** 649–655.
Bishop, J. M. (1978). *Annu. Rev. Biochem.* **47,** 35–88.

Bishop, J. M. (1982). *Sci. Am.* **246,** 80–92.

Bottenstein, J., Hayashi, I., Hutchings, S., Masui, H., Mather, J., McClure, D. B., Okasa, S., Rizzino, A., Sato, G., Serrero, G., Wolfe, R., and Wu, R. (1979). *In* "Methods in Enzymology" (W. B. Jakoby and I. H. Pastan, eds.), Vol. 58, pp. 94–109. Academic Press, New York.

Boyer, G. S., Leuchtenberger, C., and Ginsberg, H. S. (1957). *J. Exp. Med.* **105,** 195–216.

Brugge, J. S., and Erikson, R. L. (1977). *Nature (London)* **269,** 346–347.

Carrel, A. (1912). *J. Exp. Med.* **15,** 516–528.

Carrel, A. (1928). *In* "Filterable Viruses" (T. M. Rivers, ed.), pp. 97–109. Baillière, London.

Chanock, R., and Finberg, L. (1957). *Am. J. Hyg.* **66,** 291–300.

Collett, M. S., and Erikson, R. L. (1978). *Proc. Natl. Acad. Sci. U.S.A.* **75,** 2021–2024.

Cooper, G. M., Okenquist, S., and Silverman, L. (1980). *Nature (London)* **284,** 418–421.

Dulbecco, R. (1952). *Proc. Natl. Acad. Sci. U.S.A.* **38,** 747–752.

Eagle, H. (1955). *J. Biol. Chem.* **214,** 839–852.

Eagle, H. (1959). *Science* **130,** 432–437.

Emmelot, P. (1973). *Eur. J. Cancer* **9,** 319–333.

Enders, J. F., and Peebles, T. C. (1954). *Proc. Soc. Exp. Biol. Med.* **86,** 277–286.

Gross, L. (1951). *Proc. Soc. Exp. Biol. Med.* **76,** 27–32.

Ham, R. G. (1963). *Exp. Cell Res.* **29,** 515–526.

Ham, R. G. (1965). *Proc. Natl. Acad. Sci. U.S.A.* **53,** 288–293.

Harrison, R. G. (1907). *Proc. Soc. Exp. Biol. Med.* **4,** 140–143.

Healy, G. M., and Parker, R. G. (1966). *J. Cell Biol.* **30,** 531–538.

Henle, G., Deinhardt, F., and Girardi, A. (1954). *Proc. Soc. Exp. Biol. Med.* **87,** 386–393.

Hoggan, M. D., and Roizman, B. (1959). *Am. J. Hyg.* **70,** 208–219.

Hunter, T., and Sefton, B. M. (1980). *Proc. Natl. Acad. Sci. U.S.A.* **77,** 1311–1315.

Knight, B. C. J. G. (1945). *Vitam. Horm. (N.Y.)* **3,** 105–228b.

Leibovitz, A. (1963). *Am. J. Hyg.* **78,** 173–180.

Lewis, W. H., and Lewis, M. R. (1912). *Anat. Rec.* **6,** 207–211.

Ling, C. T., Gey, G. O., and Richters, V. (1968). *Exp. Cell Res.* **52,** 469–489.

Lwoff, A. (1957). *JNCI, J. Natl. Cancer Inst.* **19,** 511–528.

McCoy, T. A., Maxwell, M., and Kruse, P. F. (1959). *Proc. Soc. Exp. Biol. Med.* **100,** 115–118.

Marston, R. Q. (1958). *Proc. Soc. Exp. Biol. Med.* **98,** 853–856.

Moore, G. E., Gerner, R. E., and Franklin, H. A. (1967). *JAMA, J. Am. Med. Assoc.* **199,** 519–524.

Morgan, D. A., Ruscetti, F. W., and Gallo, R. C. (1976). *Science* **193,** 1007–1008.

Morgan, J. F., Morton, H. J., and Parker, R. C. (1950). *Proc. Soc. Exp. Biol. Med.* **73,** 1–8.

Morgan, J. F., Campbell, M. E., and Morton, H. J. (1955). *JNCI, J. Natl. Cancer Inst.* **16,** 557–567.

Murakami, H., Masui, H., Sato, G. H., Sueoka, N., Chow, T. P., and Kano-Sueoka, T. (1982). *Proc. Natl. Acad. Sci. U.S.A.* **79,** 1158–1162.

Nagle, S. C. (1968). *Appl. Microbiol.* **16,** 53–55.

Nagle, S. C., Tribble, H. R., Anderson, R. E., and Gary, N. D. (1963). *Proc. Soc. Exp. Biol. Med.* **112,** 340–344.

Nicolson, G. L. (1971). *Nature (London) New Biol.* **233,** 244–246.

Nicolson, G. L. (1974). *In* "Control of Proliferation in Animal Cells" (B. Clarkson and R. Baserga, eds.), pp. 251–270. Cold Spring Harbor Lab., Cold Spring Harbor, New York.

Parker, R. C. (1961). *In* "Methods of Tissue Culture," 3rd ed., p. 77. Harper, New York.

Pereira, H. G. (1961). *Adv. Virus Res.* **8,** 245–285.

Perucho, M., Goldfarb, M., Shimizu, K., Lama, C., Fogh, J., and Wigler, M. (1981). *Cell* **27**, 467–476.

Poiesz, B. J., Ruscetti, F. W., Mier, J. W., Woods, A. M., and Gallo, R. C. (1980a). *Proc. Natl. Acad. Sci. U.S.A.* **77**, 6815–6819.

Poiesz, B. J., Ruscetti, F. W., Gazdar, A. F., Bunn, P. A., Minna, J. D., and Gallo, R. C. (1980b). *Proc. Natl. Acad. Sci. U.S.A.* **77**, 7415–7419.

Poiesz, B. J., Ruscetti, F. W., Reitz, M. S., Kalyanaraman, V. S., and Gallo, R. C. (1981). *Nature (London)* **294**, 268–271.

Rapp, F. (1973). *In* "Tissue Culture" (P. Kruse, Jr. and M. K. Patterson, eds.), pp. 653–658. Academic Press, New York.

Rapp, F., and Melnick, J. L. (1966). *In* "Cells and Tissues in Culture" (E. N. Willmer, ed.), Vol. 3, pp. 263–316. Academic Press, New York.

Rapp, F., and Westmoreland, D. (1976). *Biochim. Biophys. Acta* **458**, 167–211.

Reddy, E. P., Reynolds, R. K., Santos, E., and Barbacid, M. (1982). *Nature (London)* **300**, 149–152.

Reissig, M., and Melnick, J. L. (1955). *J. Exp. Med.* **101**, 341–352.

Reissig, M., Howes, D. W., and Melnick, J. L. (1956). *J. Exp. Med.* **104**, 289–304.

Robbins, F. C., Enders, J. F., and Weller, T. H. (1950). *Proc. Soc. Exp. Biol. Med.* **75**, 370–374.

Rous, P., and Jones, F. S. (1916). *J. Exp. Med.* **23**, 549–555.

Ruscetti, F. W., Morgan, D. A., and Gallo, R. C. (1977). *J. Immunol.* **199**, 131–138.

Rustigian, R., Johnston, P., and Reihart, H. (1955). *Proc. Soc. Exp. Biol. Med.* **88**, 8–16.

Sefton, B. M., Hunter, T., Beemon, K., and Eckhart, W. (1980). *Cell* **20**, 807–816.

Seligman, S. J., and Rapp, F. (1959). *Virology* **9**, 143–145.

Shih, C., Padhy, L. C., Murray, M. J., and Weinberg, R. A. (1981). *Nature (London)* **290**, 261–264.

Shilo, B., and Weinberg, R. A. (1981). *Nature (London)* **289**, 607–609.

Steinhardt, E., Israeli, C., and Lambert, R. A. (1913). *J. Infect. Dis.* **13**, 294–300.

Sweet, B. H., and Hilleman, M. R. (1960). *Proc. Soc. Exp. Biol. Med.* **105**, 420–427.

Syverton, J. T. (1957). *JNCI, J. Natl. Cancer Inst.* **19**, 687–706.

Tabin, C. J., Bradley, S. M., Bargmann, C. I., Weinberg, R. A., Papageorge, A. G., Scolnick, E. M., Dhar, R., Lowy, D. R., and Chang, E. H. (1982). *Nature (London)* **300**, 143–149.

Waymouth, C. (1955). *Tex. Rep. Biol. Med.* **13**, 522–536.

Waymouth, C. (1957). *JNCI, J. Natl. Cancer Inst.* **19**, 495–504.

Weller, T. H., Witton, H. M., and Bell, E. J. (1958). *J. Exp. Med.* **108**, 843–868.

Yoshida, M., Miyoshi, I., and Hinuma, Y. (1982). *Proc. Natl. Acad. Sci. U.S.A.* **79**, 2031–2035.

Lectin-Induced Changes in Metabolic Function and Nutritional Requirements of Cultured Human Lymphocytes

Peter B. Rowe

Children's Medical Research Foundation
The University of Sydney
Camperdown, New South Wales, Australia

I. HISTORICAL PERSPECTIVE OF CELL CULTURE

One of the major long-term goals of scientists working in mammalian biology over the past 80 years or so has been to achieve the continuous clonal culture of normal cells that display, in full, the differentiated properties of the cells of their tissue of origin. As a corollary to this aim, continuous culture

51

Nutritional Factors in the Induction
and Maintenance of Malignancy

should be achieved in a completely defined medium. Unfortunately, neither of these hopes has been, as yet, fully realized, and if one surveys the history of cell culture (Waymouth, 1972), it can be seen that a series of inspired and perhaps fortuitous observations have mitigated against these achievements (Rizzino et al., 1979).

Harrison (1906), the "father" of tissue culture techniques and his contemporaries, Lewis and Lewis (1911), really commenced the critical studies of the interaction between the cells of cultured tissues and their environment. Progress was extremely slow until the dramatic demonstration in 1913 by Carrel of the potent growth-stimulating effect on tissue explants of embryo extracts added to the plasma clots that constituted the basic culture medium then in use. This observation so dominated research thought in the tissue culture field for several decades that relatively little effort was concentrated on defining the essential requirements of individual components of culture media. Eventually White (1946) and Morgan et al. (1950) developed defined media for the prolonged survival of, if not the active growth of, tissue explants. These media were based on the current knowledge of the nutritional requirements of animals, plants, and microorganisms.

At this time, the first permanent cell lines were developed (Sanford et al., 1948; Gey et al., 1952), and the course of cell culture technology was dramatically altered. Eagle's classic studies, on the amino acid and vitamin requirements of cells cultured in the presence of dialyzed serum literally changed the direction of cell culture research for the next 20 years. Eagle (1955a) demonstrated that HeLa cells and L cells required 13 "essential" amino acids (arginine, cysteine, glutamine, histidine, isoleucine, leucine, lysine, methionine, phenylalanine, threonine, tryptophan, tyrosine, and valine) and seven vitamins (biotin, folic acid, nicotinamide, pantothenic acid, pyridoxal, thiamine, and riboflavin). These observations formed the basis of the now famous minimum essential medium (MEM). Although a large number of complex artificial media were rapidly developed with the aim of achieving optimal growth of a huge range of cell types, the necessary addition of serum prevented the accurate assessment of nutritional requirements for individual cells.

II. RECENT APPROACHES TO DEFINED MEDIA

A limited number of research groups have, however, undertaken systematic identification of specific growth factors required for individual cells, although most of these cells are malignant. The major recent achievements in this area of painstaking research have probably been from the laboratories of Ham and of Sato.

The approach employed by Ham and his colleagues (see Ham and McKeehan, 1978, 1979) has been essentially a reductionist one in which the optimal concentration of a massive range of metabolites and cofactors has been examined in the presence of minimal amounts of serum with the ultimate aim of eventually removing the serum requirement.

Sato's approach has been to replace serum with a series of specific hormones and defined serum fractions for a particular cell line (Barnes and Sato, 1980a,b). As a result he has been able successfully to propagate a number of tumor cell lines in serum-free medium, although it is not clear to what extent these cells fully resemble the original clone (Barnes and Sato, 1980b). Based on work during the 1970s, Sato and his associates have listed the basic nutrient requirements for mammalian cells in culture and have also defined some of the serum factors and hormone requirements for individual cell lines (Rizzino *et al.*, 1979).

The possible functions of serum have been summarized by Ham and McKeehan (1978). In broad terms, serum (1) can serve as a source of essential nutrients, (2) can enhance nutrient availability and/or utilization, (3) can detoxify components of the defined portion of the medium, (4) can reverse the effects of proteolytic agents, (5) can alter the physical and physicochemical aspects of the culture system, (6) may contain macromolecules that have direct effects on cellular multiplication [a good example of this is the low molecular weight protein (MW 10,000– 15,000) in serum that is derived from platelets and has been shown to be a transforming growth factor for certain types of cell (Childs *et al.*, 1982)], and (7) may also promote cellular multiplication by a variety of mechanisms as yet unidentified.

Serum, of course, may be toxic to many cells. The only cells that are ever exposed to serum *in vivo* are those in the vicinity of a wound where clotting has occurred. Conversely, serum contains many substances that never come into contact with most body cells (Gospodarowicz *et al.*, 1979).

Most cells in culture and also *in vivo* release molecules that are important for their own growth. This is exemplified by the range of soluble factors released by mitogen-stimulated cultured lymphocytes (Hume and Weidemann, 1980). One of these factors, interleukin 2, is now widely used for continuous culture of normal T lymphocytes (Ruscetti and Gallo, 1981). The effects of these various growth factors may be counteracted by various serum ingredients that also complicate their identification and analysis.

III. CHARACTERISTICS OF CULTURED CELLS

An exact classification of cultured cells is extremely difficult because they do not fall uniformly into defined classes by the current relatively crude criteria. At one extreme, the "normal" cell is considered as being diploid, finite in life span, anchorage dependent, density inhibited, and nonmalignant, while the classic permanent cell line is aneuploid, immortal, not anchorage dependent, not density inhibited, and malignant. There is a large number of cell types that exhibit a varying range of these properties. For example, normal cells such as chondrocytes and various blood cells are not anchorage dependent, and keratinocytes do not show density-dependent inhibition. There are some permanent cell lines such as 3T3 (Swiss mouse fibroblasts) that are aneuploid and multiply indefinitely but are anchorage dependent and density inhibited, but not malignant by most criteria.

Cells *in vivo* live in an extraordinarily complex environment consisting of a wide range of hormonal and stromal influences that must be simulated by an *in vitro* culture medium. It may be that we will never effectively achieve long-term culture of individual cells from solid organs, for example, hepatocytes, which are the exact biological replica of their cells of origin because of our inability to reproduce exactly the controls exerted by cell–cell interactions. At this stage in the evolution of cell culture most of the established cell lines are of animal (i.e., nonhuman) origin and more importantly are derived from animal tumors.

IV. LYMPHOCYTE TRANSFORMATION

The observation by Nowell (1960) of the mitogenic effect of the lectin phytohemagglutinin (PHA), derived from the red bean (*Phaseolus vulgaris*), on short-term cultured human peripheral blood lymphocytes constituted a major breakthrough in the study of human cells. It is of interest that these proteins, which are characterized by their ability to bind selectively to specific carbohydrate-containing cell surface receptors, had been used commercially to agglutinate red cells for almost 50 years (Dorset and Henley, 1916). The study of lectins, their physical properties, the nature of their interaction with receptors on different types of cell, and the secondary cellular effects of this binding now constitutes a major discipline in biological research, particularly in immunobiology (Oppenheim and Rosenstreich, 1976).

The study of the phenomena associated with the interaction of lectins with lymphocytes in particular is now a significant field of research, as is evident from the regular publication of the deliberations of international symposia. These reports reflect the interest in almost every parameter of the biology of the lymphocyte, ranging from transport mechanisms through membrane structure, energy metabolism, metabolic pathways, enzyme induction and activation, to the exploitation of recombinant DNA technology to explore the genetic events associated with the process of lectin-induced transformation (Resch and Kirchner, 1981).

The exposure of a lymphocyte to a "mitogenic" lectin activates a great variety of metabolic events representing a classic example of the pleiotropic response. The analysis of the data acquired in experiments with this cell system is hampered first by the heterogeneity of the cell population under study and second by the absence of a defined medium for optimal culture conditions. We do not have the information about the nutrient requirements that of course may vary between different T cell subgroups, and the continued serum requirement represents another major variable. Moore and his colleagues (1967) described the use of medium RPM1 1640 for the culture of "normal" human leukocytes, and this medium, supplemented by serum, has become the accepted basis for most lymphoid culture work since then.

When a population of normal lymphocytes derived from peripheral blood, lymph nodes, thymus, spleen, or other lymphoid tissue is exposed to a mitogenic lectin, a fairly typical sequence of events occurs. Morphologically, after a lag phase of some 20–36 hours, the cell increases some three- to fivefold in volume over a total 72-hour period. This involves enlargement of both the nuclear and cytoplasmic compartments with the appearance of prominent nucleoli and increased number of cytoplasmic organelles such as mitochondria and lysosomes. Scanning electron microscopy reveals the development of a variety of membrane microprojections, most frequently fingerlike or cone-shaped microvilli, but occasionally cells display ruffled membranes and others show elongated uropods terminating in tuftlike extremities (Polliack, 1977).

Within a few minutes to a few hours, there are striking metabolic changes, as illustrated by increases in the flux of cations, anions, amino acids, nucleosides, carbohydrates, and other substrates for cellular metabolism across the plasma membrane. These changes are to some extent overshadowed by the later (> 24 hours) fluxes of metabolites associated with the more delayed marked increases in macromolecular biosynthesis. Over the course of 72 hours there is a three- to fivefold increase in the RNA, protein, and phospholipid content of the cell, while the DNA content, on the average virtually doubles. This sequence of events, with the accompanying overt morphological changes, is referred to as blastogenesis. Some of the cells actually undergo chromosome replication and cell division, but the vast majority, particularly at cell culture densities of 1.0×10^6 per milliliter or greater, revert to small lymphocytes that physically closely resemble those of the original cell population.

In this context, the experiments of Stewart *et al.* (1975) are most instructive. Irrespective of whether the cells were cultured at a density of 10^5 or 10^6 per milliliter, there was no "proliferation" in the sense of an increase in cell number over the usual 72-hour time period of most experiments. At the lower cell density there was a later (96-hour) fivefold increase in cell number. Although some have attributed the lack of cell division in higher cell density cultures to nutrient deprivation, it is evident that many other factors must be involved.

V. LYMPHOCYTE ONE-CARBON METABOLISM

We have been using lectin-transformed human peripheral blood lymphocytes in two areas of biochemical research. First, we have been investigating one-carbon metabolism, particularly as it relates to the interaction of folate derivative metabolism and *de novo* purine biosynthesis. For studies of this type the cell heterogeneity is not a significant problem in data interpretation. Second, we have been investigating possible mechanisms of gene activation as a secondary response to lectin stimulation. For these studies cell heterogeneity will ultimately provide some real difficulties in data analysis.

Lectin-induced lymphocyte transformation is associated with a variable increase in both the total and specific activities of a wide range of enzymes (for review, see Hume and Weidemann, 1980). We have demonstrated an increase in the activity of a number of human peripheral blood lymphocyte enzymes associated with one-carbon metabolism and purine nucleotide synthesis (Table I) after 72 hours of exposure to PHA. During the course of this work we observed that deletion of folic acid from the serum-supplemented standard RPM1 1640 medium resulted in a significant reduction in both cell viability and the extent of transformation. In addition, a variable number of unduly large transformed cells were observed (Rowe *et al.*, 1979). We also established that methionine was an absolute medium requirement for the survival of both "resting" cells and those exposed to PHA.

It has been long accepted that the three-carbon atom of serine is the major source of one-carbon units for most organisms. These units are used predominantly for *de novo* purine synthesis, the synthesis of dTMP from dUMP, and the methylation of phospholipids. Coupled with the

TABLE I

Changes in Enzymatic Activity in PHA-Transformed Human Peripheral Blood Lymphocytes[a]

	Activity			
	−PHA		+PHA	
Enzyme	Total[b]	Specific[b]	Total	Specific
10-Formyl tetrahydrofolate synthetase	15	150	360	1200
5,10-Methylene tetrahydrofolate dehydrogenase	9.6	96	202	673
5,10-Methenyl tetrahydrofolate cyclohydrolase	52	520	490	1633
Serine hydroxymethyl-transferase	18.5	185	200	667
Dihydrofolate reductase	2.5	25	71	236
Tetrahydrofolate methyltransferase	0.05	0.5	0.5	1.7
Thymidylate synthetase	0.10	1.0	14.0	46.7
5,10-Methylene tetrahydrofolate reductase	0.6	6.0	2.2	7.3
γ-Glutamyl carboxypeptidase	0.6	6.0	6.4	21.4
Thymidine kinase	0.3	3.0	42	140
Deoxyuridine kinase	0.3	3.0	53	176
De novo purine biosynthesis	0.35	3.5	6.3	21
HGPRT′ase	80	800	190	633
APRT′ase	149	1490	406	1353
ADOMET synthetase	0.4	4	7	23

[a] The enzyme activities were determined on the supernatant solution of homogenized lymphocytes centrifuged at 100,000 g for 1 hour (Rowe et al., 1979).

[b] Total activity is expressed as nanomoles per hour per 10^7 cells; specific activity is nanomoles per hour per milligram protein.

rapid increase in protein synthesis that occurs in response to PHA activation, it is evident that there would be a heavy demand for serine by the lymphocyte.

Serine is classically a nonessential amino acid since pathways exist for its synthesis from glucose and from glycine. Lockhart and Eagle (1959) have shown that some of the nonessential amino acids were required for the growth of low density cultures of certain types of cells. The need for nonessential amino acids could be met by serine. Eagle (1955b) also established that certain amino acids (methionine and trytophan) inhibited the growth of L cells at high medium concentrations, while others (histidine, phenylalanine, and valine) exerted no such effect.

Regan et al. (1969) have shown that the serine requirement for the growth of human bone marrow cells results from their limited capacity to synthesize serine from glucose, while Dubrow *et al.* (1973) have shown that the serine requirement for PHA-mediated transformation of blood lymphocytes, which results from the low levels of activity of the phosphorylated pathway for serine biosynthesis, can be partially met by glycine.

[3-14C]Serine is extensively incorporated into the cellular amino acid and purine and pyrimidine (thymine) nucleotide pools, nucleic acid purines and thymine, protein, and phospholipid (Table II) following lectin transformation of human peripheral blood lymphocytes. Almost 50% of the incorporated serine was cleaved and the one-carbon unit cycled via the reduced folate derivative pool for the synthesis of adenine, guanine, and thymine nucleotides. Over the course of 72 hours there was equilibration of the intracellular serine pool with the medium. The specific radioactivity of the adenine and guanine nucleotides of the acid-soluble cell fraction was twice that of the medium serine, indicating that the three-carbon atom of serine was virtually the sole source of one-carbon units for *de novo* purine synthesis, the major metabolic pathway for the total turnover of the purine nucleotide pool.

More surprisingly, perhaps, the extent of cellular transformation was a function of the medium serine concentration. The degree of transformation was reflected in the concentration-dependent incorporation of serine (Fig. 1). While the incorporation into the amino acid pool was optimal at a medium concentration of 1–2 mM, the maximal incorporation into soluble phase and nucleic acid nucleotides and into protein was achieved at a much lower level, usually between 200 and 600 μM. The

TABLE II

Incorporation of [3-14C]Serine into Lymphocytes[a–c]

Cell fraction	+PHA	−PHA
Free amino acid	22.4	5.1
Acid soluble purines	56.0	0.4
Acid soluble pyrimidine	9.4	0.3
Nucleic acid purines	240.0	0.8
Nucleic acid pyrimidines	50.4	0.6
Protein	362.0	24.0
Phospholipid	23.1	5.0

[a] From Rowe (1983).

[b] Cell cultures were exposed to [3-14C]serine, 300 μM, for 72 hours in the presence or absence of PHA.

[c] Incorporation expressed as nanomoles per 10^7 cells.

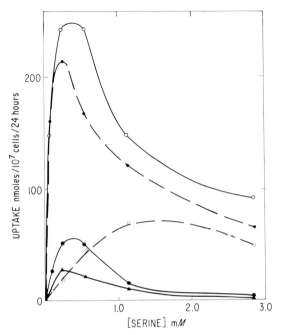

Fig. 1. Serine uptake as a function of medium serine concentration. Cells were cultured in the presence of PHA for 72 hours in HEPES buffered RPM1 1640 medium supplemented with 5% heated dialyzed fetal calf serum containing varying concentrations of serine. The cells were pulsed with [3-^{14}C]serine from 48 to 72 hours in culture. Serine incorporated into (O- -O) soluble amino acid pool, (●- -●) soluble purine nucleotides, (O————O) proteins, (●————●) nucleic acid purines, and (▲————▲) nucleic acid thymine is expressed as nanomoles per 10^7 cells.

reduced incorporation of serine both at high and low medium concentrations was reflected in the microscopic appearance of the cells and the low rates of macromolecular synthesis as measured by the incorporation of radiolabeled leucine, deoxyuridine, and uridine. Interestingly, the optimum serine concentration of 300 μM was that used by Moore *et al.* (1967) in their initial use of RPM1 1640 medium for the culture of lymphoid cells.

In the absence of serine in the medium, the cell viability was reduced from 95% to 85% and the degree of blastic transformation from 90 to 50%. This was confirmed by the decrease in all biosynthetic parameters as shown on Table III. Transformation, however, did occur, and clearly alternative sources of one-carbon units were available, but it is not yet clear from where these were derived. Methionine, histidine, glycine, choline, and tryptophan were all present in the culture medium. Only

TABLE III

RNA, DNA, Protein and Phospholipid Content of Cells Transformed with PHA ± Serine[a]

	With serine	Without serine
RNA[b]	104	50
DNA[b]	151	110
Protein[c]	840	640
Phospholipid[d]	156	117

[a] From Rowe (1983).
[b] Nanomoles of purine and pyrimidine bases per 10^7 cells.
[c] Micrograms per 10^7 cells.
[d] Nanomoles phospholipid phosphorus per 10^7 cells.

tryptophan, via the carbon-2 atom of pyrrole ring contributes to the one-carbon pool. At a medium concentration of 25 μM, only 11 nmole per 10^7 cells or 22% of the total tryptophan uptake was incorporated into the one-carbon pool over 72 hours, a very small fraction of that contributed by serine. In the absence of serine from the medium, this contribution from tryptophan was halved.

Formate, at the relatively high medium concentration of 2.5 mM could correct for some of the effects of serine deficiency. The maximum availability of one-carbon units as assessed by the incorporation of deoxyuridine into DNA and of leucine into protein was delayed by some 20–24 hours and never attained the levels observed in serine-containing medium (Fig. 2). The addition of hypoxanthine, thymidine, and glycine (at high concentration) had no additional corrective effect.

It would appear that the synthesis of serine from glycine was the rate-limiting step. Serine hydroxymethyltransferase total activity usually increased tenfold with PHA transformation (Table I), but in the absence of serine the increase was only fourfold although the specific activity increase was unaffected (Table IV). This phenomenon was also observed with the activity of other folate pathway enzymes, suggesting that there was considerable selectivity in the effects of serine deprivation on protein synthesis.

The analysis of one-carbon metabolism in the course of PHA-mediated lymphocyte transformation emphasizes the need for the careful nutritional assessment of the ever-increasing number of mammalian cell lines in order to ensure that they are not growing under conditions of metabolic imbalance. It also raises the question of the mechanism of amino acid toxicity, which in the case of serine is clearly quite complex.

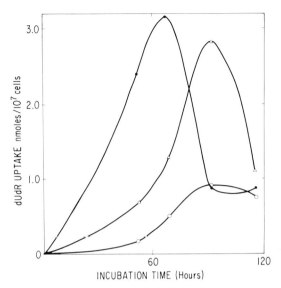

Fig. 2. Deoxyuridine (dUdR) incorporation into DNA of cultured human lymphocytes as a function of time of exposure to PHA. Cells were transformed in (●) complete RPM 1640, (○) serine-free RMP1 1640, and (△) serine-free RPM1 1640 containing 2.5 m*M* sodium formate and 1.0 m*M* glycine and pulsed for 4 hours with 4 μ*M* [³H]dUdR at the designated time points. All media were supplemented with 5% heated dialyzed fetal calf serum. (From Rowe, 1983.)

TABLE IV

Transformation Linked Changes in Enzymatic Activity, Effect of Serine Deficiency

	Activity[a]		
		With PHA	
Enzyme	Without PHA	Without serine	With serine
10-Formyl tetrahydrofolate synthetase	17 (170)	85 (485)	407 (925)
5,10-Methylene tetrahydrofolate dehydrogenase	12 (120)	65 (348)	259 (589)
5,10-Methylene tetrahydrofolate reductase	1 (10)	2 (11.6)	4 (9.5)
Serine hydroxymethyltransferase	19 (190)	80 (434)	207 (472)
Thymidylate synthetase	0.03 (0.3)	1.3 (6)	3.2 (7.3)
HGPRT'ase	23 (230)	46 (222)	55 (120)

[a] Activity is expressed as nanomoles per hour per 10⁷ cells. Values in parentheses are specific activity expressed as nanomoles per milligram of protein.

REFERENCES

Barnes, D., and Sato, G. (1980a). *Anal. Biochem.* **102,** 255–270.
Barnes, D., and Sato, G. (1980b). *Cell* **22,** 649–655.
Carrel, A. (1913). *J. Exp. Med.* **17,** 14–19.
Childs, C. B., Proper, J. A., Tucker, R. F., and Moses, H. L. (1982). *Proc. Natl. Acad. Sci. U.S.A.* **79,** 5312–5316.
Dorset, M., and Henley, R. R. (1916). *J. Agric. Res.* **6,** 333–336.
Dubrow, R., Pizer, L. I., and Brody, J. I. (1973). *JNCI, J. Natl. Cancer Inst.* **51,** 307–311.
Eagle, H. (1955a). *Science* **122,** 501–504.
Eagle, H. (1955b). *J. Biol. Chem.* **214,** 839–853.
Gey, G. O., Coffman, W. D., and Kubicek, M. T. (1952). *Science* **122,** 501–504.
Gospodarowicz, D., Vlodsavsky, I., Greenberg, G., and Johnson, L. K. (1979). *In* "Hormones and Cell Culture" (R. Ross and G. Sato, eds.), pp. 5561–5592. Cold Spring Harbor Lab., Cold Spring Harbor, New York.
Ham, R. G., and McKeehan, W. L. C. (1978). *In* "Nutritional Requirements of Cultured Cells" (H. Katsuta, ed.), pp. 63–1165. University Park Press, Baltimore, Maryland.
Ham, R. G., and McKeehan, W. L. (1979). *In* "Methods in Enzymology" (W. B. Jakoby and I. H. Pastan, eds.), Vol. 58, pp. 44–93. Academic Press, New York.
Harrison, R. G. (1906). *Proc. Soc. Exp. Biol. Med.* **4,** 140–143.
Hume, D., and Weidemann, M. (1980). "Mitogenic Lymphocyte Transformation." Elsevier/North-Holland, Amsterdam.
Lewis, M. R., and Lewis, W. H. (1911). *Anat. Rec.* **5,** 277–293.
Lockhart, R. Z., Jr., and Eagle, H. (1959). *Science* **129,** 252–254.
Moore, G. E., Gerner, R. E., and Franklin, H. A. (1967). *JAMA, J. Am. Med. Assoc.* **199,** 87–92.
Morgan, J. F., Morton, H. J., and Parker, R. C. (1950). *Proc. Soc. Exp. Biol. Med.* **73,** 1–8.
Nowell, P. C. (1960). *Cancer Res.* **20,** 462–467.
Oppenheim, J. J., and Rosenstreich, D. L., eds. (1976). "Mitogens in Immunobiology." Academic Press, New York.
Polliack, A. (1977). "Normal, Transformed and Leukemic Leukocytes." Springer Verlag, Berlin and New York.
Regan, J. D., Vodopick, H., Takeda, S., Lee, W. H., and Faulcon, F. M. (1969). *Science* **163,** 1452–1453.
Resch, K., and Kirchner, H., eds. (1981). "Mechanisms of Lymphocyte Activation." Elsevier/North-Holland, Amsterdam.
Rizzino, A., Rizzino, H., and Sato, G. (1979). *Nutr. Res.* **37,** 369–378.
Rowe, P. B. (1983). *In* "Proceedings of Chemistry and Biology of Pteridines Symposium, St. Andrews, 1982" (J. A. Blair, ed.) (in press). de Gruyter, Berlin.
Rowe, P. B., Tripp, E., and Craig, G. (1979). *In* "Chemistry and Biology of Pteridines" (R. L. Kisliuk and G. M. Brown, eds.), pp. 587–592. Elsevier/North-Holland, Amsterdam.
Ruscetti, F. W., and Gallo, R. C. (1981). *Blood* **57,** 379–394.
Sanford, K. K., Earle, W. R., and Likely, G. D. (1948). *JNCI, J. Natl. Cancer Inst.* **9,** 229–246.
Stewart, C. C., Cramer, S. F., and Steward, P. G. (1975). *Cell. Immunol.* **16,** 237–250.
Waymouth, C. (1972). *In* "Growth, Nutrition and Metabolism of Cells in Culture" (G. H. Rothblat and V. J. Cristofalo, eds.), Vol. 1, pp. 11–47. Academic Press, New York.
White, P. R. (1946). *Growth* **10,** 231–289.

5

Fragile Chromosomes

Grant R. Sutherland

Cytogenetics Unit
Department of Histopathology
The Adelaide Children's Hospital
North Adelaide, South Australia, Australia

I. INTRODUCTION

Chromosome abnormalities are seen in most malignant cells, indeed chromosomal damage or breakage and subsequent rearrangement is probably one of the primary events in the induction of some malignancies (Radman *et al.*, 1982). An understanding of the mechanisms involved in chromosome breakage could provide insights into cellular processes of malignant transformation. Chromosomal fragility occurs, apparently nonspecifically and sporadically at a very low level, in all individuals. It is seen at higher levels and with some specificity in the chromosome instability syndromes and at much higher levels at a specific locus in carriers of heritable fragile sites. The chromosomal fragility that occurs at fragile sites is the only type for which a biochemical basis is at least partly known.

Nutritional Factors in the Induction
and Maintenance of Malignancy

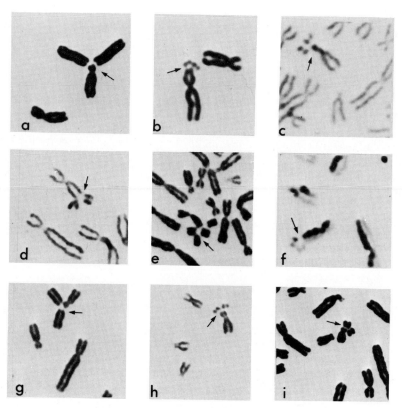

Fig. 1. Multiradial figures produced by fragile sites. (a) Triradial at 2q13. (b) Triradial at 6p23. (c) Triradial at 9p21. (d) Triradial at 9q23. (e) Pentaradial at 10q23. (f) Triradial at 10q25. (g) Triradial at 11q13. (h) Triradial at 16p12. (i) Triradial at 20p11. (From Sutherland, 1983.)

II. THE HERITABLE FRAGILE SITES

Fragile sites are morphological features of chromosomes that were defined by Sutherland (1979a) as specific points that are liable to show the following features:

1. A nonstaining gap of variable width that usually involves both chromatids
2. Always at exactly the same point on the chromosome in an individual or kindred
3. Inherited in a Mendelian codominant fashion
4. Exhibits fragility by the production of acentric fragments, deleted chromosomes, triradial figures, etc.

The triradial (or multiradial) figure is the most spectacular cytogenetic manifestation of the fragile site (Fig. 1) and also an essential manifestation for confirmation of a lesion as a fragile site rather than some other phenomenon causing chromosome damage. While the nature of a fragile site, in terms of chromosome structure, is unknown, it presumably represents a segment of chromosome that does not undergo normal compaction for mitosis.

To date 15 fragile sites have been detected, and these are shown in the partial ideogram (Fig. 2) and partial karyotype (Fig. 3). These fragile sites can be classified into three groups. The first group, the folate-sensitive fragile sites, contains all except two of the known sites which each come into separate categories.

Group 1. The folate-sensitive fragile sites are those at 2q13, 6p23, 7p11, 8q22, 9p21, 9q32, 10q23, 11q13, 11q23, 12q13, 16p12, 20p11, and

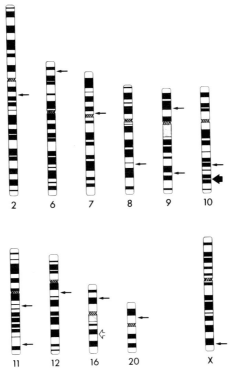

Fig. 2. The known fragile sites. Group 1, small arrows, at 2q13, 6p23, 7p11, 8q22, 9p21, 9q32, 10q23, 11q13, 11q23, 12q13, 16p12, 20p11, and Xq27; Group 2, open arrow, 16q22; Group 3, broad arrow, 10q25. (From Sutherland et al., 1983.)

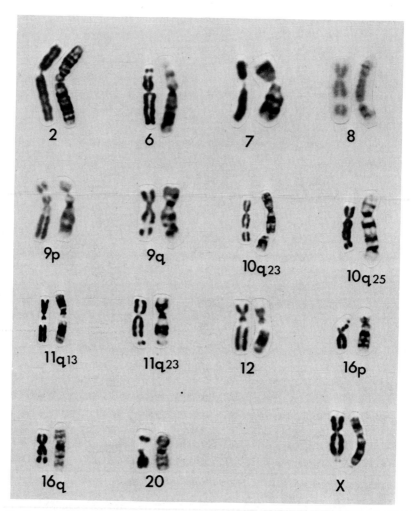

Fig. 3. Partial karyotype showing the fragile sites. The left chromosome of each pair is unbanded and the right G-banded. (Pair number 8 courtesy Dr. N. B. Kardon, pair number 7 courtesy Dr. G. C. Webb; from Sutherland, 1983.)

Xq27. They are termed folate sensitive because removal of folic acid (and thymidine) from culture medium was the first factor found to be essential for their demonstration in lymphocyte culture.

Group 2. This group contains only the fragile site at 16q22. This fragile site is not dependent upon conditions of tissue culture (Sutherland, 1979a), but its expression is reportedly enhanced by the addition of distamycin A to lymphocyte cultures (Schmid *et al.*, 1980). If the findings of Croci (1983) are confirmed, then this fragile site may be regarded as a bromodeoxyuridine (BrdU) requiring fragile site similar to the one in Group 3.

Group 3. This group contains only the fragile site at 10q25. This common fragile site was independently discovered by Scheres and Hustinx (1980) and Sutherland *et al.* (1980) and shown to be a polymorphism present in one in 40 members of the Australian population sample studied (Sutherland, 1982). This fragile site is unique in that its expression is dependent upon the presence of BrdU or bromodeoxycytidine (BrdC) in lymphocyte cultures some hours prior to harvest.

Of all the fragile sites only the one at Xq27 (the fragile X) has been proved to be of clinical significance in that it is associated with, if not the cause of, one form of X-linked mental retardation (Sutherland, 1982b). However, none of the folate-sensitive fragile sites have been seen in homozygotes and it has been suggested that they could be deleterious in this situation (Sutherland, 1979b). On the other hand, heterozygotes for the autosomal folate-sensitive fragile sites have been found to be ten times more common among the mentally retarded than among neonates, but this data is very limited, and more information is required before it can be asserted that such heterozygotes (most of whom are intellectually normal) are at increased risk of mental retardation (Sutherland, 1983).

III. THE BIOCHEMISTRY OF FRAGILE SITE EXPRESSION

A number of factors have been shown to be important in fragile site expression since Sutherland (1977) showed that they were expressed in lymphocyte cultures only if the cells were grown in medium 199 and not in a range of other commercially available culture media. Sutherland (1979a) subsequently demonstrated that fragile site expression will only occur if the culture medium is free of folic acid and thymidine, that it is enhanced by a culture medium pH of greater than 7.3, that in the presence of folic acid it can be induced by the folate antagonist methotrexate, and that the folic acid precursor folinic acid or the thymidine analog BrdU will suppress it in folate-free medium (Sutherland, 1979a). Addition of fluorodeoxyuridine (FudR), an inhibitor of the enzyme thymidylate synthetase, will induce expression in the presence of folic acid but not thymidine (Glover, 1981). Methionine has been shown to be essential for fragile site expression even in folic acid-free medium (Howard-

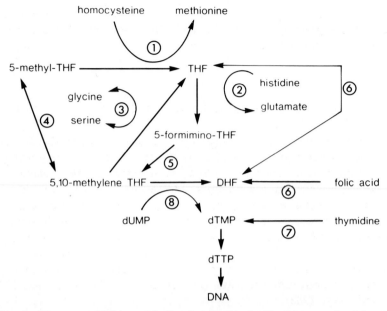

Fig. 4. The areas of folate metabolism involved in fragile site expression (after Erbe, 1975; Scott and Weir, 1981). The enzymes controlling the various reactions are (1) methionine synthetase, (2) glutamate formiminotransferase, (3) serine hydroxymethyltransferase, (4) methylene-THF reductase, (5) formimino-THF cyclodeaminase, (6) dihydrofolate reductase, (7) thymidine kinase, and (8) thymidylate synthetase. THF, tetrahydrofolate; DHF, dihydrofolate; dUMP, uridine monophosphate; dTMP, thymidine monophosphate; dTTP, thymidine triphosphate. (From Sutherland, 1983.)

Peebles and Pryor, 1981; Sutherland, 1983), but the reasons for this may be indirect in that cell cycle times are greatly increased in the absence of methionine and the effect of methionine deprivation can be overcome by FudR induction (Glover and Howard-Peebles, 1983).

All available data suggest the areas of metabolism involved are those shown in Fig. 4 and that any perturbation of conditions of tissue culture that lead to a relative deficiency of thymidine monophosphate toward the end of S phase will result in fragile site expression. Even though it now seems clear that this is the area of metabolism involved, it is not clear how it is involved. Why is it that in some cells the fragile site is only expressed on one chromatid? Analogously, in two homozygotes for the fragile site at 10q25, the fragile site was more often expressed on one chromosome than on both (Sutherland, 1981), even though environmental conditions that surrounded the homologous chromosomes during DNA synthesis must be more similar to each other than in different cells. One possibility is that in conditions appropriate for expression of fragile sites they are expressed in close to 100% of cells at the completion of S phase, but are gradually repaired during G_2 phase. This could account for expression in a single chromatid, since presumably the repair events would be independent for each chromatid, but expression, if it does occur during S phase, would not be.

IV. "SPONTANEOUS" CHROMOSOMAL FRAGILITY

Chromosome breakage in lymphocyte cultures has been a recognized phenomenon for many years, and some genetic toxicology testing is based upon increases of particular types of chromosome damage after exposure to potentially toxic agents. Chromosome breakage is difficult to quantitate cytogenetically, partly because of difficulties in distinguishing between chromosomal gaps and breaks. Chromosomal breakage in proliferating cell systems, which include PHA-stimulated lymphocyte cultures, is followed by the formation of micronuclei, which can be easily scored in interphase cells and provide a reliable approach to quantitation of chromosome breakage (Heddle *et al.*, 1978; Beek *et al.*, 1980; Obe and Beek, 1982).

In proliferating lymphocyte cultures, micronucleus frequency has been found to reach a peak after 5 days (Fig. 5), and fragile site carriers

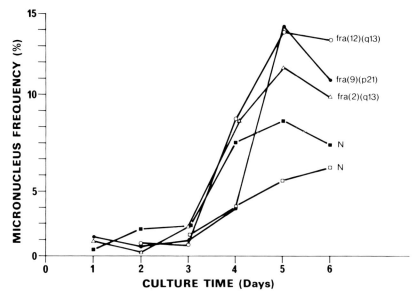

Fig. 5. Micronucleus frequencies in lymphocytes from carriers of fragile sites (fra) and controls (N) cultured in folic acid and thymidine-deficient medium and harvested at different times. (Data from Beek *et al.*, 1983.)

TABLE I

Frequency of Micronuclei in 5-Day Lymphocyte Cultures[a,b]

		Medium supplement		
Fragile site	Nil	Folic acid (5 mg/liter)	Thymidine (10 mg/liter)	Ham's F10
fra(2)(q13)	11.7			2.4
fra(6)(p23)	12.2			2.3
fra(9)(p21)	14.4			
fra(12)(q13)	13.8			
fra(X)(q27)	9.2	1.8	1.2	
Control				
1	6.6	1.7	0.9	
2	6.5	0.2	0.6	
3	4.4	0.4	0	
4	1.0	0	0	
5	3.6	0.2	0.6	

[a] In medium deficient in and supplemented with folic acid and thymidine or in Ham's F10 from fragile site carriers and controls.
[b] Data from Beek et al. (1983) and Jacky et al. (1983). Values in percentages.

have been found to have higher frequencies of micronucleus formation (Table I) than do appropriate controls without fragile sites (Beek et al., 1983) when the cultures are grown under conditions of folic acid and thymidine deprivation suitable for fragile site expression. When these components are present in the culture medium, only low micronucleus frequencies are seen in cultures from fragile site carriers and controls (Table I). This difference in micronucleus frequency seen for all individuals studied, whether fragile site carriers or controls, between cells cultured in the absence or presence of folic acid or thymidine suggests that the same mechanisms that control fragile site expression might also be involved in the manifestation of "spontaneous" chromosomal breakage. This means that the study of fragile sites may be able to be used as a model for the study of spontaneous chromosome breakage that is the primary event in at least some forms of carcinogenesis.

V. THE CHROMOSOME INSTABILITY SYNDROMES

There are a number of rare genetic diseases, mostly inherited in an autosomal recessive manner, in which there is an increase in various types of chromosomal breakage (Hecht and McCaw, 1977). In all these disorders there is a marked predisposition to develop different types of cancers.

In Bloom syndrome, which predisposes mainly to nonlymphocytic leukemias, the chromosome breakage is nonrandom and is usually shown by the presence of quadriradials involving homologous chromosomes. The rate of spontaneous sister chromatid exchange is also markedly increased. Patients with Fanconi anemia have an increased risk of developing leukemia, squamous cell carcinomas, and hepatic adenomas, and have an increase in apparently random chromatid breakage (Fig. 6); sister chromatid exchange is normal. In ataxia telangiectasia there is a marked increase in malignancies of the lymphoreticular system

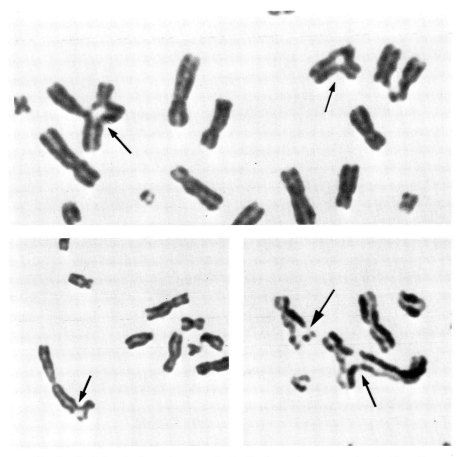

Fig. 6. Partial metaphases from a patient with Fanconi anemia and, coincidentally, a fragile site at 10q25 (large arrow). Note asymmetric chromatid exchange figures (small arrows) which are typical of the chromosome damage seen in this disorder.

and increased breakage of the chromosome, rather than chromatid, type that is apparently at random, although clones of cells with a translocation involving a break at 14q11-12 are frequently seen in such patients. There are also a number of other chromosome instability syndromes that predispose to cancer but that are not as well documented as the ones mentioned here.

None of the chromosome instability syndromes, or other syndromes involving defects of DNA repair that have been reported not to show chromosomal instability, have been studied to determine whether the type of chromosome breakage that they manifest can be affected by varying the concentrations of folic acid and thymidine in the medium in which the cells are cultured for chromosome studies. This should be done and could be approached directly by chromosome examination or indirectly by determination of micronucleus frequencies.

VI. CONCLUSIONS

Various types of chromosome fragility have been reviewed, and two of them, the one associated with heritable fragile sites and at least one form of "spontaneous" chromosome breakage, have been shown to be greatly influenced by concentrations of folic acid and thymidine in tissue culture medium. Since chromosome breakage is probably the primary event in the genesis of some forms of cancer, it is not improbable that these compounds may be found to be important in protecting against malignant transformation at the cellular level.

ACKNOWLEDGMENTS

Financial support for this work has been provided by grants from the National Health and Medical Research Council of Australia, The Channel 10 Children's Medical Research Foundation, and the Adelaide Children's Hospital Research Trust. I thank Dr. P. B. Jacky for helpful discussions during the preparation of this chapter.

REFERENCES

Beek, B., Klein, G., and Obe, G. (1980). *Biol. Zentralbl.* **99**, 73–84.
Beek, B., Jacky, P. B., and Sutherland, G. R. (1983). *Ann. Genet.* **26**, 5–9.
Croci, G. (1983). *Am. J. Hum. Genet.* **35**, 530–532.
Erbe, R. W. (1975). *N. Engl. J. Med.* **293**, 753–757.
Glover, T. W. (1981). *Am. J. Hum. Genet.* **33**, 234–242.
Glover, T. W., and Howard-Peebles, P. N. (1983). *Am. J. Hum. Genet.* **35**, 117–122.

Hecht, F., and McCaw, B. K. (1977). *Prog. Cancer Res. Ther.* **3**, 105–123.

Heddle, J. A., Benz, R. D., and Countryman, P. J. (1978). *In* "Mutagen-Induced Chromosome Damage in Man" (H. J. Evans and D. C. Lloyd, eds.), pp. 191–200. Yale Univ. Press, New Haven, Connecticut.

Howard-Peebles, P. N., and Pryor, J. C. (1981). *Clin. Genet.* **19**, 228–232.

Jacky, P. B., Beek, B., and Sutherland, G. R. (1983). *Science* **220**, 69–70.

Obe, G., and Beek, B. (1982). *Chem. Mutagens* **7**, 337–400.

Radman, M., Jeggo, P., and Wagner, R. (1982). *Mutat. Res.* **98**, 249–264.

Scheres, J. M., and Hustinx, T. W. (1980). *Am. J. Hum. Genet.* **32**, 628–629.

Schmid, M., Klett, C., and Nierderhofer, A. (1980). *Cytogenet. Cell Genet.* **28**, 87–94.

Scott, J. M., and Weir, D. G. (1981). *Lancet* **2**, 337–340.

Sutherland, G. R. (1977). *Science* **197**, 265–266.

Sutherland, G. R. (1979a). *Am. J. Hum. Genet.* **31**, 125–135.

Sutherland, G. R. (1979b). *Am. J. Hum. Genet.* **31**, 136–148.

Sutherland, G. R. (1981). *Am. J. Hum. Genet.* **33**, 946–949.

Sutherland, G. R. (1982). *Am. J. Hum. Genet.* **34**, 753–756.

Sutherland, G. R. (1983). *Int. Rev. Cytol.* **81**, 107–143.

Sutherland, G. R., Baker, E., and Seshadri, R. S. (1980). *Am. J. Hum. Genet.* **32**, 542–548.

Sutherland, G. R., Jacky, P. B., Baker, E., and Manuel, A. (1983). *Am. J. Hum. Genet.* **35**, 432–437.

Variations in Chromatin Structure and Nucleosomal DNA Repeat Length with Nutritional Manipulation

C. Elizabeth Castro and

J. Sanders Sevall

Department of Cellular and Molecular Biology
Southwest Foundation for Research and Education
San Antonio, Texas

I. INTRODUCTION

Nutrient regulation of genetic processes has been a classic tool with which molecular biologists defined the first models

Nutritional Factors in the Induction
and Maintenance of Malignancy

of gene expression in prokaryotes. Nutrient regulation of certain genomic processes occurs in higher organisms. An understanding of how nutritional factors affect genetic activities will lead toward an understanding of how aberrant genetic activity, such as malignant transformation, may be affected by nutrient variation.

The first portion of this chapter briefly describes nutritional variation as a tool for studying mechanisms of genetic regulation in both prokaryotic and eukaryotic systems. The second portion focuses on fundamental characteristics of the eukaryotic genome, such as DNA structure, chromosomal proteins, and levels of organization of chromatin structure. Chromatin structure will be emphasized since we have demonstrated that nutritional variation, particularly a lipogenesis-inducing diet, can alter the higher level of chromatin organization, as well as the fundamental unit of chromatin organization, the nucleosome.

II. NUTRITIONAL VARIATION AS A TOOL FOR ELUCIDATING MOLECULAR MECHANISMS OF REGULATION

A. In Prokaryotes

Nutritional variation of growth media has been a major tool that molecular biologists have exploited in studying the mechanisms of gene expression in *Escherichia coli*. The phenomenon of enzyme induction gave rise to the operon model and characterization of the molecular mechanism by which lactose can induce the cell to synthesize the transport enzymes. The mechanism involves a lactose-binding protein, the *lac* repressor, which allosterically alters its binding affinity toward the genomic regulatory region. As lactose levels are increased, the affinity that the lactose-binding protein has toward DNA is decreased, derepressing the transcription of the lactose operon regions coding for enzymes that metabolize lactose.

If glucose, a more efficient energy nutrient, is added to a lactose growth medium, *Escherichia coli* respond by inhibiting the transcription of genes for enzymes needed in catabolism of lactose and other non-glucose energy-yielding substrates. This phenomenon is termed catabolite repression, and the exact mechanism is unknown. However, the presence of glucose causes a decrease in the level of cyclic AMP. Cyclic AMP stimulates the initiation of transcription of many operons (genes) in bacteria by modulating the DNA affinity of a cyclic AMP-binding protein (Perlman and Pastan, 1974). One exact site of binding on the

DNA for the cyclic AMP-binding protein has been shown to be next to the *lac* repressor-binding site within the lactose operon. How this DNA-binding protein can increase the rate of initiation of mRNA transcription has been hypothesized as destabilization of the DNA helix for increased RNA polymerase entry (Dickson *et al.*, 1975).

Nutrition can modulate the enzymatic machinery in bacteria by positive and negative control mechanisms at the level of transcription of the DNA. These mechanisms are controlled by levels of metabolites that reflect the nutritional environment of growth media. Hence, modulation of the genetic apparatus by nutritional stimulus is a major factor regulating the response of bacteria to particular growth media.

B. In Eukaryotes

The plasticity of the genetic apparatus to nutritional environment is not unique to bacteria. In *Saccharomyces cerevisiae,* the expression of the genetic system for the utilization of galactose as a primary carbon source induces a permease activity and the tightly linked *GAL 1, GAL 7, GAL 10* gene cluster (Douglas and Condie, 1954; Douglas and Hawthorne, 1964). The induction is greater than tenfold in the presence of an appropriate sugar (Douglas and Hawthorne, 1966).

The regulation of the inducible gene products in *Saccharomyces cerevisiae* is more complicated than found in bacteria. All of the galactose genes or cluster of genes are unlinked (Mortimer and Hawthorne, 1969) except for *GAL 1, GAL 10,* and *GAL 7* genes (Douglas and Hawthorne, 1964; Bassel and Mortimer, 1971) and the tight linkage of *GAL 81* and *GAL 4* (Douglas and Hawthorne, 1966). The regulation of the *GAL 1, GAL 10,* and *GAL 7* genes occurs at the RNA level (Hopper and Rowe, 1978; Hopper *et al.*, 1978). These genes, whose induction is regulated at the RNA level, have been identified by a "differential plaque hybridization" that utilizes multiple nitrocellulose filter replicas of plaque plates produced from a λ phage yeast hybrid pool as hybridization templates for cDNA probes (St. John and Davis, 1979). This technology uses recombinant DNA procedures for the isolation of a larger number of genes regulated by nutritional modulation. The isolated DNA sequences will allow an in-depth analysis of the physical structure, transcriptional, and posttranscriptional regulation of expression of these genes.

In higher eukaryotes, a number of genes have been identified for which nutrient regulation, or at least nutrient involvement, occurs. Two such phenotypic genes of liver are serum transferrin and serum albumin. Transferrin gene expression in chicks is regulated by dietary iron deficiency (McKnight et al., 1980). The level of liver transferrin mRNA sequences increases two- to threefold, while the circulating level of transferrin increases two- to fourfold when chicks are fed an iron-defi-cient diet. When iron stores are replenished by the administration of iron-saturated ferritin, the rate of transferrin synthesis, as well as the level of transferrin mRNA, returns to control values within 2 to 3 days. The synthesis of rat serum albumin also is regulated by nutritional state. After 9 days of protein-free feeding, albumin synthesis falls from 15 to 8% of total liver protein synthesis (Pain et al., 1978). Concomitantly, the level of albumin mRNA is about 50% that of control rats. A short-term fast also decreases the content of total cytoplasm albumin mRNA by 40% per gram of rat liver (Yap et al., 1978). Feeding a lipogenic diet for 5 days decreases the amount of albumin mRNA by almost 30% of that of rats fed a complete basal diet (Sevall and Castro, 1983). Whether the de-creased level of albumin mRNA is due to decreased transcription of the albumin gene or decreased stability of the message is not known at present.

Several genes coding for metabolic "housekeeping" functions have been shown to be regulated directly or indirectly (via hormone interac-tion) by dietary alteration. The gluconeogenic enzyme phosphoenol-pyruvate carboxykinase (PEPCK) (EC 4.1.1.32) is inducible at the mRNA level by epinephrine, norepinephrine, dibutyryl-cAMP, or glucagon (Watford et al., 1982), but glucose feeding or insulin decrease the amount of PEPCK mRNA (Beale et al., 1982; Andreone et al., 1982).

The synthesis of a number of enzymes participating in the lipogenic pathway is modulated by dietary substrates. The levels of enzymatic induction of acetyl-CoA carboxylase (EC 6.4.1.2) (Nakanishi et al., 1976), fatty acid synthetase (Finkelstein et al., 1979; Alberts et al., 1975), and ATP citrate lyase (Finkelstein et al., 1979) are proportional to the popula-tion of immunoprecipitable polysomes bearing nascent polypeptide chains. The induction of synthesis varies from fourfold for acetyl-CoA carboxylase (Nakanishi et al., 1976) to greater than tenfold for ATP cit-rate lyase and fatty acid synthetase (Finkelstein et al., 1979) for rats fasted for 2 days and then fed a high carbohydrate, fat-free diet for 3 days. Induction of the lipogenic enzyme 6-phosphogluconate dehydrog-enase (EC 1.1.1.44) in rat liver by fasting and refeeding a high carbohy-drate, fat-free diet is accompanied by a fivefold increase in translatable mRNA compared with fasted rats (Hutchison and Holten, 1978).

When purified mRNAs are obtained for the inducible lipogenic en-zymes, such as for avian fatty acid synthetase (Zehner et al., 1980), full-length complementary DNA (cDNA) can be synthesized and used to isolate specific genes. An isolated gene model will allow one to define regulatory mechanisms that are nutritionally controlled. A battery of genes for a pathway of metabolism, such as for the inducible lipogenic enzymes, would facilitate the study of coordinated gene regulation. Coordinated regulation of lipogenic enzymes may bear directly on the malignant state, as Thompson and Smith (1982) have demonstrated that a human breast cell line SKBr3, derived from transformed tissue, lacks such regulation.

III. CHARACTERISTICS OF THE EUKARYOTIC GENOME

A. Structure of DNA

The genomic structure of higher eukaryotes is fundamentally different from bacteria. The content of DNA per eukaryotic cell ranges from 10 to 1000 times greater in size than their bacterial genomes. However, the structure of the DNA is fundamentally the same, although it is understood that the structure may be polymorphic and heterogeneous (Zimmerman, 1982). The sequence organization of the eukaryotic DNA is characterized by sequence classes that are repetitive, whereas the bacterial genome is characterized as being a unique sequence. The organization of the repetitive sequences may influence the structure and the genetic activity of the eukaryotic chromosomes (Jelinek and Schmid, 1982). Common to prokaryotic and eukaryotic DNA is the topological perspective of DNA structure (Bauer and Vinograd, 1974). The fundamental rules of topological orientation of the DNA fiber dictate how the DNA turns and twists in the eukaryotic genome and may correlate with a number of genetic processes. A more detailed account of DNA topology follows in Section III,C.

B. Chromosomal Proteins

A major difference in higher eukaryotes is the compartmentalization of the DNA in the nucleus of the cell. Associated with the DNA in the nucleus are nuclear proteins that are thought to carry out the genetic metabolism of the cell (Sevall, 1983). Just how much protein is associated with the nucleus is difficult to determine, since low salt washes can remove loosely associated protein or nuclear sap proteins (Peters and Comings, 1980; Bidney and Reeck, 1978). Hence, chromatin composition generally is reported as protein:DNA ratios of "purified" chromatin (interphase chromosomes). Purified chromatin is that which is obtained

TABLE I

Chemical Composition of Rat Liver Chromatin

$\dfrac{\text{Histone (mg)}}{\text{DNA (mg)}}$	$\dfrac{\text{Nonhistone (mg)}}{\text{DNA (mg)}}$	$\dfrac{\text{RNA (mg)}}{\text{DNA (mg)}}$	Type of diet	References
1.10	0.61	0.03	—	van den Broek *et al.* (1973)
1.00	0.67	0.04	—	Marushige and Bonner (1966)
1.20	1.00	0.10	—	Spelsberg and Hnilica (1971)
0.89	1.13	0.07	Chow	Castro and Sevall (1982)
0.89	2.73	0.13	Lipogenic	Castro and Sevall (1982)
1.20	4.01	0.12	Protein-free	Castro and Sevall (1982)
1.18	1.24	—	Lysine deficient	Canfield and Chytil (1978)
1.05	0.79	—	Control (0.8% lysine)	Canfield and Chytil (1978)

by low salt, isotonic centrifugation of nuclear material after nuclear membrane disruption. Table I contains protein:DNA mass ratios from chromatin isolated from rat liver. The ratios are characteristically a 2:1 mass ratio. The nuclear proteins can be further fractionated into basic proteins (histones) and acidic proteins (nonhistones). Table I indicates little variability of histone levels in the nucleus, whereas the nonhistone proteins show considerable variability of levels within the nucleus.

1. Histone Proteins

The histones have been extensively studied and reviewed (Isenberg, 1979). These basic proteins are represented by five major protein molecules: H1, H2a, H2b, H3, and H4 (Fig. 1). These are found in all eukaryotes. In inactive nucleated erythrocytes from birds, fish, and amphibians a sixth histone, H5, has been identified. Within each class of histones, the molecules may vary.

Histone H1 is by far the most variable in amino acid composition and sequence of the major histone classes. The histone H4 is the most conserved of all proteins. The conserved sequence also exhibits marked asymmetries in the distributions of charged and apolar amino acid residues. Histones H2a, H2b, and H3 have nonallelic variants that are related by simple amino acid substitutions (Franklin and Zweidler, 1977). The patterns of nonallelic variants may change during embryogenesis (Newrock *et al.*, 1977) or can exist in the same organism (West and Bonner, 1980). All the histone species undergo a series of protein modifications including acetylation (Dixon *et al.*, 1975), phosphorylation (Ruiz-Carrillo *et al.*, 1975), methylation (Delange *et al.*, 1969, 1973), condensation with ubiquitin (Goldknopf and Busch, 1978; Busch and Goldknopf, 1981), and poly(adenosine 5'-diphosphate) ribosylation (Wong *et al.*, 1977; Giri *et al.*, 1978). The precise function of modification of the histone is not clear. However, the modification events can affect the way in which histones interact with each other and other nuclear proteins. Histones H2a, H2b, H3, and H4 can interact with each other in very specific ways (D'Anna and Isenberg, 1973, 1974a,b; Skandrani *et al.*, 1972; Kornberg and Thomas, 1974; Roark *et al.*, 1974; Weintraub *et al.*, 1975; Lewis, 1976a,b,c; Nicola *et al.*, 1978). There are three strong interactions leading to the formation of two dimers (H2a–H2b and H3–

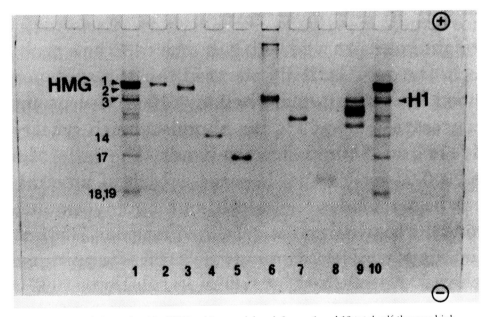

Fig. 1.   Polyacrylamide (20%) acid-urea slab gel. Lanes 1 and 10 total calf-thymus high mobility group (HMG) proteins (10 μg); lane 2 HMG1, (1 μg); lane 3 HMG 2 (1 μg); lane 4 HMG 14 (1 μg); lane 5 HMG 17 (2 μg); lane 6 HMG 3 (2 μg); lane 7 HMG 8 (1 μg); lane 8 ubiquitin (1 μg); lane 9 pig thymus whole histone (4 μg). HMG 3 and HMG 8 are degradation products of HMG 1 and histone H1. [With permission from Nicolas and Goodwin, 1982. Copyright: Academic Inc. (London) Ltd.]

H4) and one tetramer (H3$_2$–H4$_2$). There are two weak interactions, H2a–H4 and H2b–H3, and one intermediate interaction, H2a–H3 (for a review, see McGhee and Felsenfeld, 1980). X-ray crystallography has confirmed the general structure of the histone complex as two each of H2a, H2b, H3, and H4 (Dubochet and Noll, 1978; Wachtel et al., 1981; Lattman et al., 1982).

2. Nonhistone Proteins

Excluding the histones, all other proteins associated with eukaryotic chromosomes are grouped together under the general classification name of the nonhistone proteins (NHP). The tremendous diversity of these proteins with respect to size, charge, solubility, and function has hindered the study of the NHP. A correlation between genetic activity and the ratios of NHP to DNA have stimulated interest in the NHP and their role in transcription (Elgin and Weintraub, 1975). The constancy of the overall composition of NHP with successive or increasing ionic salt extracts (Comings and Harris, 1976; Bidney and Reeck, 1978; Comings and Tack, 1973) imply multiple functions of the NHP in a dynamic process. Characterization of these proteins now involve groups or families of proteins that are purified by physical properties or associated with nuclear organelles (Peters and Comings, 1980).

The high mobility group or HGM proteins are a group of NHP that are extracted from chromatin in 0.35 M NaCl and migrate rapidly on polyacrylamide gels (Fig. 1). Well-characterized mammalian HMG proteins constitute a small group called HMG1, HMG2, HMG14, and HMG17. They are abundant and occur in all tissues at some stage in development, but their proportions are not fixed. HMG1 can interact with histone H1 (Shooter et al., 1974; Smerdon and Isenberg, 1976), which may have consequences in understanding the functions of HMG1. HMG14 and HMG17 are preferentially associated with transcribed genes (Weisbord and Weintraub, 1979; Goodwin et al., 1979; Bakayev et al., 1979; Weisbrod et al., 1980; Albanese and Weintraub, 1980).

Classes of nuclear NHP associated with cellular organelles of mammalian cells are the nuclear lamina and matrix proteins. A subnuclear fraction composed of peripheral lamina and pore complexes has been isolated. Three major polypeptides with molecular weights between 60,000 and 80,000 and a major high molecular weight polypeptide (150,000–200,000) have been observed. A meshwork located internally, and designated the nuclear matrix, has a polypeptide composition similar to the pore complex–lamina preparations (Detke and Keller, 1982; Shelton et al., 1982). The function of these organelles is an area of intense investigation. It appears that the nuclear matrix has a central role in DNA replication and transcription.

3. Effect of Nutritional Variation on Chromosomal Proteins

We have measured the concentration of histone and nonhistone chromosomal proteins in nuclei of rats fed a complete diet, a lipogenic diet, or a protein-free, low carbohydrate diet. The mass amount of histones relative to DNA is similar for nuclei of all three groups (Table I). The histone : DNA ratio apparently remains stable under a variety of metabolic conditions, including chronic lysine deficiency (Canfield and Chytil, 1978), in weanling rat pups of zinc-deficient dams (Duerre et al., 1977), and in pregnant rats after protein restriction (Ravi and Ganguli, 1980). In contrast to the stability of the histones : DNA ratio, the mass amount of NHP : DNA is altered by dietary variation (Table I). When rats are fed a lipogenic diet or a protein-free, low carbohydrate diet there is a 2.4- or 3.5-fold increase in the NHP : DNA ratio, relative to that of stock-fed rats (Castro and Sevall, 1982). Canfield and Chytil (1978) demonstrated that the mass ratio of NHP to DNA in liver chromatin from lysine-deficient rats is higher than that for control rats. The biological significance of diet-induced increases in NHP remains to be determined and probably is based on the multiplicity of functions of these chromosomal proteins. The multitude of functions exhibited by NHP, including specific DNA-binding properties in moderate-salt extractable NHP (Berent and Sevall, 1982), has been reviewed by Sevall (1983).

C. Chromosome Structure

Nuclear DNA is packaged with the help of histones such that it is accessible for binding of polymerases and effector molecules. The various levels of chromatin organization are summarized in Table II (Feinberg and Coffey, 1982). The basic structural unit is the nucleosome. The full nucleosome can be released from the nucleus by the initial cut with micrococcal nuclease (for review, see McGhee and Felsenfeld, 1980). As nuclease digestion proceeds, stable nucleosome components are generated, the first being a 160–170 bp DNA fragment with bound histone H1, termed a chromatosome (Simpson, 1978). A nuclease-stable fragment of 146 bp of DNA and an octamer consisting of two each of the four core histones, H2A, H2B, H3, and H4 is then generated. Two molecules of HMG14 and/or HMG17 can be bound to a monosome (Albright et al., 1980; Sandeen et al., 1980; Mordian et al., 1980). The major sites of interaction are near the ends of the DNA associated with the histone octamer. The H1 minus core nucleosomal particle is cylindrical with a diameter of 11 nm and a height of 5.5 nm (Finch et al., 1981; Bentley et al., 1981). The DNA is wound around the cylindrical core from one to two left-handed superhelical turns.

TABLE II

Higher-Order Structure of DNA[a]

Structure (unit)	Number of base pairs	Dimension	Packing ratios[b]	Linking number[c]	Number of nucleosomes
Double helix (turn)	10.4	3.2 nm (32 Å) pitch 2.0 nm (20 Å) diameter	1	+1	—
Nucleosome (core)					
−H1	146	11 × 11 × 5.5 nm	5	−1.75	1
+H1	166			−2.0	1
Fibril (core + linker)	200	10 nm diameter	5.7	?	
Fiber (turn)	1,200	10 nm pitch 30 nm diameter	40	−6	6
Gene (intron, exon)	1,000 10,000	?	?	?	50
Loop					
− Histones	30,000	10–30 μm	100–500	150–500	0
+ Histones	100,000	0.2–1.0 μm			150–500
Metaphase chromatid	$0.5–2.4 \times 10^8$	1–10 μm length 0.5 μm diameter	8000–10,000	?	0.25×10^6
Interphase nucleus	7×10^9	10 μm diameter	?	?	3.5×10^7

[a] Reprinted with permission from Feinberg and Coffey (1982).
[b] Length of DNA in the unit structure, fully extended, divided by the axial length of structure.
[c] Number of times one edge of DNA helix crosses the other edge in the B helix.

The second level of chromatin organization is characterized by the "thick fiber" with a 25.0–30.0 nm diameter. Morphological studies on the electron microscope implicate the requirement for histone H1 (Thoma et al., 1979). The general model has a continuous coiling of the nucleofilament that is termed a solenoid with 607 nucleosomes per turn (Finch and Klug, 1976; Thoma et al., 1979; Suau et al., 1979; Thoma and Koller, 1981). Physical studies indicate that the nucleosomal disk is parallel with the axis of the solenoid, with H1 being involved in the higher-order packing of the nucleosomes (McGhee et al., 1980). An alternative model also supported by electron microscopy of the 25 nm fiber is a repeating globular supernucleosomal unit originally termed a superbead (Renz et al., 1977; Straetling et al., 1978; Meyer and Renz, 1979). Physical analyses of such superbeads have not been done.

The next level of structure is the formation of these 25 nm fibers into loops (Benyajati and Worcel, 1976; Paulson and Laemmli, 1977) or domains (Igo-Kemenes and Zachau, 1977). The loops are found in both interphase and metaphase chromosomes and are attached at their base to nonhistone proteins of the nuclear envelope, also referred to as the matrix, lamina, nuclear membrane ghost, cage, or, for the metaphase chromosome, the scaffold. Three lines of experimental approaches help to formulate the domain model (Igo-Kemenes et al., 1982). Centrifugation studies with lysed mouse cells (Ide et al., 1975; Nakane et al., 1978), hamster (Hartwig, 1978), and HeLa cells (Cook and Brazell, 1975) reveal supercoiled circular DNA structures with a characteristic biphasic response of sedimentation rates to increasing concentrations of intercalating agents. Electron microscopic investigations on interphase nuclei (Riley et al., 1975; Murray and Davies, 1979; Lepault et al., 1980) suggest that most chromatin is located in large domains in contact with the nuclear envelope. In metaphase chromosomes of HeLa cells, a radial loop model (where the loops radiate from a central scaffold) has been proposed for loop organization (Paulson and Lammli, 1977; Marsden et al., 1980). Alternately, electron microscopic studies of metaphase chromosome structure indicate that fiber–fiber contacts, rather than a shape-maintaining backbone or scaffold (Labhart et al., 1982), are required for higher-order structure. Restriction nuclease and micrococcal nuclease digestion of rat liver nuclei (Igo-Kemenes et al., 1977) can be interpreted in terms of the domain model.

The DNA loops appear to be functionally important. A single DNA loop is replicated as a unit and may be equivalent to a replicon (a unit of replication) (Vogelstein et al., 1980; Pardoll et al., 1980). DNA of the same length as a loop (30–40 × 10^3 bp) appears to become preferentially sensitive to DNase I during germ activation (Schrader et al., 1981). The nuclear matrix has been reported to be enriched in repetitive DNA sequences (Razin *et al.*, 1979), although these observations are being re-evaluated (Basler *et al.*, 1981; Kuo, 1982). The nature of the proteins involved in the formation of domains is far from clear. Specific mRNAs appear to be associated with the protein matrix of the DNA loop (Ross *et al.*, 1982). If domains are functional units, their specific structure, possible rearrangements, and activation may play a role in gene regulation.

The final level of structural organization is the condensation of the interphase chromatin to form the metaphase chromosome (Feinberg and Coffey, 1982). The organization of the loops into the highly structured metaphase chromosome is a full area of study and has yet to be determined (see above). It is clear that the metaphase chromosome loop contains the characteristic structure of the interphase loop (Gazit *et al.*, 1982). Over 90% of the metaphase chromosome volume is occupied by nucleosome volume. The formation of nucleosomes, fibrils, and loops produces topological problems for the DNA molecule. A topological perspective of DNA structure is listed in Table II (Feinberg and Coffey, 1982). The linking number is defined as the number of times the closed edge of the double helix crosses the other edge (Crick, 1976; Gellert, 1981; Record *et al.*, 1981). The relaxed double helix contributes $+1$ (right-handed turns) to the linking number per 10.4 bp. The different structures of released DNA may strongly influence the linking number of relaxed DNA. The linking number of DNA relaxed while in the form of a string of nucleosomes (a fiber) is less than the linking number of the same DNA in a relaxed double-stranded ring, which is consistent with a left-handed wrapping of the DNA outside the protein. Experimentally, each nucleosome, containing about 200 bp, contributes only -1 to the linking number (Germond *et al.*, 1975). The structural form of the DNA would be one complete coil (supercoil) of the DNA per nucleosome. However, physical studies have shown two complete turns of the DNA per nucleosome actually occurs. This is termed the "linking-number paradox." One theory postulates modifying the geometric states of the DNA by altering the writhe (twist) of the axis curve of the DNA as it goes around the histones (Finch *et al.*, 1977; Peck and Wang, 1981; Rhodes and Klug, 1981). Another theory is that the 25–30 nm fiber is organized with the nucleosomes in a zigzag pattern rather than a simple coil or solenoid (Worcel, 1981). There may be a more complex order to the loop domain than simple coiling (Feinberg and Coffey, 1982). These topological constraints can have a profound effect on the structure of the loop and may, in fact, regulate the DNA function.

The ultrastructure of transcribing chromatin has been extensively studied. There is general agreement that nucleosomal structures are absent from highly active gene regions. Biochemical studies with the mouse ribosomal genes revealed that template active or potentially active genes lack a nucleosomal configuration (Davis *et al.*, 1982). Contrary to this, the amplified structural gene dihydrofolate reductase, as shown by nuclease digestation experiments, derives the characteristic nucleosome repeat length expected for the presence of nucleosomes (Barsoum *et al.*, 1982). Hence, specific genomic loops may have a characteristic structural organization depending on their metabolic function. What regulates the altered chromatin structure of the template active loops remains a major area of intense research. Undermethylation of deoxycytosine is correlated with active gene regions (Razin and Riggs, 1980; Ehrlich and Wang, 1981; Andrews *et al.*, 1982). Altered structural regions leading to nuclease-sensitive chromosomal sites are attributed to altered DNA structure (Panayotatos and Wells, 1981; Lilley, 1981; Larsen and Weintraub, 1982). The HMG proteins confer a nuclease sensitivity conformation to template active regions of chromatin (Weintraub and Groudine, 1976; Weisbrod and Weintraub, 1979; Weisbrod *et al.*, 1980; Levy-Wilson and Dixon, 1978). Although recent analysis has raised some questions concerning the specificity of these proteins, more recently, minor chromosomal proteins can interact with specific sites at the 5' end of template active genes (Berent and Sevall, 1982).

Effect of Nutritional Variation on Alteration of Chromatin Structure

We investigated whether higher-level chromatin organization is alterable by nutritional variation (Castro and Sevall, 1980). Rats were fed a complete, stock diet or one of a number of semisynthetic diets in which one of the energy-yielding components were omitted or deficient (Table III). When nuclear chromatin from rats fed a complete diet is digested with micrococcal nuclease, 50.3% of the chromatin was rendered acid soluble in agreement with others (Sollner-Webb and Felsenfeld, 1975; Axel, 1975). However, the amount of chromatin that is disgested to acid solubility by micrococcal nuclease from rats fed six semisynthetic diets varies with the nature of dietary variation (Fig. 2). When rats are fed a lipogenic diet, 71% of chromatin is solubilized by micrococcal nuclease, whereas only 39% is solubilized if rats are fed a protein-free, low carbohydrate diet (Fig. 3). These observations indicate that the higher-order configuration of rat liver chromatin may be alterable by diet. Lipogenesis, in particular, modifies the higher-order structure of rat liver chro-

TABLE III

Composition of Diets[a,b]

Component	Diet 1, high carbohydrate/ fat-free	Diet 2, low carbohydrate/ high fat	Diet 3, low carbohydrate/ high protein	Diet 4, high carbohydrate/ low protein	Diet 5, high carbohydrate/ protein-free	Diet 6, low carbohydrate/ protein-free
Casein, vitamin-free[c]	30	30	64	8	0	0
d-(+)-dextrose[c]	60	19	18	72	72	18
Salt mixture[c]	4	4	4	4	4	4
Alphacel, non-nutritive bulk[c]	4	20	4	4	12	67
Vitamin mixture[c]	2	2	2	2	2	2
Corn oil[d]	0	25	8	10	10	15
Total energy value (kcal/100 g)	368	429	408	418	386	215
Carbohydrate energy value (kcal/100 g)	248	84	80	296	296	80

[a] From Castro and Sevall (1980). © *J. Nutr.* American Institute of Nutrition.
[b] Composition in grams per 100 grams of food.
[c] ICN Nutritional Biochemicals, Cleveland, Ohio.
[d] CPC International Inc., Englewood Cliffs, New Jersey.

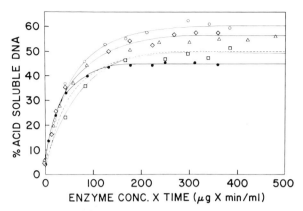

Fig. 2. Micrococcal nuclease digestion of nuclei from animals fed experimental diets. Diet 2: ◇, 170 μg DNA/ml, 74 units nuclease/ml; △, 170 μg DNA/ml, 100 units nuclease/ml. Diet 3: ⊔, 205 μg DNA/ml, 70 units nuclease/ml. Diet 4: ○, 182 μg DNA/ml, 70 units nuclease/ml. Diet 5: ●, 220 μg DNA/ml, 74 units nuclease/ml. Digestion of control nuclei, dashed line. (From Castro and Sevall, 1980. © *J. Nutr.* American Institute of Nutrition.)

matin. The structural alteration effected by lipogenesis may be interpreted as a localized, specific unwinding of template active chromatin, or a generalized, nonspecific unwinding of chromatin.

Nucleosomal repeat length, i.e., the length of the 146 bp stable core particle, plus the linker length of DNA, has been measured in the nuclei of rats fed a lipogenic diet; a protein-free, low carbohydrate diet; or a complete stock diet (Castro, 1983). After a 5-day feeding period, liver

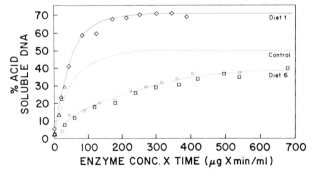

Fig. 3. Micrococcal nuclease digestion of nuclei from animals fed diet 1 and diet 6. Diet 1: △, 190 μg DNA/ml, 35 units nuclease/ml; ◇, 150 μg DNA/ml, 71 units nuclease/ml. Diet 6: ☐, 217 μg DNA, 60 units nuclease/ml; ○, 217 μg DNA/ml, 73 units nuclease/ml. (From Castro and Sevall, 1980. © *J. Nutr.* American Institute of Nutrition.)

C. Elizabeth Castro and J. Sanders Sevall

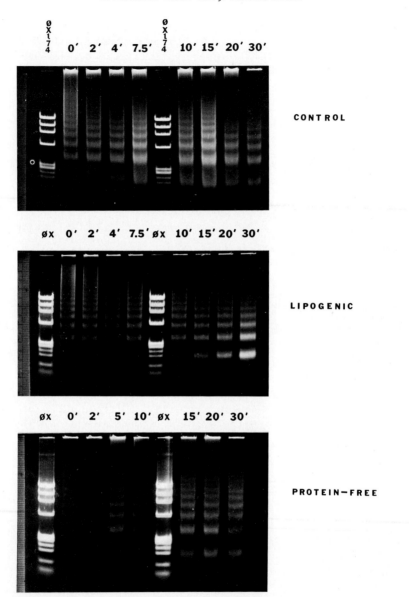

Fig. 4. Purified DNA fragments generated by incubation with micrococcal nuclease for the time (minutes) indicated at the top of each lane. Lane labeled ∅X contains 4 µg of 0X174 RF DNA digested with *Hae*III restriction enzyme. (From Castro, 1983. © *J. Nutr.* American Institute of Nutrition.)

nuclei were purified and mildly incubated with micrococcal nuclease until 5–6% of the chromatin was acid soluble. Mild incubation conditions were selected because more transcriptionally active DNA is released under these conditions (Bloom and Anderson, 1979). A time course of digestion with micrococcal nuclease for 0–30 minutes generated chromatin digestion products that were purified and sized by electrophoresis.

Deproteinized DNA oligomers produced from very mild digestion of nuclei from rats fed a complete stock diet; a lipogenic diet; or a protein-free, low carbohydrate diet are shown in Fig. 4. For each diet, the length of the nucleosomal repeat length decreases as incubation time with micrococcal nuclease increases. At each time point measured there are differences in repeat length between chromatin of lipogenic rats and protein-free or stock-fed rats. Regardless the calculation method used (Tables IV or V), nucleosome repeat length for rats fed a lipogenic diet is

TABLE IV

Nucleosomal Repeat Length (bp) Calculated from Length of Oligomeric DNA Divided by Oligomer Number[a–c]

Incubation time with micrococcal nuclease (minutes)	Diet		
	Stock	Lipogenic	Protein-free
0	222.8 ± 6.9a (21)	200.6 ± 4.0b (31)	210.9 ± 5.9c (17)
2	216.3 ± 3.9a (23)	195.4 ± 4.4b (29)	205.8 ± 6.0c (19)
4	212.1 ± 3.6a (22)	194.0 ± 4.2b (26)	N.D.[d]
7.5	210.8 ± 5.2a (23)	191.2 ± 4.2b (29)	N.D.
10	206.7 ± 5.3a (24)	188.9 ± 4.7b (25)	207.3 ± 7.4a (18)
15	206.1 ± 5.0a (25)	186.0 ± 4.5b (26)	206.4 ± 7.1a (19)
20	205.4 ± 5.6a (20)	188.5 ± 3.6b (23)	203.8 ± 5.7a (11)
30	200.8 ± 4.9a (24)	188.5 ± 3.1b (21)	200.7 ± 4.0a (23)

[a] From Castro (1983). © J. Nutr. American Institute of Nutrition.
[b] Mean (bp) ± S.D. Number in parentheses is the number of electrophoretic oligomeric bonds > mononucleosome used in calculation.
[c] Means within a row followed by the same letter are not different (P = 0.05).
[d] N.D., not determined.

consistently 6–10% shorter than that of rats fed the stock diet or the protein-free, low carbohydrate diet. The nucleosome repeat length for rats fed the stock diet or the protein-free, low carbohydrate diet are virtually identical after 10–30 minutes of incubation with micrococcal nuclease.

A 6–10% difference in nucelosome repeat length in nuclei of lipogenic rats may have important biological significance. A difference of the same magnitude (6%) is seen when transcriptionally active chromatin of chicken liver is compared with the more inactive chicken erythrocyte chromatin (Morris, 1976). In other instances, a shorter nucleosome repeat length is observed in transcriptionally active cells (Spadafora et al., 1976; Thomas and Thompson, 1977). Repeat length decreases also as malignant Friend erythroleukemic cells become progressively more malignant (Leonardson and Levy, 1980).

The size distribution of oligonucleosomal products generated by micrococcal nuclease is shown in Fig. 5 for rats fed a stock diet, a lipogenic

TABLE V

Nucleosomal Repeat Length (bp) Calculated by the Slope of Regression Lines[a–d]

Incubation time with micrococcal nuclease (minutes)	Diet		
	Stock	Lipogenic	Protein-free
0	239.1 ± 3.6a $r = 1.00$	204.7 ± 3.4b $r = 1.00$	214.4 ± 5.7b $r = 1.00$
2	223.0 ± 4.4a $r = 1.00$	201.5 ± 4.6b $r = 1.00$	211.9 ± 8.4c $r = 1.00$
4	219.8 ± 5.2a $r = 1.00$	195.2 ± 9.1b $r = 1.00$	N.D.[e]
7.5	212.1 ± 6.4a $r = 1.00$	197.2 ± 4.7b $r = 1.00$	N.D.
10	214.5 ± 10.0a $r = 1.00$	194.5 ± 8.5b $r = 1.00$	209.3 ± 13.6a $r = 1.00$
15	212.0 ± 7.1a $r = 1.00$	192.7 ± 7.1b $r = 1.00$	220.5 ± 1.3c $r = 1.00$
20	210.4 ± 5.3a $r = 1.00$	194.0 ± 5.6b $r = 1.00$	216.1 ± 4.0a $r = 1.00$
30	206.1 ± 1.7a $r = 1.00$	192.6 ± 4.4b $r = 1.00$	206.8 ± 2.8a $r = 1.00$

[a] From Castro (1983). © J. Nutr. American Institute of Nutrition.
[b] Mean (bp) ± S.D.
[c] Means within a row followed by the same letter are not different ($P = 0.01$).
[d] r = coefficient of correlation.
[e] N.D., not determined.

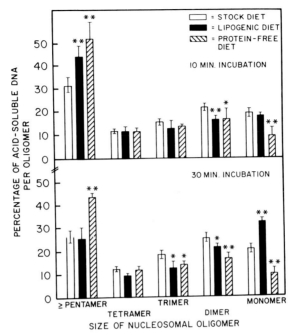

Fig. 5. Percentage of total input DNA found in different nucelosome classes after incubation with micrococcal nuclease for indicated time. In each case, the statistical difference is relative to value of stock-fed treatment within each size class. * $P = 0.05$, ** $P = 0.01$. (From Castro, 1983. © *J. Nutr.* American Institute of Nutrition.)

diet, or a protein-free, low carbohydrate diet (Castro, 1983). The percentage of input DNA digested by micrococcal nuclease to mononucleosome (monomer), dinucleosome (dimer), trinucleosome (trimer), tetranucleosome (tetramer), and pentanucleosome (pentamer) was measured. After 10 minutes, the slowest rate of digestion of DNA to monomer occurs in rats fed the protein-free diet.

After 30 minutes, about 44% of DNA from rats fed a protein-free diet is still in large oligomers, whereas only about 26% of DNA from rats fed the other two diets is pentamer size (Fig. 5). The percentage distribution of monomer is greatest in DNA of lipogenic rats, coincident with a decreased nucleosome repeat length.

IV. PERSPECTIVE

The eukaryotic nucleus faces what may seem an insurmountable obstacle, that of packaging over 2 m of helical, double-stranded DNA into an approximate volume of 10 μm^3 (Berlin *et al.*, 1982). Accomplishing this feat requires specific chromosomal proteins, such as the histones H2a, H3b, H3, H4, and H1, as well as several successive levels of chromosomal organization. The manner in which chromatin is oriented and organized within the confines of the interphase nucleus must influence a multitude of genomic processes.

It is not surprising that the nucleus, as well as its contents, is responsive to nutritional variation. Indeed, the first model of gene regulation in prokaryotes, the *lac* model, was defined by utilization of substrate from growth medium. In eukaryotic organisms, we observe that nutritional variation can alter the higher-order arrangement of chromatin as measured by the amount of chromatin rendered accessible to micrococcal nuclease. A lipogenesis-inducing diet renders greater than 70% of nuclear chromatin accessible to micrococcal nuclease, whereas a protein-free, low carbohydrate diet renders less than 40% accessible. Micrococcal nuclease makes initial cuts at linker regions of DNA. Lipogenesis apparently causes internucleosomal linking DNA to be more accessible to micrococcal nuclease. In addition, lipogenesis decreases the length of the nucleosomal repeat distance by as much as 11%. The decreased nucleosomal repeat length may be due to endonucleolytic activity of micrococcal nuclease after the initial cut is made. This finding substantiates that the internucleosomal linking DNA is more available to micrococcal nuclease.

What are mechanisms by which a nutritional variation, such as lipogenesis, can mediate an alteration of chromatin structure or a decrease in nucleosomal repeat length? One manner may be that of changing the topological constraints on the DNA in localized regions or along long stretches of molecule. If one could demonstrate that nutritional environment directly or indirectly (via hormone interaction) exerts an effect on superhelicity or relaxation of the DNA molecule, there would be a clearer understanding of nutrient–genome interaction. Such an effect on the topology of DNA might be mediated enzymatically by nutrient-related changes in topoisomerase (I or II), an enzyme that removes or adds linking numbers to the DNA, which could be observed as a condensation or decondensation of chromatin (for review, see Sevall, 1983).

Another mechanism of nutritionally mediated alteration in chromatin structure may be through the variation of the secondary structure of DNA, which again would alter the topology of the DNA. The nuclear structural proteins, such as HMG protein or histones H1, H3, and H2a and H2b, that have protein variants could be involved in such structural modulation due to their internucleosomal location, as well as their intimate contact with the nucleosomal core particle. These proteins are well characterized, and techniques are available to study them in defined nutritional systems.

Dynamic events within the genome may, in some instances, result in malignant transformation. The malignantly transformed condition may be either maintained or challenged by the certain environmental determinants. Nutritional state is one of these environmental determinants. It is to our advantage to understand fundamental interactive processes between the genetic machinery and the nutritional state of the nucleus.

ACKNOWLEDGMENTS

Supported in part by the Oree Meadows Perryman Molecular Genetics Laboratory for Cancer Research Grant from Meadows Foundation, Inc., Dallas, Texas, and by Department of Health and Human Services Grants 1 R01 AM28 162-02 to CEC and 1 R01 AM2852-02 to JSS.

REFERENCES

Albanese, I., and Weintraub, H. (1980). *Nucleic Acids Res.* **8**, 2787–2805.

Alberts, A. W., Strauss, A. W., Hennessy, S., and Vagelos, P. R. (1975). *Proc. Natl. Acad. Sci. U.S.A.* **72**, 3956–3960.

Albright, S. C., Wiseman, J. M., Lang, R. A., and Garrard, W. T. (1980). *J. Biol. Chem.* **255**, 3673–3684.

Andreone, T. L., Beale, E. G., Bar, R. S., and Granner, D. K. (1982). *J. Biol. Chem.* **257**, 35–38.

Andrews, G. K., Dziadek, M., and Tamaok, T. (1982). *J. Biol. Chem.* **257**, 5148–5153.

Axel, R. (1975). *Biochemistry* **14**, 2921–2925.

Bakayev, V. V., Schmatchenko, V. V., and Georgiev, P. (1979). *Nucleic Acids Res.* **7**, 1525–1540.

Barsoum, J., Levinger, L., and Varshavsky, A. (1982). *J. Biol. Chem.* **257**, 524–5282.

Basler, J., Hastie, N. D., Pietras, D., Matsui, S. I., Sandberg, A. A., and Bereznscy, R. (1981). *Biochemistry* **20**, 6921–6929.

Bassel, J., and Mortimer, R. J. (1971). *J. Bacteriol.* **108**, 179–183.

Bauer, W., and Vinograd, J. (1974). In "Basic Principles in Nucleic Acid Chemistry" (P. O. P. Ts'o, ed.), Vol. 2, pp. 135–216, pp. 265–303. Academic Press, New York.

Beale, E. G., Hartley, J. L., and Granner, D. K. (1982). *J. Biol. Chem.* **257**, 2022–2028.

Bentley, G. A., Finch, J. T., and Lewit-Bentley, A. (1981). *J. Mol. Biol.* **145**, 771–784.

Benyajati, C., and Worcel, A. (1976). *Cell* **9**, 393–407.

Berent, S. L., and Sevall, J. S. (1982). *J. Cell Biol.* **95**, Abstr. 10021.

Berlin, J., Castro, C. E., Franklin, B., and Sevall, J. S. (1982). *Nutr. Res.* **2**, 51–63.

Bidney, D. L., and Reeck, G. R. (1978). *Biochim. Biophys. Acta* **521**, 753–761.

Bloom, K. S., and Anderson, J. N. (1979). *J. Biol. Chem.* **254**, 10532–10539.

Busch, H., and Goldknopf, I. L. (1981). *Mol. Cell. Biochem.* **40**, 173–187.

Canfield, L. M., and Chytil, F. (1978). *J. Nutr.* **108**, 1336–1342.

Castro, C. E. (1983). *J. Nutr.* **113,** 557–565.

Castro, C. E., and Sevall, J. S. (1980). *J. Nutr.* **110,** 105–116.

Castro, C. E., and Sevall, J. S. (1982). *J. Nutr.* **112,** 1203–1211.

Comings, D. E., and Harris, D. C. (1976). *J. Cell Biol.* **70,** 440–452.

Comings, D. E., and Tack, L. O. (1973). *Exp. Cell Res.* **82,** 175–191.

Cook, P. R., and Brazell, I. A. (1975). *J. Cell Sci.* **19,** 261–279.

Crick, F. H. C. (1976). *Proc. Natl. Acad. Sci. U.S.A.* **73,** 2639–2643.

D'Anna, J. A., Jr., and Isenberg, I. (1973). *Biochemistry* **12,** 1035–1043.

D'Anna, J. A., Jr., and Isenberg, I. (1974a). *Biochemistry* **13,** 2098–2104.

D'Anna, J. A., Jr., and Isenberg, I. (1974b). *Biochem. Biophys. Res. Commun.* **59,** 542–547.

Davis, A. H., Reudelhuber, T. L., and Garrard, W. T. (1982). *J. Cell Biol.* **95,** Abstr. 3019.

Delange, R. J., Fambrough, D. M., Smith, E. L., and Bonner, J. (1969). *J. Biol. Chem.* **244,** 319–334.

Delange, R. J., Hooper, J. A., and Smith, E. L. (1973). *J. Biol. Chem.* **248,** 3261–3274.

Detke, S. and Keller, J. M. (1982). *J. Biol. Chem.* **257,** 3905–3911.

Dickson, R. C., Abelson, J., Barnes, W. M., and Reznikoff, W. S. (1975). *Science* **187,** 27–35.

Dixon, G. H., Candido, E. P. M., Honda, B. M., Louie, A. J., Macleod, A. R., and Sung, M. T. (1975). *Ciba Found. Symp.* [N.S.] **28,** 229–258.

Douglas, H. C., and Condie, F. (1954). *J. Bacteriol.* **68,** 662–670.

Douglas, H. C., and Hawthorne, D. C. (1964). *Genetics* **19,** 837–844.

Douglas, H. C., and Hawthorne, D. C. (1966). *Genetics* **54,** 911–916.

Dubochet, J., and Noll, M. (1978). *Science* **202,** 280–286.

Duerre, J. A., Ford, K. M., and Sandstead, H. H. (1977). *J. Nutr.* **107,** 1082–1093.

Ehrlich, M., and Wang, R. Y. H. (1981). *Science* **212,** 1350–1357.

Elgin, S. C. R., and Weintraub, H. (1975). *Annu. Rev. Biochem.* **44,** 725–774.

Feinberg, A. P., and Coffey, D. S. (1982). *In* "The Nuclear Envelope and the Nuclear Matrix" (G. G. Maul, ed.), pp. 293–305. Alan R. Liss, Inc., New York.

Finch, J. T., and Klug, A. (1976). *Proc. Natl. Acad. Sci. U.S.A.* **73,** 1897–1901.

Finch, J. T., Lutter, L. C., Rhodes, D., Brown, R. S., Rushton, B., Levitt, D. H., and Klug, P. (1977). *Nature (London)* **269,** 29–36.

Finch, J. T., Rhodes, D., Brown, R. S., Richmond, T., Rushton, B., Lutter, L. C., and Klug, A. (1981). *J. Mol. Biol.* **145,** 757–769.

Finkelstein, M. B., Auringer, M. P., Halper, L. A., Linn, T. C., Singh, M., and Srere, P. A. (1979). *Eur. J. Biochem.* **99,** 209–216.

Franklin, S. G., and Zweidler, A. (1977). *Nature (London)* **266,** 273–275.

Gazit, B., Cedar H., Lerer, I., and Voss, R. (1982). *Science* **217,** 618–650.

Gellert, M. (1981). *Annu. Rev. Biochem.* **50,** 879–910.

Germond, J. E., Hirt, B. Oudet, P., Gross-Bellard, M., and Chambon, P. (1975). *Proc. Natl. Acad. Sci. U.S.A.* **72,** 1343–1847.

Giri, C. P., West, M. H. P., Ramirez, M. L., and Smulson, M. E. (1978). *Biochemistry* **17,** 3495–3500.

Goldknopf, I. L., and Busch, H. (1978). *In* "The Cell Nucleus," (H. Busch, ed.), Vol. 6, Part C, pp. 149–180. Academic Press, New York.

Goodwin, G. H., Mathew, C. G. P., Wright, C. A., Venkov, C. D., and Johns, E. W. (1979). *Nucleic Acids Res.* **7,** 1815–1835.

Hartwig, M. (1978). *Acta Biol. Med. Ger.* **37,** 421–432.

Hopper, J. E., and Rowe, L. B. (1978). *J. Biol. Chem.* **253,** 7566–7569.

Hopper, J. E., Broach, J. R., and Rowe, L. B. (1978). *Proc. Natl. Acad. Sci. U.S.A.* **75,** 2878–2882.

Hutchison, J. S., and Holten, D. (1978). *J. Biol. Chem.* **253**, 52–57.

Ide, T., Nakane, M., Anzai, K., and Andoh, T. (1975). *Nature (London)* **258**, 445–447.

Igo-Kemenes, T., and Zachau, H. G. (1977). *Cold Spring Harbor Symp. Quant. Biol.* **42**, 109–118.

Igo-Kemenes, T., Greil, W., and Zachau, H. (1977). *Nucleic Acids Res.* **4**, 3387–3400.

Igo-Kemenes, T., Hörz, W., and Zachau, H. (1982). *Ann. Rev. Biochem.* **51**, 89–121.

Isenberg, I. (1979). *Annu. Rev. Biochem.* **48**, 159–192.

Jelinek, W. R., and Schmid, C. W. (1982). *Annu. Rev. Biochem.* **51**, 813–844.

Kornberg, R. D., and Thomas, J. O. (1974). *Science* **184**, 865–868.

Kuo, M. T. (1982). *Biochemistry* **21**, 321–326.

Kuo, M. T., Iyer, B., and Schwartz, R. J. (1982). *Nucleic Acids Res.* **10**, 4565–4579.

Labhart, P., Koller, T., and Wunderli, H. (1982). *Cell* **30**, 115–121.

Larsen, A., and Weintraub, H. (1982). *Cell* **29**, 609–622.

Lattman, E., Burlingame, R., Hatch, C., and Moudrianakis, E. N. (1982). *Science* **216**, 1016–1018.

Leonardson, K. E., and Levy, S. B. (1980). *Nucleic Acids Res.* **8**, 5317–5331.

Lepault, J., Bram, S., Escaig, J., and Wray, W. (1980). *Nucleic Acids Res.* **8**, 265–278.

Levy-Wilson, B., and Dixon, G. H. (1978). *Nucleic Acids Res.* **5**, 4155–4162.

Lewis, P. N. (1976a). *Can. J. Biochem.* **54**, 641–649.

Lewis, P. N. (1976b). *Can. J. Biochem.* **54**, 963–970.

Lewis, P. N. (1976c). *Biochem. Biophys. Res. Commun.* **68**, 329–335.

Lilley, D. M. (1981). *Nucleic Acids Res.* **9**, 1271–1289.

McGhee, J. D., and Felsenfeld, G. (1980). *Annu. Rev. Biochem.* **49**, 1115–1156.

McGhee, J. D., Rau, D. C., Charney, E., and Felsenfeld, G. (1980). *Cell* **22**, 87–96.

McKnight, G. S., Lee, D. C., Hemmaplardh, D., Finch, C. A., and Palmiter, R. D. (1980). *J. Biol. Chem.* **255**, 144–147.

Marsden, M. P. F., and Laemmli, U. K. (1980). *Cell* **17**, 849–858.

Marushige, K., and Bonner, J. (1966). *J. Mol. Biol.* **15**, 160–174.

Meyer, G. F., and Renz, M. (1979). *Chromosoma* **75**, 177–184.

Mordian, J. K. W., Paton, A. E., Bumick, G. J., and Olins, D. E. (1980). *Science* **209**, 1534–1536.

Morris, N. R. (1976). *Cell* **9**, 627–632.

Mortimer, R. K., and Hawthorne, D. C. (1969). *In* "The Yeasts" (A. H. Rose and J. S. Harrison, eds.), pp. 385–460. Academic Press, New York.

Murray, A. B., and Davies, H. G. (1979). *J. Cell Sci.* **35**, 59–66.

Nakane, M., Ide, T., Anzai, K., Ohara, S., and Andoh, T. (1978). *J. Biochem. (Tokyo)* **84**, 145–157.

Nakanishi, S., Tanabe, T., Horikawa, S., and Numa, S. (1976). *Proc. Natl. Acad. Sci. U.S.A.* **73**, 2304–2307.

Newrock, K. M., Alfageme, C. R., Nardi, R. V., and Cohen, L. H. (1977). *Cold Spring Harbor Symp. Quant. Biol.* **42**, 421–431.

Nicola, N. A., Fulmer, A. W., Schwartz, A. M., and Fasman, G. D. (1978). *Biochemistry* **17**, 1779–1785.

Nicolas, R. H., and Goodwin, G. H. (1982). *In* "The HMG Chromosomal Proteins" (E. W. Johns, ed.), p. 56. Academic Press, London.

Pain, V. M., Clemens, M. J., and Garlick, P. J. (1978). *Biochem. J.* **172**, 129–135.

Panayotatos, N., and Wells, R. D. (1981). *Nature (London)* **289**, 466–470.

Pardoll, D. M., Vogelstein, B., and Coffey, D. S. (1980). *Cell* **19**, 527–536.

Paulson, J. R., and Laemmli, U. K. (1977). *Cell* **12**, 817–828.

Peck, L. J., and Wang, J. C. (1981). *Nature (London)* **292,** 375–378.
Perlman, R. L., and Pastan, I. (1974). *Curr. Top. Cell. Regul.* **3,** 117–134.
Peters, K. E., and Comings, D. E. (1980). *J. Cell Biol.* **86,** 135–155.
Ravi, R. T., and Ganguli, N. C. (1980). *J. Nutr.* **110,** 1144–1151.
Razin, A., and Riggs, A. D. (1980). *Science* **210,** 604–610.
Razin, S. U., Mantieva, U. L., and Georgiev, G. P. (1979). *Nucleic Acids Res.* **7,** 1713–1735.
Record, M. T., Jr., Mazur, S. J., Melancon, P., Roe, J. H., Shanner, S. L., and Unger, L. (1981). *Annu. Rev. Biochem.* **50,** 997–1024.
Renz, M., Nehls, P., and Hozier, J. (1977). *Proc. Natl. Acad. Sci. U.S.A.* **74,** 1879–1883.
Rhodes, D., and Klug, A. (1981). *Nature (London)* **292,** 378–380.
Riley, D. E., Keller, J. M., and Byers, B. (1975). *Biochemistry* **14,** 3005–3013.
Roark, D. E., Georghegan, T. E., and Keller, G. H. (1974). *Biochem. Biophys. Res. Commun.* **59,** 542–547.
Ross, D. A., Yen, R. W., and Chae, C. B. (1982). *Biochemistry* **21,** 764–771.
Ruiz-Carrillo, A., Wangh, L. J., and Allfrey, V. P. (1975). *Science* **190,** 117–128.
St. John, T. P., and Davis, R. W. (1979). *Cell* **16,** 443–452.
Sandeen, G., Wood, W., and Felsenfeld, G. (1980). *Nucleic Acids Res.* **8,** 3757–3778.
Schrader, W. T., Birnbaumer, M. E., Hugh, M. R., Weigel, N. L., Grody, W., and O'Malley, B. W. (1981). *Recent Prog. Horm. Res.* **37,** 583–597.
Sevall, J. S. (1983). *In* "Chromosomal Nonhistone Proteins" (L. S. Hnilica, ed.), Vol. 1, pp. 25–46. CRC Press, Boca Raton, Florida.
Sevall, J. S., and Castro, C. E. (1983). In preparation.
Shelton, K. R., Guthrie, V. H., and Cochran, D. L. (1982). *J. Biol. Chem.* **257,** 4328–4332.
Shooter, K. V., Goodwin, G. H., and Johns, E. W. (1974). *Eur. J. Biochem.* **47,** 263–270.
Simpson, R. T. (1978). *Biochemistry* **17,** 5524–5592.
Skandrani, E., Mizon, J., Sautiere, P., and Biserte, G. (1972). *Biochimie* **54,** 1267–1272.
Smerdon, M. J., and Isenberg, I. (1976). *Biochemistry* **15,** 4242–4247.
Sollner-Webb, B., and Felsenfeld, G. (1975). *Biochemistry* **14,** 2915–2920.
Spadafora, C., Bellard, M., Compton, J. L., and Chambon, P. (1976). *FEBS Lett.* **69,** 281–285.
Spelsberg, T. C., and Hnilica, L. S. (1971). *Biochim. Biophys. Acta* **228,** 202–211.
Straetling, W. H., Mueller, U., and Zentgraf, H. (1978). *Exp. Cell Res.* **117,** 301–311.
Suau, P., Bradbury, E. M., and Baldwin, J. P. (1979). *Eur. J. Biochem.* **97,** 593–602.
Thoma, F., and Koller, T. (1981). *J. Mol. Biol.* **149,** 709–733.
Thoma, F., Koller, T., and Klug, A. (1979). *J. Cell Biol.* **83,** 403–427.
Thomas, J. O., and Thompson, R. J. (1977). *Cell* **10,** 633–640.
Thompson, B. J., and Smith, S. (1982). *Biochim. Biophys. Acta* **712,** 217–220.
van den Broek, H. W. J., Nooden, L. D., Sevall, J. S., and Bonner, J. (1973). *Biochemistry* **12,** 229–236.
Volgelstein, B., Pardoll, D. M., and Coffey, D. S. (1980). *Cell* **22,** 79–85.
Wachtel, E. J., Gilon, C., and Sperling, R. (1981). *Nucleic Acids Res.* **9,** 3605–3619.
Watford, M., Cameron, D. K., and Hanson, R. W. (1982). *Int. Symp. Isolation, Characterization Use Hepatocytes, 1982* p. 17. Abstract.
Weintraub, H., and Groudine, M. (1976). *Science* **193,** 848–856.
Weintraub, H., Paiter, K., and van Leute, F. (1975). *Cell* **6,** 85–110.
Weisbrod, S., and Weintraub, H. (1979). *Proc. Natl. Acad. Sci. U.S.A.* **76,** 630–634.
Weisbrod, S., Groudine, M., and Weintraub, H. (1980). *Cell* **19,** 289–301.
West, M. H. P., and Bonner, W. M. (1980). *Biochemistry* **19,** 3238–3245.
Wong, N. C. W., Poirier, G. G., and Dixon, G. H. (1977). *Eur. J. Biochem.* **77,** 11–21.
Worcel, A. (1981). *Proc. Natl. Acad. Sci. U.S.A.* **78,** 1461–1465.

Yap, S. H., Strair, R. K., and Shafritz, D. A. (1978). *J. Biol. Chem.* **253**, 4944–4950.

Zehner, Z. E., Mattick, J. S., Stuart, R., and Wakil, S. J. (1980). *J. Biol. Chem.* **255**, 9519–9522.

Zimmerman, B. (1982). *Annu. Rev. Biochem.* **51**, 395–428.

7

Cytogenetic Studies of a Family with a Hereditary Defect of Cellular Folate Uptake and High Incidence of Hematologic Disease

Diane C. Arthur,* Thomas J. Danzl,† and

Richard F. Branda**

Departments of Laboratory Medicine/Pathology and Pediatrics*
Department of Laboratory Medicine/Pathology†
Department of Medicine, Division of Hematology**
University of Minnesota Hospitals
Minneapolis, Minnesota

** Present address: Department of Medicine, University of Vermont, Burlington, Vermont 05401.

Nutritional Factors in the Induction
and Maintenance of Malignancy

I. INTRODUCTION

Folate compounds are essential for normal nucleic acid metabolism since they participate as cofactors in both purine and pyrimidine synthesis. Consequently, this nutrient is required by all dividing cells. Deficiency of the vitamin folic acid or defective cellular metabolism of folate compounds commonly result in impaired production of blood cells and serious hematologic disease. Studies of patients with megaloblastic anemia due to folate deficiency suggest that the underlying mechanism is impaired elongation of newly initiated DNA fragments due to a reduced amount of deoxyribonucleoside triphosphate necessary for gap filling (Hoffbrand *et al.*, 1976). This mechanism could also account for the chromosome abnormalities observed in these patients. Chromosomal breaks, gaps, despiralization, and increased sister chromatide exchanges (SCE) that disappear after vitamin replacement have been reported (Heath, 1966; Menzies *et al.*, 1966; Knuutila *et al.*, 1978). That normal folic acid metabolism is necessary for the integrity of human chromosomes is further supported by reports that methotrexate, a folic acid antagonist, causes chromosomal abnormalities *in vivo* (Jensen and Nyfors, 1979), and folate-deficient medium enhances expression of heritable fragile sites on human chromosomes in cultured lymphocytes (Sutherland, 1979).

There is also evidence to suggest that abnormalities of folate metabolism contribute to teratogenesis and possibly carcinogenesis. Clinical folate deficiency and inhibitors of folate metabolism, such as nitrous oxide, methotrexate, and diphenylhydantoin are associated with fetal abnormalities and wastage (Laurence *et al.*, 1981; Lane *et al.*, 1980; Sieber and Adamson, 1975; Smith, 1977). Moreover, uterine cervical dysplasia was found to progress to carcinoma *in situ* in folate-deficient women also taking oral contraceptives, but not in their folate-sufficient counterparts (Butterworth *et al.*, 1982). Finally, malignancies have developed in patients receiving methotrexate for nonmalignant conditions (Sieber and Adamson, 1975).

To further investigate the possible relationship of abnormal folate metabolism, chromosomal defects, and the development of serious hematologic disorders, we have done cytogenetic studies in a unique family with a hereditary defect of cellular folate uptake, high incidence of hematologic diseases, and a history of chromosomal abnormalities.

II. MATERIALS AND METHODS

A. Patients

The patient population consisted of the six children of a man who had been treated for severe aplastic anemia at the University of Minnesota Hospitals. Family history, diagnostic studies, and clinical course of this man (the proband) have been previously published (Branda *et al.*, 1978). Briefly, he was a member of a large kindred who had an unusually high incidence of severe anemia, pancytopenia, and leukemia. Among four generations, 32 individuals had hematologic disease, and 17 of these 32 died of their disease. Several of the affected individuals were reported to have chromosomal abnormalities, particularly hypodiploidy. The proband was found to have a defect of cellular folate uptake by stimulated lymphocytes and bone marrow cells, and treatment with high doses of oral folate caused marked improvement of his aplasia. In addition, five other family members manifested the same defect of folate uptake. The proband died in 1980 of respiratory failure due to unexplained chylous pleural effusion and ascites.

Six of the proband's seven children were available for cytogenetic studies, three males and three females ranging in age from 2 to 18 years. None of them were on medication or smoking cigarettes at the time of the study, and none had known exposures to toxins. It is of interest that the eldest son has been leukopenic in the past, that he has developed lymphedema of his lower extremities as had his father, and that he was admitted to the hospital for treatment of cellulitis of his leg at the time blood was drawn for these studies.

B. Controls

The five younger children (patients 1–5) and three concurrent controls (controls 1–3) were studied initially. The controls included the patients' mother, age 41 years, and two known normal healthy cytogenetic technologists, a 23-year-old female and 35-year-old male. None of the controls were on medications, smoked cigarettes, or had known exposures to toxins. The oldest son (patient 6) was studied subsequently, and the same 35-year-old male technologist also served as his concurrent control (control 4).

C. Cytogenetic Studies

The cytogenetic studies were done on cultured lymphocytes from 10 ml heparinized peripheral blood from each patient and control.

1. Mitotic Index

Phytohemagglutinin-stimulated lymphocytes were cultured for 72 hours at 37°C in folate-supplemented (Dulbecco's modified Eagle medium [MEM], 4 mg folate/liter) and unsupplemented (Roswell Park Memorial Institute Medium 1603, 0.01 mg folate/liter) media with 10% fetal calf serum. As usual in our laboratory, the cultures were then synchronized with methotrexate and harvested according to a modification of the technique of Yunis *et al.* (1978). Slides were stained with a 1 : 1 mixture of Harleco Wright Stain–Fisher Wright stain. Mitotic index was expressed as the percent of nuclei in metaphase per 800 total nuclei counted.

2. Spontaneous Chromosomal Breakage

To avoid introducing breakage with methotrexate, cultures were set up as for mitotic index, but were not synchronized. After 72 hours in culture, the cells were exposed to Colcemid for 30 minutes and harvested in the usual fashion. Slides were stained as above, and chromosome and chromatid breaks were scored in 50 metaphases from each patient and control who had sufficient cell growth.

3. G-Banded Chromosome Analysis

The same slides used for mitotic index and breakage studies were destained as needed and restained for G bands using the Wright's technique of Sanchez *et al.* (1973). Twenty metaphases per patient were fully analyzed at the microscope, and several photokaryotypes were prepared for each.

4. Sister Chromatid Exchange (SCE)

The method used for SCE was similar to that described by Perry and Wolff (1974). Phytohemagglutinin-stimulated lymphocytes were cultured in folate-supplemented medium (see above) and also unsupplemented medium (Medium 199/Earle's Base, K. C. Biological, Inc., 0.01 mg folate/liter) for 24 hours before adding 10^{-5} M bromodeoxyuridine. Cultures were harvested at 72 hours after 1 hour exposure to Colcemid. The slides were allowed to age at least 4 days before staining with Hoechst 33258, exposure to light (General Electric 160 W E-Z Merc mercury vapor lamp) and counterstaining with Giemsa. The number of SCE was recorded in 20 mitoses for each patient and control. Individual patients were compared to controls in each of the two media, as were the controls and patients as a group, using the Mann Whitney rank sum statistic. In addition, SCE data for control and patient groups were compared between the two media using the paired t test.

D. Other Studies

Complete blood counts, white cell differential counts, and serum and red cell folate levels were done on each patient and the mother using routine laboratory techniques.

TABLE I

Hematologic Characteristics and Folate Measurements

Subject	Hemoglobin (g/dl)	RBC $10^6/mm^3$	MCV[a]	MCH[b]	MCHC[c]	WBC $(10^9/liter)$	Platelet $(10^9/l)$	Folate (ng/ml) Serum[d]	Folate (ng/ml) RBC[e]
Patient 1	13.5	4.87	79.5	27.7	34.8	10.2	228	14.3	522
Patient 2	12.0	4.27	80.8	28.3	35.0	6.2	256	25.0	573
Patient 3	14.3	4.72	87.4	30.3	34.7	6.1	228	10.9	488
Patient 4	13.8	4.27	90.5	32.4	35.7	3.1	156	29.5	843
Patient 5	13.7	4.12	93.9	33.3	35.5	3.8	164	46.0	997
Patient 6	14.6	4.56	94.7	32.0	33.8	8.8	122	6.9	380

[a] MCV, mean corpuscular volume.
[b] MCH, mean corpuscular hemoglobin.
[c] MCHC, mean corpuscular hemoglobin concentration.
[d] Serum folate normal range, 3.50–15 ng/ml.
[e] RBC folate normal range, 160–600 ng/ml.

III. RESULTS

The results of the hematologic studies and folate measurements from the six patients are shown in Table I. Hemoglobin, red cell counts, and red cell indices were all within normal limits. Patients 4 and 5 had white blood cell counts below the normal range for their ages (4.8 to 10.8 × 10^9/ liter).

Results of the cytogenetic studies are summarized in Table II. None of the six children nor their mother (Control 3) had numerical or structural chromosome abnormalities in the 20 cells analyzed with G banding. Mitotic indices in patients 1 and 5 were considerably lower than those of controls and siblings, both in folate-sufficient and deficient media. Mitotic indices of all but control 1 and patient 5 were actually higher in the low folate media RPMI 1603. None of the patients had increased spontaneous chromosomal breakage when compared to controls or established laboratory norms. Although the numbers are small, there is a suggestion from these data that chromosomal breakage is generally higher in low-folate than folate-supplemented media.

The SCE data are given in Table II and also shown in Fig. 1. When individual patients were compared to concurrent controls, patients 1, 5, and 6 had significantly lower SCE ($p<0.05$) in Dulbecco's MEM; patients 1, 2, and 6 had significantly lower SCE ($p < 0.05$) in Medium 199. Group data revealed the patients had significantly lower SCE ($p<0.05$) than

TABLE II

Cytogenetic Studies

Subject	Sex/age (years)	Mitotic index (% mitoses/800 nuclei)		Chromosomal breakage (no. breaks/50 cells)		Sister chromatid exchange				G-banded karyotype
		Dulbecco[a]	1603[b]	Dulbecco	1603	Dulbecco		199[c]		
						Mean ± S.D.	Range	Mean ± S.D.	Range	
Control 1	M/35	4.75	3.63	1	3	8.85 ± 3.15	4–15	10.65 ± 2.92	5–15	46,XY
Control 2	F/23	2.50	5.25	2	2	8.50 ± 2.31	4–13	9.80 ± 3.83	5–22	46,XX
Control 3	F/41	1.75	4.25	No mitoses	3	7.26 ± 3.45	0–16	11.15 ± 2.54	5–16	46,XX
Control 4	M/35[d]	2.88	5.25	3	3	10.20 ± 5.03	4–20	12.50 ± 4.52	6–25	46,XY
Patient 1	M/2	1.00	2.13	2	1[e]	5.85 ± 2.35	0–11	6.95 ± 2.89	2–11	46,XY
Patient 2	M/6	4.13	6.38	1	4	7.10 ± 2.38	3–13	7.65 ± 2.74	4–13	46,XY
Patient 3	F/15	2.00	3.75	0[f]	0	7.90 ± 2.38	4–13	8.15 ± 2.46	4–14	46,XX
Patient 4	F/12	1.63	4.88	0	2	7.85 ± 2.58	3–13	7.70 ± 2.96	4–15	46,XX
Patient 5	F/9	0.63	0.25	0	2	6.40 ± 2.96	1–12	9.10 ± 3.24	2–18	46,XX
Patient 6	M/18	4.88	7.25	3	4	7.70 ± 3.20	3–14	8.00 ± 3.77	2–20	46,XY

[a] Dulbecco's modified Eagle medium (4.0 mg folate/liter).
[b] Roswell Park Memorial Institute Medium 1603 (0.01 mg folate/liter).
[c] Medium 199, K.C. Biological, Inc. (0.01 mg folate/liter).
[d] Same as Control 1.
[e] Only 20 metaphases counted.
[f] Only 10 metaphases counted.

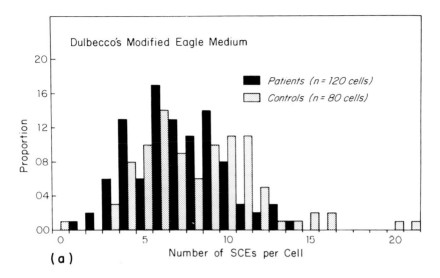

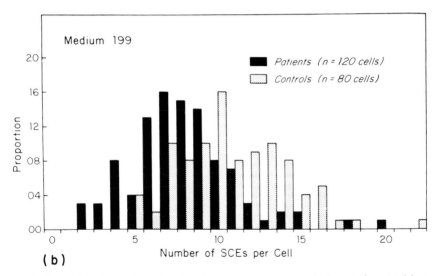

Fig. 1.   Distribution of SCE in patients and concurrently studied controls in (a) folate-supplemented Dulbecco's MEM and (b) folate-deficient Medium 199.

controls in both Dulbecco's and Medium 199. In Dulbecco's medium, the mean SCE for patients was 7.13 and for controls 8.61. In Medium 199, the mean SCE were 7.93 and 11.05, respectively. Numbers of SCE were also compared between the two media. Although the patients as a group showed slightly higher SCE in the folate-deficient Medium 199, the difference was not statistically significant. The controls, however, had significantly higher ($p=0.026$) SCE in the folate-deficient Medium 199.

IV. DISCUSSION

We have previously described a large kindred with a hereditary defect of cellular folate uptake by lymphocytes and bone marrow cells and a high incidence of anemia, pancytopenia, and leukemia. This kindred provides an unusual opportunity to investigate the interrelationship of folate metabolism, chromosomal abnormalities, and the development of serious hematologic disease. Therefore, we have done detailed cytogenetic analyses of six children from one family of the kindred. The father of these children had severe aplastic anemia that was also characterized by megaloblastic changes in the remaining bone marrow cells. He was found to have defective cellular uptake of folate, and his aplasia improved markedly with high doses of oral folic acid (Branda *et al.,* 1978).

Because several members of this kindred affected with hematologic disease had been found in the past to have chromosomal aneuploidy, we analyzed 20 G-banded metaphases from each of the six children. All had normal diploid karyotypes. No numerical or structural chromosome abnormalities were observed, nor was increased breakage noted.

Two of the patients (patients 1 and 5 in Table II) had very low mitotic indices in both folate-deficient and -supplemented media. These results could be due to an abnormality of lymphocyte responsiveness to the mitogen phytohemagglutinin in these patients. Alternatively, the cell cycle time of the lymphocytes from these patients may be different from normal, and thus we could have missed the wave of mitoses that follows release from the methotrexate block using our routine synchronization technique. A third possible explanation for the reduced *in vitro* proliferation of cells from some family members is increased methotrexate toxicity. This last mechanism may be particularly relevant in this family. An inherited defect of cellular folate metabolism might cause lymphocytes from affected family members to be unusually sensitive to methotrexate (which is a folic acid antagonist).

Previous cytogenetic studies of patients with megaloblastic anemia have shown increased chromosomal breakage and SCEs (Heath, 1966; Menzies *et al.,* 1966; Knuutila *et al.,* 1978). Our studies of spontaneous chromosomal breakage revealed our patients were within normal limits when compared to concurrent controls and laboratory norms in both folate-sufficient and -deficient media; thus we do not have evidence that these patients have increased chromosomal fragility. However, five of the nine subjects studied had more spontaneous chromosomal breaks in the unsupplemented medium RPMI 1603 than in the supplemented medium. Moreover, SCE of controls and patients were consistently increased in lymphocytes incubated in folate-deficient medium as compared to the folate-supplemented medium. This statistically significant difference indicates that interchanges of DNA are more likely to occur in folate-deficient medium. Our data confirm and extend those reported in the literature. The exact mechanism by which folate lack enhances chromosomal instability is unknown. Hoffbrand and associates have reported a reduction in the rate of DNA replication fork movement and inhibition of the gap-filling step and/or joining of Okazaki pieces, resulting in DNA with persistent single-stranded regions in lymphocytes from folate-deficient patients (Hoffbrand et al., 1976; Wickremasinghe and Hoffbrand, 1980). These single-stranded regions may be more susceptible to breakage and SCE formation.

Although the precise nature of the DNA lesion(s) that lead to the formation of SCE is currently unknown, SCE are believed to be a sensitive indicator of mutagenesis (Latt et al., 1980; Perry and Evans, 1975; Wolff, 1978). They are also increased in the congenital chromosome instability syndrome, Bloom syndrome (Chaganti et al., 1974). Based on these findings and that of elevated SCE in bone marrow from patients with megaloblastic anemia (Knuutila et al., 1978), we expected that some of our patients would have increased SCE levels. To the contrary, patients 1, 5, and 6 had significantly lower SCE in Dulbecco's MEM than concurrent controls, and patients 1, 2, and 6 had significantly lower SCE in Medium 199. The importance of lower than normal (or expected) numbers of SCEs is unclear. We do not think our results can be explained by the younger ages of the patients as compared to controls because age alone should not influence SCE (Morgan and Crossen, 1977). The controls were not exposed to agents, such as cigarette smoke, medications, or known toxins, which might increase their level of SCE (Latt et al., 1980; Lambert et al., 1978). We considered the possibility that our patients had decreased SCE because their cells were unusually susceptible to the relatively toxic culture conditions used for SCE and were thus unable to repair the DNA damage adequately during replication to be measured as SCE. This situation has been described among patients with Fanconi anemia (Cervenka et al., 1981). However, this explanation also seems unlikely because our patients had many more mitoses that had completed second and third rounds of replication than those with Fanconi anemia.

We postulate that the reduced number of SCEs observed in these family members may be related to the serious hematologic diseases affecting this kindred. Decreased SCE and prolonged cell cycle times (with reduced mitotic indices) have been found in some patients with leukemia (Stoll *et al.*, 1982; Raposa, 1982). Moreover, in one disease, chronic myelogenous leukemia, the number of SCE progressively decrease as the disease accelerates (Stoll *et al.*, 1982). Since several kindred members had leukemia or preleukemic conditions, it seems possible that an underlying hereditary defect of cellular metabolism may account for the decreased SCE, low mitotic indices, and ultimate development of serious hematologic diseases. In addition, several of our patients had surprisingly high serum and red cell folate levels, suggesting that this metabolic defect may also somehow involve folate homeostasis. Unfortunately, at present, there is little direct evidence to substantiate these speculations, and the exact relationship between the cytogenetic defects, folate abnormalities, and hematologic diseases in this perplexing kindred remains to be elucidated.

ACKNOWLEDGMENTS

Supported by grants from the American Cancer Society (CH-220 and IN-13) and the National Institutes of Health (CA 28234). Dr. Branda is the recipient of a Research Career Development Award (CA 00657).

REFERENCES

Branda, R. F., Moldow, C. F., MacArthur, J. R., Wintrobe, M. M., Anthony, B. K., and Jacob, H. S. (1978). *N. Engl. J. Med.* **298,** 469–475.
Butterworth, C. E., Hatch, K. D., Gore, H., Mueller, H., and Krumdieck, C. L. (1982). *Am. J. Clin. Nutr.* **35,** 73–82.
Cervenka, J., Arthur, D., and Yasis, C. (1981). *Pediatrics* **67,** 119–127.
Chaganti, R. S. K., Schonberg, S., and German, J. (1974). *Proc. Natl. Acad. Sci. U.S.A.* **71,** 4508–4512.
Heath, C. W. (1966). *Blood* **27,** 800–815.
Hoffbrand, A. V., Ganeshaguru, K., Hooton, J. W. L., and Tripp, E. (1976). *Clin. Haematol.* **5,** 727–745.
Jensen, M. K., and Nyfors, A. (1979). *Mutat. Res.* **64,** 339–343.
Knuutila, S., Helminen, E., Vuopio, P., and de la Chapelle, A. (1978). *Hereditas* **89,** 175–181.
Lambert, B., Lindblad, A., Nordenskjold, M., and Werelius, B. (1978). *Hereditas* **88,** 147–149.
Lane, G. A., Nahrwold, M. L., Tait, A. R., Taylor-Busch, M., and Cohen, P. J. (1980). *Science* **210,** 899–901.
Latt, S. A., Schrock, R. R., Loveday, K. S., Dougherty, C. P., and Shuler, C. F. (1980). *Adv. Hum. Genet.* **10,** 267–330.

Laurence, K. M., James, N., Miller, M. H., Tennant, G. B., and Campbell, H. (1981). *Br. Med. J.* **282,** 1509–1511.

Menzies, R. C., Crossen, P. E., Fitzgerald, P. H., and Gunz, F. W. (1966). *Blood* **28,** 581–594.

Morgan, W. F., and Crossen, P. E. (1977). *Mutat. Res.* **42,** 305–312.

Perry, P., and Evans, H. J. (1975). *Nature (London)* **258,** 121–125.

Perry, P., and Wolff, S. (1974). *Nature (London)* **261,** 156–158.

Raposa, T. (1982). *In* "Sister Chromatid Exchange," (A. A. Sandberg, ed.), pp. 579–617. Alan R. Liss, Inc., New York.

Sanchez, O., Escobar, J. J., and Yunis, J. J. (1973). *Lancet* **2,** 269.

Sieber, S. M., and Adamson, R. H. (1975). *Adv. Cancer Res.* **22,** 57–155.

Smith, D. W. (1977). *Am. J. Dis. Child.* **131,** 1337–1339.

Stoll, C., Oberling, F., and Roth, M. P. (1982). *Cancer Res.* **42,** 3240–3243.

Sutherland, G. R. (1979). *Am. J. Hum. Genet.* **31,** 125–135.

Wickremasinghe, R. G., and Hoffbrand, A. V. (1980). *J. Clin. Invest.* **65,** 26–36.

Wolff, S. (1978). *In* "Mutagen-Induced Chromosome Damage in Man" (H. J. Evans and D. C. Lloyd, eds.), pp. 208–215. Yale Univ. Press, New Haven, Connecticut.

Yunis, J. J., Sawyer, J. R., and Ball, D. W. (1978). *Chromosoma* **67,** 293–307.

Virus-Induced Folates and Folate Enzymes: Formation and Incorporation into Viral Particles

Lloyd M. Kozloff

Department of Microbiology
University of California
San Francisco, California

Nutritional Factors in the Induction
and Maintenance of Malignancy

I. INTRODUCTION

A. Phage Genes, Phage Assembly, and the Nutritional Status of the Infected Cell

In eukaryotic cells, the physiological and biochemical activities of many gene products were recognized long before the chromosomal genes were identified or mapped. This sequence of discovery is rapidly changing, especially in studies of transformed cells, but in bacteria and most notably in viruses formal gene identification has preceded biochemical identification of the gene products. For *Escherichia coli* T4 bacteriophage, fine genetic mapping has led to the characterization of genes as belonging to certain functional areas long before any biochemical role could be assigned to individual gene products. Our current interest is to define the chemical roles of each gene product in the assembly of a complex molecular structure, such as T4. In general terms, the question is how the linear arrangement of the information in genes leads to the formation of complex biological ultrastructure. Further, there is the question in these systems of whether the environment, including the nutritional status of the medium, might influence the assembly process. This question was not relevant as long as self-assembly was thought to be controlled by the amino acid sequences of the individual products and then by product–product interaction. If, however, cellular metabolites other than those involved in protein synthesis or energy production do play a role in assembly, then one can examine the effect of nutritional status of the infected cell on the assembly process.

B. The Assembly of the T4 Tail Structure and the Infection of the Host Cell

The T4 bacteriophage particle, a double-stranded DNA virus, has a well-known tadpole shape with a complex tail through which the DNA contained within the head is delivered into the host cell. The intact tail structure contains a terminal hexagonal-shaped flat, solid-appearing baseplate. Upon interaction with the host cell, there is a dramatic morphological alteration to a thinner star-shaped structure with a central opening large enough to permit the exit of the DNA (Fig. 1). This conformational alteration is easily triggered, and the hexagonal baseplate has been called a "metastable" structure by Crowther *et al.* (1977), since no energy is required for this morphological change.

The assembly pathway of this "metastable" structure has been outlined by Kikuchi and King (1975). Using various conditional lethal phage

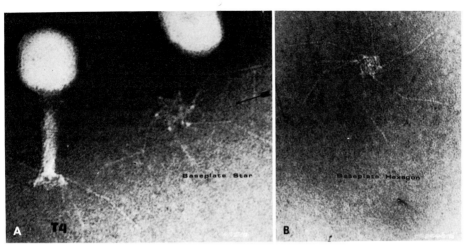

Fig. 1. (A) Electron micrographs of intact *E. coli* bacteriophage T4 and a detached baseplate which has changed into the "star" configuration with an open central hole. × 424,000. (B) A free baseplate in the intact hexagonal configuration. × 460,000. These electron micrographs were taken by H. Fernandez-Moran.

mutants, they were able to identify various intermediates and to construct a sequence in which two main substructures were assembled independently. The baseplate was found to be formed by the addition of six outer arms or wedges around a central hub as shown in Fig. 2. The wedges were formed by the sequential interaction of eight gene products. The pathway for the formation of the central hub was also branched, and only three gene products (gP5, gP27, and gP29) were identified at that time in the final structure. An additional three gene products (gP26, gP28, and gP51) were required but their precise role was not defined. Interestingly, the six wedges were shown to form a hexagonal structure in the absence of a hub, although this structure apparently was never converted into an active baseplate.

One important question is how these two main substructures bind together to form a reasonably stable form. This is a significant variation from the normal requirements for assembly of substructures, such as joining the head and tail, since no freedom for later structural change needs to be incorporated at the "neck" juncture, but conformational plasticity does have to be permitted in the baseplate.

This chapter reports that the assembly of baseplate involves the incorporation into the structure of a unique polyglutamyl form of folic acid. Searches for folate-binding proteins have led to the discovery that the baseplate contains two enzymes, dihydrofolate reductase and thymidy-

STRUCTURE AND ASSEMBLY OF
T4 BACTERIOPHAGE BASEPLATE

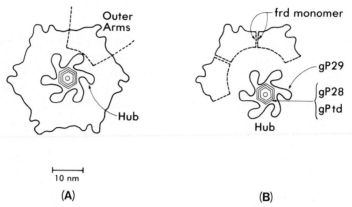

Fig. 2. (A) Division of the hexagonal baseplate into hub and outer wedge structure, based on the optical imaging analysis of electron micrographs by Crowther *et al.* (1977). (B) Presumed interaction of the hub structure with the outer wedges.

late synthase, both of which normally require folate for their catalytic action. Finally, investigations into folyl polyglutamyl formation in infected cells has revealed that two enzymes involved in forming the new phage folate, a carboxypeptidase and a folyl polyglutamyl synthetase, are also incorporated into the baseplate as key structural elements. It should be emphasized that, in the phage structure, there is no evidence that any of these enzymes or the folate itself participates in any typical catalytic reaction.

II.   FOLATES IN PHAGE PARTICLES

A.   Identification of the Phage Folate

Analysis of phage preparations for their folate content was stimulated by the finding that some unidentified electron acceptor compound was a normal constituent of the tail of *E. coli* bacteriophage T4B (Kanner and Kozloff, 1964). These initial analyses led to the report in 1965 that a small amount of folyl polyglutamate was a required component of the phage tail (Kozloff and Lute, 1965). A useful probe in investigating the role of the folate compound was a γ-glutamyl exopeptidase from hog kidney, which specifically cleaved the large folyl polyglutamates to a smaller size. Treatment with this purified enzyme was found to inactivate live phage particles, but still allowed virus attachment and host cell killing. The inactivated phage could not inject their DNA into the host cell. These results were the first evidence that the folate was involved in baseplate functioning, even though at that time the baseplate structure itself was poorly understood.

Later analytical work (Kozloff *et al.*, 1970a; Nakamura and Kozloff, 1978) clearly showed that the phage compound was dihydropteroyl polyglutamate most likely containing six glutamate residues. The definitive experiment (Kozloff *et al.*, 1970c) confirming that the phage compound was a pteroyl hexaglutamate is shown in Fig. 3. In this experiment, extracts were made of separate cultures of nonpermissive host

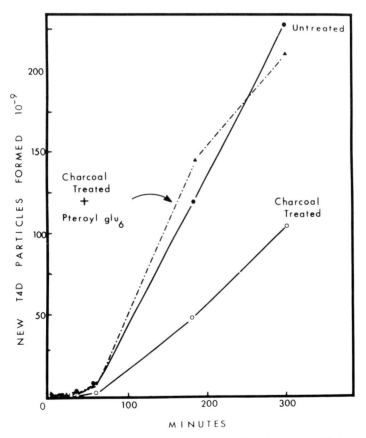

Fig. 3. The reconstitution of the rate and amount of T4 phage assembly by synthetic pteroyl hexaglutamate in *in vitro* complementation systems, using charcoal-treated extracts prepared with two different T4 baseplate wedge amber mutants, gene 7 and gene 10.

bacteria infected with two different T4 amber mutants, in gene 7 or in gene 10. These two gene products are both required to form the outer wedges of the hexagonal baseplate. These two extracts contained complete heads, complete central tail hubs, and all of the other tail components except those blocked by the specific amber mutation. When mixed, the two extracts complemented each other forming new wedges and then rapidly forming complete new infectious phage particles. If endogenous folate compounds were partially removed by a charcoal treatment, then the rate and amount of phage formation was decreased. When chemically synthesized pteroyl hexaglutamate was added to the charcoal-treated extracts, then the rate and amount of phage formation was completely restored. Neither pteroyl pentaglutamate nor pteroyl heptaglutamate restored phage assembly to normal, and the addition of either of these two compounds inhibited phage assembly below that of the charcoal-treated control. This experiment showing that folate can be removed from a wedge extract is in agreement with the proposal to be presented later that the folate is initially bound to baseplate wedges and only later to the hub.

B. Amount and Location of Phage Folate

Analysis of phage preparations gave values of two to five folate molecules per phage particle (Kozloff and Lute, 1965; Kozloff *et al.*, 1970a). These are minimal values, since phage preparations always contain some incomplete or damaged particles, and the most likely value, in accordance with the symmetry of the baseplate, is six folates per phage particle.

Isolation of various incomplete T4 tail structures (Kozloff *et al.*, 1970a) and the determination of their relative folate content per milligram of protein led to the conclusion that the baseplate was the structure containing the folate. Additional probes, such as antibody against the pteroyl residue or the polyglutamate portion of the molecule, indicated that these portions of the molecule were all buried within the baseplate structure (Kozloff *et al.*, 1970a, 1979).

C. Folates in Other Phages

No systematic search for folates in phages other than the closely related *E. coli* T2, T4, and T6, which have similar tails and baseplates, has been carried out. However, we have isolated and purified two phages that attack *Pseudomonas syringae* (Kozloff, 1981). Both of these phages are somewhat smaller than T4, but both have T4-like tails and baseplates.

When exposed to the hog kidney glutamyl carboxypeptidase, both phages were irreversibly inactivated. One can conclude that both have a pteroyl polyglutamate as a critical structural element. It should be noted that *P. syringae* is evolutionarily quite distant from *E. coli*, since their DNAs have only about 1% homology. One suspects that the hexagonal baseplates widely observed on other phages might all contain a pteroyl polyglutamate, but the identification of their chemical nature still must be carried out before we can even speculate about the evolutionary origin of this use of folate.

III. FOLATE-REQUIRING ENZYMES IN PHAGE PARTICLES

A. Dihydrofolate Reductase

With the identification of the phage folate compound as a dihydropteroyl hexaglutamate, phage particles were examined for the presence of viral-induced proteins that could be binding the folate compound in the tail structure. The binding constant of dihydrofolate compounds for the enzyme dihydrofolate reductase (the phage gene is called *frd*) is high, and this enzyme was known to be induced by phage infection (Mathews, 1967). No *frd* enzymatic activity was found in purified intact phage particles, but gentle denaturing treatments with urea or formamide revealed a weak reductase activity (Kozloff *et al.*, 1970b). The presence of this enzyme in phage particles and its essential nature to this particle were confirmed in a variety of experiments that bear directly on its function during virus assembly and during phage infection.

These experiments include (a) phage inactivation by antisera prepared against homogeneous phage-induced dihydrofolate reductase (Mathews *et al.*, 1973), (b) experiments showing that mutations in the *frd* gene changed the heat stability of T4 particles (Kozloff *et al.*, 1975c), and (c) the correlation of phage viability with some of the enzymological properties of dihydrofolate reductase (Kozloff *et al.*, 1970b). For example, T4 was inactivated by NADPH (but not by NADH) and was partially reactivated upon subsequent incubation with NADP. It should be emphasized that studies with phage mutants have shown that, although coded for by a phage gene, enzymatic activity of the particle-bound dihydrofolate reductase was not required for phage assembly.

The evidence pointed to the baseplate as the site of the dihydrofolate reductase. Isolated baseplates, when treated with urea, did show dihydrofolate reductase activity that was 40-fold increased on a weight basis over that found in whole phage particles. It is not surprising that any dihydrofolate reductase activity would be poorly expressed when the enzyme was incorporated into a complex structure such as a baseplate. In whole phage particles, the dihydropteroyl group would be almost permanently bound to the active site of the dihydrofolate reductase molecules and would not be expected to be more than the number of folate molecules. Since two to five folate molecules per particle have been found in different phage preparations, possibly six potentially active dihydrofolate reductase catalytic sites could be available in each phage particle. The catalytic activities found have always been considerably below that expected for this number of dihydrofolate reductase molecules (Kozloff et al., 1977).

Two recent reports from the laboratory of C. K. Mathews on the chemical nature of the phage dihydrofolate reductase and its location have been important in assigning a role to this molecule in phage assembly. Mosher and Mathews (1979) have found that dihydrofolate reductase is a component of the outer wedges of the baseplate. This enzyme had not previously been detected in wedges, and only the use of labeled antibody aided its detection in analytical gels made from purified wedges. Additionally, Purohit et al. (1981) have reported that phage dihydrofolate reductase exists as a dimer of two 20,000 dalton monomers. This observation, together with the finding (1) of only a maximal of six folates per particle and (2) of only three thymidylate synthase dimers (see later) supports the view that there are only three dihydrofolate reductase dimers per phage particle. An attractive possibility is that each wedge contains one dihydrofolate reductase monomer (Fig. 2) and that the lateral binding of the individual wedges to each other is enhanced by the formation of dihydrofolate reductase dimers.

B. Thymidylate Synthase

Thymidylate synthase, induced by a phage gene called *td*, was shown by Capco and Mathews (1973) to be a phage component. Phage infectivity was neutralized by antiserum against the purified homogenous enzyme and the transfer of the *td* gene from phage T6 to T4 resulted in T4 particles with altered heat sensitivity. This last observation implied that thymidylate synthase was a component of the baseplate, since the baseplate is the most heat-labile component of the phage particle. This last observation was amplified in further studies of thymidylate synthase mutants (Kozloff et al., 1975b). These results established that the *td* gene product was a phage structural component and pointed to the baseplate as the most likely substructure for its location. Careful measurements of thymidylate synthase activity in wild-type phage preparations showed small levels of activity, and no activity was found in preparations of particles containing the *td* amber mutation. Treatment of particles with denaturing agents analogous to those used to expose the buried dihydrofolate reductase activity destroyed all thymidylate synthase activity as might have been expected from the lability of the latter molecule.

While these results indicated that the thymidylate synthase molecule was in the baseplate, they did not indicate the number of thymidylate synthase molecules nor whether the enzyme was a wedge or hub component. A highly sensitive chase labeling procedure in complementation experiments devised to detect minor components of the baseplate hub resolved these questions (Kozloff, 1981; Kozloff and Zorzopulos, 1981). These experiments showed that the hub contained a small amount of a previously undetected component of molecular weight of 29,000. Since thymidylate synthase monomers have this size, and since no 29,000 MW component has been found in baseplate wedges, it seems quite likely that thymidylate synthase is a hub component. The number of thymidylate synthase monomers in the hub was calculated relative to the amount of the other hub components. Given that the hexagonal hubs contained six molecules each of gP29, gP27, and gP5 (see Fig. 4, and Table II later), there appeared to be about one-half as much thymidylate synthase, or three to four monomers. Since this enzyme normally forms dimers, one might expect that there would be at least two complete molecules or four monomers. This value agrees only reasonably well with the number of folate molecules found per particle and the proposed three dihydrofolate reductase dimers (six monomers) in the wedges. All the analytical results, even with the uncertainties in the measurements, imply that there are six dihydropteroyl hexaglutamates, three dihydrofolate reductase dimers in baseplate wedges, and most likely two thymidylate synthase dimers in the hub baseplate of each T4 particle.

IV. FOLYL POLYGLUTAMATE SYNTHESIS IN INFECTED CELLS

A. Sulfa Drug Inhibition of Phage Assembly

The requirement for dihydropteroyl hexaglutamate to assemble the baseplate led to studies to determine which phage genes might be involved in the formation of this compound (Kozloff *et al.*, 1973; Kozloff and Lute, 1973). One approach was to decrease the total folate pool in cells by the addition of sulfa drugs to the complete broth media. This experiment has been presented briefly elsewhere (Kozloff and Lute, 1982), but the relation to the nutritive status of the infected cells is worth

TABLE I

Sulfadiazine Inhibition of Plaque Formation by T4 Baseplate Hub Mutants[a]

Phage	Broth only / Broth + sulfadiazine
T4 (wild type)	0.84 ± 0.08
5 amber	0.81 ± 0.12
25 amber	0.93 ± 0.10
26 amber	0.81 ± 0.20
51 amber	0.96 ± 0.02
27 amber	0.23 ± 0.14
28 amber	0.04 ± 0.03
29 amber	0.10 ± 0.06
td amber	0.70 ± 0.04

[a] Phage stocks were plated on E. coli CR63, the permissive host strain, at 37°C on broth plates in the presence or absence or 1 mM sulfadiazine. At least two separate experiments were carried out for each mutant; for wild-type T4 eight separate measurements were made.

elaboration: Table I shows the effect of sulfadiazine on plaque formation by T4 baseplate hub mutants. In these experiments, 1 mM sulfadiazine (or sulfathiazole, which gave similar results) was added to the standard broth medium for plating bacteriophage stocks. The rationale for this type of experiment is that the T4 amber mutants do produce a mutant gene product in the permissive host cells, but these proteins have a substituted amino acid so that they function less efficiently. Thus these mutants may show a marked change in ability to produce phage if this decrease in efficiency of this gene product can be exaggerated by decreasing the concentration of any precursor which this gene product further processes. Plaque production by wild-type T4 and three hub mutants were unaffected, but three other hub mutants were markedly inhibited by sulfadiazine, the 28 amber was most sensitive, the 29 amber was somewhat less sensitive, and the 27 amber was also somewhat sensitive. The inhibitions were completely reversed by the addition of p-amino benzoate. Results described below indicate how the gene 28 and gene 29 products are involved in phage folate formation. The role of the 27 product in folate metabolism is still undefined. It sbould be noted that plaque formation by mutants in thymidylate synthase and dihydrofolate reductase genes were not sensitive to sulfadiazine. Detailed analysis of the effect of the sulfa compound on virus growth showed that the latent period was not altered but that the virus burst size was markedly decreased presumably because not enough of the pteroyl hexaglutamate required for assembly was formed (Kozloff, 1981).

B. Folyl Polyglutamyl γ-Carboxypeptidase—T4D Gene Product 28

In complementation experiments using the sensitive ^{14}C chase labeling technique, T4D gP28 was shown to be a component of the central hub of the baseplate and to have a molecular size of 24,000 (Kozloff and Zorzopulos, 1981). This component had not been detected previously (Kikuchi and King, 1975), probably because of its relatively small size and because of the small amount present in the phage baseplate. Besides the direct analytical evidence, there was evidence that properties of assembled phage particles reflected the nature of the gene 28 product. For example, T4 gene 28 mutant particles had altered host ranges, heat sensitivities, and adsorption rates (Kozloff and Lute, 1982). Perhaps most unexpected and revealing was the inability of T4D 28ts particles to infect any E. coli K12 strain at any temperature, although this mutant grew well on E. coli B. The failure of gene 28 mutants to infect K12 strains was shown by gene rescue experiments to be a defect in the injection mechanism itself, rather a defect in another step of the infection process.

In addition to serving as a component of the baseplate, the gene 28 product was also shown to be a cleavage enzyme or carboxypeptidase attacking the γ-glutamyl bonds in folyl polyglutamates. In E. coli B infected with T4D 28am, i.e., in the absence of the 28 product, as described above, large folyl polyglutamate compounds accumulated, amounting to as much as 8% of the total folates (Nakamura and Kozloff, 1978). When an assay was devised to measure peptidase activity, it was found that gene 28 product was a γ-glutamyl carboxypeptidase (Kozloff and Lute, 1982), which could be readily distinguished from an endogenous host carboxypeptidase. The virus-induced enzyme had a pH optimum of 6.0–6.5, while the host enzyme had a pH optimum of about 8.0. The characterization of the gene 28 product is quite preliminary, and the enzyme appears to be quite labile (Kozloff and Lute, 1982).

Determination of the amount of 28 product in phage particles is based on the radioautography after polyacrylamide gel electrophoresis (PAGE) analysis of labeled T4 baseplate hubs. Compared to the amounts of the major hub components, there appeared to be only three molecules of gP28 per particle. These three molecules appear to effect baseplate function and especially the changes involved in the hexagon to star transition which occurs during injection. Since single amino acid changes in the 28 product caused drastic changes in the ability to infect K12 strains, it appears that the 28 product is located on the distal surface of the baseplate and either directly interacts with the host cell itself or influences the interaction of the other phage tail components with the host cell. It should be noted that phage particles themselves have a weak carboxypeptidase activity, indicating again that the active site of the 28 product is exposed sufficiently to be able to bind a folyl polyglutamate substrate. This proposal for the location of the 28 product catalytic site is also supported by the finding (a) that antisera to baseplates inactivated the catalytic activity of phage particles and (b) that pyrimethamine, a folate analog, inhibited the carboxypeptidase activity of phage particles.

C. Folyl Polyglutamyl Synthetase—T4D Gene Product 29

The increase in the relative amount of folates containing six glutamate residues that occurs in cells infected with wild-type T4D suggested that phage infection was inducing a new folyl polyglutamate synthetase. This view was also supported by the observation that in cells infected with T4D 28am, a carboxypeptidase-minus mutant, folates not found in uninfected host cells containing 12–14 glutamate residues accumulated. Efforts to detect phage induction of a new synthetase were initially unsuccessful because of the presence of both the host- and the phage-induced carboxypeptidase. However, a modification of the assay procedure of Shane (1980) so that extracts of uninfected or infected cells were incubated for only 30 seconds, did show that T4D infection induced a threefold increase in the rate of addition of labeled glutamates to the folate substrate (Table II). The T4D gene 29 product was found to be

TABLE II

Folyl Polyglutamyl Synthetase Activity after T4D Infection[a]

Extract	Synthetase activity (nanomoles glutamate protein incorporated in 30 seconds)
Uninfected B	0.13–0.19
T4D infected B	0.38–0.44
T4D 29⁻ infected B	0.13–0.15
T4D 28⁻ infected B	0.62–0.75
T4D 27⁻ infected B	0.58

[a] Reaction mixture contained 5 mM ATP, 0.1 mM FH$_4$, 10 mM MgCl$_2$, 0.2 M KCl, 0.2 M TRIS pH 9.2, 0.25 M[^{14}C]glutamate, and cell extract.

the synthetase, since infection of restrictive cells with a gene 29 amber mutant did not result in any increase in synthetase activity, while infection with all other phage mutants tested, including mutants in genes 27 and 28, did result in increased levels of synthetase activity. Further, recent experiments have shown that the synthetase activity and the 29 product chromatograph identically on Sephadex columns. The enzymatic characterization of this synthetase has just been started so there is little information about the nature of the products or of other properties of the enzyme. It is, however, known that gP29 has a molecular weight of 77,000 (Kikuchi and King, 1975), which would be appropriate for an enzyme that needed binding sites for glutamate, the folate substrate and ATP.

The amount of gene 29 product in the baseplate has been estimated by Crowther *et al.* (1977) as six molecules per baseplate. This value is in accord with later estimates of the stoichiometry of the baseplates constituents (Kozloff, 1981). There is convincing evidence that the 29 product is a component of the central hub. Since the hub, like the final baseplate, has a sixfold symmetry, the presence of six molecules would be appropriate. The actual linkage of the 29 product to the other hub components is not certain. Our proposal is that the 29 product, and probably the 28 product, bind to the distal three glutamates of the pteroyl hexaglutamates (see Fig. 1 and Fig. 5, later). A synthetase, and a folyl carboxypeptidase, would be expected to have an affinity for glutamate residues linked via their γ-carboxyl groups. This would provide additional stability to the wedge–hub bonding.

Finally, there is some suggestive evidence that the ATP-binding site of the synthetase may be exposed on the distal surface of the hub. Male and Kozloff (1973) reported that ATP, and to a lesser extent AMP, but not ADP, inhibited phage absorption. This nucleotide-binding specificity is that found in synthetases and is a possibility that needs further investigation.

V. FOLATES AND FOLATE ENZYMES IN THE T4 PHAGE

Folyl Polyglutamate Formation and the Baseplate Assembly Pathway

An outline of the role of T4-induced gene products in forming the phage folate compound is shown in Fig. 4. Host enzymes synthesize the pteroyl triglutamate, which is the major form of folate in the uninfected cell. Although small amounts of the larger polyglutamates are present in the uninfected cell, T4 infection causes a relative increase in the amount

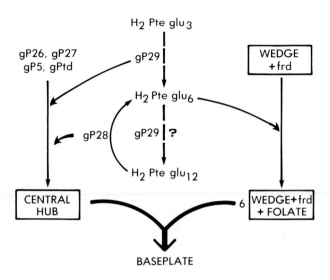

Fig. 4. Role of folate and folate enzymes in assembly of T4 baseplates.

of hexaglutamyl form of folate (Nakamura and Kozloff, 1978). Presumably, gP29 acts on the host folates to increase the amount of the hexaglutamyl compound. However, the additions of successive glutamyl residues to folate is apparently uncontrolled, and, in the absence of cleavage activity, very large folyl polyglutamates containing 12–14 glutamate residues have been found to accumulate. However, normally gP28 functions as a carboxypeptidase cleaving these large folyl polyglutamates back to the hexaglutamyl form. It should be emphasized that both the 28 and 29 gene products function catalytically to make the phage folate compound, but then both are also incorporated into the baseplate hub structure where they no longer act as typical enzymes.

It seems highly likely that the phage folate is bound to the active site on the dihydrofolate reductase on a wedge substructure. Only after the folate is bound can the wedges then bind to the hub. How then does the folate compound act to promote wedge–hub interaction and later in the baseplate structural morphological transition? With the identification of thymidylate synthase, gP28 and gP29 as hub components, a reasonable hypothesis can now be advanced. First, it should be emphasized that there is a strict requirement for hexaglutamyl form in phage assembly. Possibly the penta or hepta compounds can be incorporated into the baseplate, but they do not lead to viable phage particles. Recently,

Kisliuk *et al.* (1979) have reported that polyglutamyl forms of folate bind tightly to the T2 phage-induced thymidylate synthase and that the binding is largely through the γ-glutamyl portion of the molecule. Maximum affinity to thymidylate synthase was found with folates containing 2–3 glutamyl residues. This observation has led to the suggestion illustrated in Fig. 5. The dihydropteroyl group of the folate is thought to be tightly bound within the active site of the dihydrofolate reductase. The relatively free polyglutamyl oligopeptide can bind to components in the hub, particularly to the thymidylate synthase molecules, but also to gP28 and gP29. Both the synthetase and the carboxypeptidase have recognition sites for γ-glutamyl peptides and would be expected to bind to this portion of the folate compound. The length of the folate compound shown in Fig. 5 is insufficient to reach from the wedges (as shown in Fig. 2) to these elements of the hub. Possibly, two glutamyl residues bind to each of these three hub components. The number of chemical bonds that can be formed between these components, as

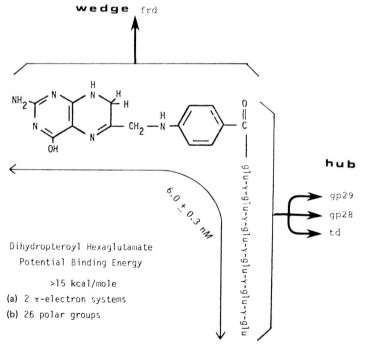

Fig. 5. Structural features of dihydropteroyl hexaglutamate relative to its function in the phage baseplate.

shown in Fig. 5, offers considerable stability to such a structure. Finally, the use of folate to serve as a link between wedge and hub would also fit both sequential nature of the assembly pathway and would provide a unique means of linking these subunits.

Table III both summarizes these facts and our proposal and relates these discoveries to the physiology of phage growth and function. Folate appears to be the critical element of the tail structure, which acts in an unusual fashion to link viral substructures together. When the nutritional status of the host cell is altered (as in the presence of a sulfa drug) viral production is inhibited. The presence of four enzymes in the baseplate, one in the wedge and three in the hub, is not only related to the assembly process, but to other features of the infectious process. A significant amount of the viral genome is devoted to making these enzymes, and they serve a dual purpose, both to make the folate compound and then to play a structural role in assembly and then infection. Here we have only fragmentary information, but we can relate these newly discovered features to the physiological role of the baseplate. These features include the fact that the carboxypeptidase (gP28) plays a role in host cell recognition and later in DNA injection. T4 mutants in gene 28, for example, do not inject their DNA into certain *E. coli* cells, which are otherwise perfectly suitable hosts for T4. The synthetase, gP29, also appears to have its catalytic binding site for ATP exposed on the bottom of the baseplate. These properties of baseplate components suggest to us that, during infection, phage attachment leads to release of cell nucleotides such as ATP (or NADPH which could react with dihydrofolate reductase) that bind to the baseplate enzymes. The binding of these cofactors to these

TABLE III

Functions of T4 Phage-Induced Folate and Folate Enzymes in the Baseplate Structure

Baseplate component	Proposed function
Folate	Links together the two main baseplate substructures—wedges to hub
Dihydrofolate reductase and thymidylate synthase	Main proteins in wedge and hub binding the folate
Hub carboxypeptidase, gene product 28	Binds to folate glutamate residues and aids host cell recognition
Hub folyl polyglutamyl synthetase, gene product 29	Binds to folate glutamate residues and contains site for recognizing nucleotides
All components	Have conformational plasticity to aid hexagon to star transition

enzymes is presumed to lead to induced conformational changes in these molecules. These conformational changes then disturb the binding of these enzymes to the cross-linking folate compound, and the baseplate spontaneously rearranges from the hexagon into the star form. This proposal is energetically attractive, but numerous technically difficult measurements still must be made to see if it is correct in general principle if not in every detail.

ACKNOWLEDGMENTS

The preparation of this manuscript was aided by Public Health Service Research Grant Aid 18370 from the National Institute of Allergy and Infectious Diseases.

REFERENCES

Capco, G. R., and Mathews, C. K. (1973). *Arch. Biochem. Biophys.* **158**, 736–743.
Crowther, R. A., Lenk, E. V., Kikuchi, Y., and King, J. (1977). *J. Mol. Biol.* **116**, 489–523.
Kanner, L. C., and Kozloff, L. M. (1964). *Biochemistry* **3**, 215–223.
Kikuchi, Y., and King, J. (1975). *J. Mol. Biol.* **99**, 695–716.
Kisliuk, R. L., Gaymont, Y., Baugh, C. M., Galivan, J. H., Maley, G. F., and Maley, F. (1979). *In* "Chemistry and Biology of Pteridines" (R. L. Kisliuk and G. M. Brown, eds.), pp. 431–436. Elsevier/North-Holland, New York.
Kozloff, L. M. (1981). *In* "Bacteriophage Assembly" (M. Dubrow, ed.), pp. 327–342. Alan R. Liss, Inc., New York.
Kozloff, L. M., and Lute, M. (1965). *J. Mol. Biol.* **12**, 780–792.
Kozloff, L. M., and Lute, M. (1973). *J. Virol.* **11**, 630–636.
Kozloff, L. M., and Lute, M. (1982). *J. Virol.* **40**, 645–656.
Kozloff, L. M, and Zorzopulos, J. (1981). *J. Virol.* **40**, 635–644.
Kozloff, L. M., Crosby, L. K., Lute, M., Rao, N., Chapman, V. A., and DeLong, S. S. (1970a). *J. Virol.* **5**, 736–739.
Kozloff, L. M., Verses, C., Crosby, L. K., and Lute, M. (1970b). *J. Virol.* **5**, 740–753.
Kozloff, L. M., Crosby, L. K., and Lute, M. (1970c). *J. Virol.* **6**, 754–759.
Kozloff, L. M., Lute, M., and Baugh, C. (1973). *J. Virol.* **11**, 637–641.
Kozloff, L. M., Crosby, L. K., and Lute, M. (1975a). *J. Virol.* **16**, 1391–1400.
Kozloff, L. M., Crosby, L. K., and Lute, M. (1975b). *J. Virol.* **16**, 1409–1419.
Kozloff, L. M., Crosby, L. K., Lute, M., and Hall, D. D. (1975c). *J. Virol.* **16**, 1401–1408.
Kozloff, L. M., Crosby, L. K., and Lute, M. (1977). *J. Virol.* **23**, 637–644.
Kozloff, L. M., Crosby, L. K., and Baugh, C. M. (1979). *J. Virol.* **32**, 497–506.
Male, C. J., and Kozloff, L. M. (1973). *J. Virol.* **11**, 840–847.
Mathews, C. K. (1967). *J. Biol. Chem.* **242**, 4083–4086.
Mathews, C. K., Crosby, L. K., and Kozloff, L. M. (1973). *J. Virol.* **12**, No. 1, 74–78.
Mosher, R. A., and Mathews, C. K. (1979). *J. Virol.* **31**, 94–103.
Nakamura, K., and Kozloff, L. M. (1978). *Biochim. Biophys. Acta* **540**, 313–319.
Purohit, S., Bestwick, R. K., Lasser, G. W., Rogers, C. M., and Mathews, C. K. (1981). *J. Biol. Chem.* **256**, 9121–9125.
Shane, B. (1980). *J. Biol. Chem.* **255**, 5655–5662.

Growth-Regulating Effects of Naturally Occurring Metabolites of Folate and Ascorbate on Malignant Cells

Cecile Leuchtenberger* and Rudolf
Leuchtenberger*

Department of Cytochemistry
Swiss Institute for Experimental Cancer Research
Epalinges, Switzerland

I. INTRODUCTION

In spite of the fact that the interrelationship between nutritional factors and malignant growth has been studied for a

---

*Present address: Hirzbodenpark 18, 4052 Basel, Switzerland.

Nutritional Factors in the Induction
and Maintenance of Malignancy

considerable time (for a recent survey, see National Research Council, 1982), the main emphasis in prevention and therapy of human cancer has been placed on chemical compounds. This approach has become particularly pertinent regarding induction of malignant growth because of the increasing recognition that chemical compounds, such as those present in tobacco smoke and in polluted air, play an important role in carcinogenesis. Furthermore, the availability and beneficial application of synthetic chemical antimetabolites has led to the concept that in addition to surgery and radiation, antimetabolites are at present the most favorable approach in the treatment of the diverse forms of human cancer. The principal goal in applying these antimetabolites of wide diversity in chemical composition is the destruction of the cancer cells without affecting the metabolism of the normal cells, a task that at present encounters many difficulties. Actually, the nonselective effects of antimetabolites on normal and cancerous cells is not too surprising when we take into consideration the fact that the cancer cell develops not *de novo*, but is an aberrant form of a normal cell, which still has the major part of its normal genetic make-up. While at the present time our limited knowledge regarding malignant growth does not permit a characterization of all the differences between normal and malignant cells, there are at least two fundamental differences that appear to be nearly specific for malignant cells.

1. In contrast to the differentiated embryonic and adult normal cell, the malignant cell displays a tendency to dedifferentiation.
2. In contrast to normal cells, which display a limited division and noninvasion, regardless of whether cell division occurs in embryonic or adult tissues, the malignant cell has the capacity to continue division without limitation and to invade not only the adjacent normal tissue, but also distant tissues by the hematogenous or lymphogenous route.

The question of whether the stable behavior regarding division and differentiation and the absence of invasiveness by dividing normal cells might be controlled by growth-regulating naturally occurring metabolites, and that there may be an aberration in occurrence and/or activity of such factors preceding and/or accompanying malignant growth, has led us to assess this concept experimentally.

This chapter deals with two types of experimental studies in this direction.

1. Experimental studies carried out by us nearly 40 years ago, which are concerned with the effects of folic acid and allied compounds on spontaneous breast cancers in mice.
2. Experimental studies, carried out by us during the last decade,

which are concerned with effects of vitamin C or L-cysteine on carcinogenesis of cultured animal and human lung tissues, and the effects of vitamin C or L-cysteine on cultured human breast cancer, before and after exposure to marijuana or tobacco smoke.

II. STUDIES ON THE EFFECTS OF FOLIC ACID AND ALLIED COMPOUNDS ON GROWTH OF SPONTANEOUS BREAST CANCERS IN MICE

The investigation of the effect of folic acid and allied compounds on animal tumors was stimulated by our experimental studies disclosing the inhibitory activity of yeast extract on growth of transplanted and spontaneous malignant tumors in mice (Lewisohn *et al.*, 1941a,b). These results aroused our interest in the importance of dietary factors, especially those of the vitamin B complex, in carcinogenesis. Furthermore, the finding by Pollack *et al.* (1942) of a high folic acid content in cancer tissues suggested a possible relationship of folic acid to cancer. The observations of Loo and Williams (1945) on the significant and striking differences between the behavior of folic acid in the livers of normal and cancer-bearing rats further supported this concept. After having observed that intravenous injections of a folic acid concentrate and of a crystalline *Lactobacillus casei* factor inhibited the growth of a transplanted tumor (sarcoma 180) in female Rockland mice (Leuchtenberger *et al.*, 1944), studies were undertaken to examine the long-term influence of folic acid and allied substances on growth of spontaneous breast cancers in mice. Eight hundred mice of different inbred strains carrying spontaneous breast cancers with confirmed malignancy were used. The mice were matched according to strain, age, and size of tumors, and divided in nontreated groups (controls) and groups treated with folic acid or allied compounds, such as liver *L. casei* factor, and xanthopterin. The mice of treated groups were injected intravenously daily with different doses of the compounds for a period of 2 months or more. The behavior of the tumors as well as the survival time of each treated animal was assessed and compared with those of matched untreated controls. Post mortem examinations, macroscopically and microscopically, were carried out for each animal, paying special attention to the presence of metastases in the lungs and other organs. In Table I data are presented that were obtained in consecutive experiments after repeated intravenous (iv) injections of folic acid, xanthopterin, and liver *L. casei* factor (R. Leuchtenberger *et al.*, 1945; R. Leuchtenberger, 1947; C. Leuchtenberger, 1947; Lewisohn *et al.*, 1946; Lewisohn, 1947). As can be seen from the data, there are significant differences between mice carrying

TABLE I

Influence of Repeated Intravenous Injections of Folic Acid,[a] Xanthopterin, and Liver *L. casei* Factor on Mice Carrying Spontaneous Breast Cancers[b]

No. of mice	Substance	Dose (μg)	No. of injections	No. of mice without tumor "healed mice"	No. of mice with new tumors	No. of mice with lung metastases		Range of survival time (days)	
						Healed mice	Nonhealed mice	Healed mice	Nonhealed mice
143	Folic acid	5	20–69	50 (35%)	10 (7%)	0	15 (16%)	132–225	85–132
145	Xanthopterin	100–200	20–69	5 (3.5%)	28 (19.7%)	0	42 (30%)	130–193	87–95
70	Liver *L. casei* factor	5–100	20–69	1 (1.4%)	23 (33%)	0	22 (33%)		55–75
205	—			5 (2.4%)	44 (21%)	0	70 (35%)	120–180	60–80

[a] Fermentation *L. casei* factor.

[b] Mice used are strain A, Rockland, Bagg. There were 4 consecutive experiments for each group.

spontaneous breast cancers after repeated iv injections of folic acid, xanthopterin, and liver *L. casei* factor and matched controls receiving no treatment. While mice after xanthopterin or liver *L. casei* factor do not show any significant differences regarding regression of the breast cancer, occurrence of new tumors, lung metastases, and survival time, mice treated with folic acid (fermentation *L. casei* factor) disclose significant alterations in all these features. In comparison with the control group and the groups treated with either xanthopterin or liver *L. casei* factor, mice treated with fermentation *L. casei* factor show a significant increase in frequency of "healed" mice, a significant decrease in frequency of new tumors and in frequency of lung metastases. Furthermore, there is also a significant increase in survival time after treatment with the fermentation *L. casei* factor, even in the nonhealed mice.

An additional number of nonhealed mice treated with folic acid for periods from 10 to 44 days were sacrificed, and the microscopical appearance of the tumor was compared with that of nontreated matched controls. In Figs. 1 and 2, size and microscopical appearance of breast cancers are presented before and after treatment with folic acid. As can be seen, there are significant differences not only regarding size, but also regarding microscopical appearance before and after treatment with folic acid (R. Leuchtenberger, 1947).

Comparing the therapeutic influence of folic acid with those of other vitamin B compounds on mice carrying spontaneous breast cancers, it is evident that only the fermentation *L. casei* factor was effective (Table I). This effect was not only observed in living mice, but extensive post mortem studies on all mice (macroscopically and microscopically) confirmed the marked growth inhibitory influence of this form of folic acid on the breast cancers.*

On the basis of these examinations, it is justified to state that tumors of folic acid-treated mice undergo considerable changes during the course of the treatment. Before healing is accomplished, the tumors pass, rather uniformly, through several stages.

In the first stage, during the first 2 or 3 weeks of treatment, more or less generalized necrobiosis with dissolution of the tumor pattern is seen, leading either to cheesy necrosis or occasionally to liquefaction. In the later stages, absorption and repair set in, resulting after several weeks either in the formation of a fibrous node, a scar, or a small inert cyst. In some cases even complete absorption with almost no trace of the former tumor is observed.

---

*Editor's note: It is of interest to note that the fermentation *L. casei* factor has the chemical structure of pteroyl triglutamate in contrast to the liver *L. casei* factor which is a monoglutamate (see Lewisohn *et al.*, 1976).

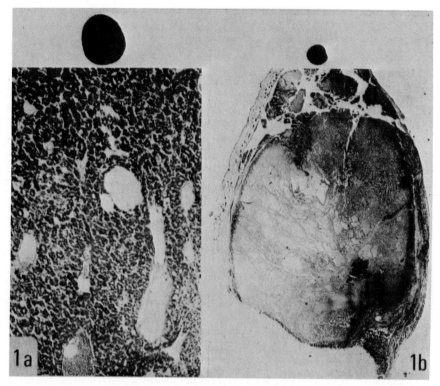

Fig. 1. Sizes and microscopic appearances of a spontaneous breast carcinoma of a mouse, before and after treatment with 44 intravenous injections of 5 µg of folic acid (*L. casei* factor). (a) Before treatment. Dense, mainly duct type of tumor. (b) After treatment. The "tumor" at the death of the animal was still of fair size. However, the bulk is changed into a cyst filled with homogeneous eosinophilic matter. In the wall of the cyst are remnants of tumor tissue. In contrast to microscopic pictures after rapid destruction, this is sometimes the final stage in slower, more low-grade destruction. (a) × 64. (b) × 17. Telly. Hematoxylin and eosin.

In the untreated controls some of the early changes described above were seen occasionally. However, complete destruction or disappearance of a tumor occurred in only about 2.5% of the controls.

Concerning the possible mode of action, the findings suggest a combination of varied interactions, namely, a direct action on the parenchyma, stroma, and tumor bed, and an indirect action, involving the general defense mechanism of the host. Vascular phenomena do not seem to be the decisive factor in initiating the destruction of these tumors. For an exact analysis of the mechanism involved in these processes, particularly those producing the early changes, many more studies have to be carried out.

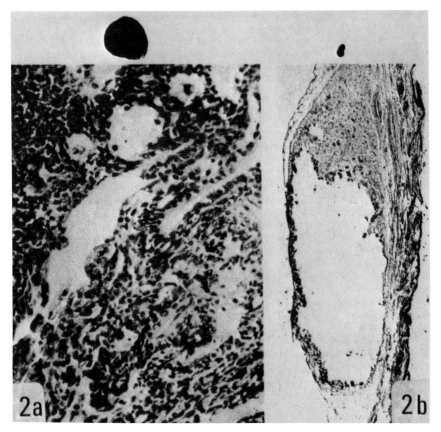

Fig. 2. Sizes and microscopic appearances of a spontaneous breast carcinoma of a mouse, before and after treatment with 47 intravenous injections of 5 μg of folic acid (*L. casei* factor). (a) Before treatment. Dense, partly spongy type of cancer. (b) After treatment. The mouse appeared clinically healed after 23 intravenous injections of 5 μg of folic acid, but received an additional 24 intravenous injections. The animal remained healthy for another 11 months. Postmortem examination revealed a cyst. In the upper pole hyalinized connective tissue containing a few lymphoid cells and lime salt deposits. Such calcified matter appears also in the other linings of the cyst wall. (a) × 125. (b) × 30, Telly. Hematoxylin and eosin.

III. STUDIES ON THE EFFECTS OF VITAMIN C OR L-CYSTEINE ON CARCINOGENESIS BEFORE AND AFTER EXPOSURE TO MARIJUANA OR TOBACCO SMOKE

These experimental studies are an outgrowth of our long-standing interest in the interrelation between cigarette smoking and human lung cancer. We developed special model systems in mice that imitate as closely as possible the human habit of cigarette smoking, as well as exposure of cell cultures to fresh smoke. Cell cultures are a necessary complementary tool to investigations on animals, because they permit an examination of the sequence of events in cells and tissues, not only in living cultures, but also in fixed and stained cultures *in situ*. Furthermore, cytological and quantitative cytochemical studies, such as microfluorometry (Leuchtenberger and Leuchtenberger, 1970b), make it possible on all cultures to examine such important features as behavior of chromosomes, DNA content in single cells, or cell parts *in situ* (Leuchtenberger and Leuchtenberger, 1970b, 1976; Leuchtenberger *et al.*, 1973a,b). Cell cultures are also a particularly favorable model system for assessing carcinogenesis and the possible preventive and/or growth regulating influence of naturally occurring metabolites.

We observed that long-term inhalation of cigarette smoke by mice, or exposure of cultures from animal or human lung tissues to puffs of fresh smoke (whole smoke or gas vapor phase) accelerates carcinogenic changes in the lung (Leuchtenberger and Leuchtenberger, 1970a, 1974). Our observation that the gas vapor phase evoked as many or more abnormalities in the DNA metabolism of cells as did the particulate matter of tobacco smoke has also been reported by Styles (1976) in an extensive study on different mammalian cell cultures. Searching for constituents responsible for the carcinogenic effects of cigarette smoke, it was also found that, while the tar content of tobacco smoke did not correlate, the degree of sulfhydryl (SH) reactivity and of NO content of tobacco smoke correlated positively with the capacity of the smoke to enhance atypical growth and malignant transformation of hamster lung cultures (Leuchtenberger *et al.*, 1974, 1976a,c; Davies *et al.*, 1975). Furthermore, there seemed to be a relationship between high SH reactivity of the smoke, decrease in lysosomes, and the subsequent malignant transformation (Davies *et al.*, 1975; Leuchtenberger and Leuchtenberger, 1977b). These results and reports that cigarette smoke inhibits SH-dependent enzyme systems (Lange, 1961; Powell and Green, 1972) and that lysosomal damage may be implicated in carcinogenesis (Allison and Paton, 1965; Allison, 1969) have led us to suggest that one of the steps in the sequential carcinogenic alterations of hamster and human lung cultures is a disturbance of SH equilibrium and lysosomes in cells, caused by SH-reactive constituents of the smoke (Leuchtenberger *et al.*, 1974, 1976c; Davies *et al.*, 1975). To assess the relevance of this concept, it seemed of interest to determine if lung cell cultures can be protected against the SH reactivity of the smoke by thiols. L-Cysteine was chosen because it is known to react with cigarette smoke (Fenner and Braven, 1968; Leuchtenberger *et al.*, 1974, 1976a) and to afford protection against the potent inhibitory effect of the gas vapor phase of cigarette smoke on the SH enzyme glyceraldehyde-3-phosphate dehydrogenase (Powell and Green, 1972).

The effect of vitamin C was also studied because a decrease in vitamin C level has been found in human cigarette smokers (Pelletier, 1975), and vitamin C has been reported to block NO compounds (Mirvish, 1975), i.e., constituents known to be present in the gas vapor phase of tobacco smoke. Furthermore, in our own studies, addition of vitamin C to normal media had a stimulating effect on lysosome formation and led to a significantly longer survival time of cultures prepared from adult normal human lung (Leuchtenberger and Leuchtenberger, 1977a).

Since in the last decade there has been not only a marked increase in the habit of smoking of tobacco but also of marijuana cigarettes, the effect of vitamin C on tobacco and marijuana smoke-exposed animal and human lung and human breast cancer cultures was assessed (Leuchtenberger et al., 1976b, 1979; Leuchtenberger and Leuchtenberger, 1977a,b; Leuchtenberger and Ozzello, 1983; Leuchtenberger, 1982).

The following essential results obtained in lung cultures after exposure to smoke without and with vitamin C or L-cysteine are briefly summarized:

1. Both tobacco and marijuana smoke accelerated carcinogenesis in animal and human lung cultures, whereby the abnormalities in cell division, chromosomes, and genetic material (DNA) were much more marked after exposure to marijuana smoke than to tobacco smoke (Leuchtenberger et al., 1973a,b, 1976b, 1979; Leuchtenberger and Leuchtenberger, 1976, 1977b).

2. The carcinogenic effects were markedly reduced when vitamin C or L-cysteine were added to the lung cultures, although the effect of vitamin C was much less marked on marijuana smoke-exposed cultures than on tobacco smoke-exposed ones (Leuchtenberger and Leuchtenberger 1976, 1977b; Leuchtenberger et al., 1976b, 1979).

In view of the preventive influence of vitamin C or L-cysteine on the development of tobacco or marijuana smoke carcinogenesis in cultures of animal and human lung, the question arose whether vitamin C or L-cysteine may also have growth-regulating effects on an established cultured human breast cancer cell line, such as SK-Br-3 (Fogh and Trempe, 1975; Leuchtenberger et al., 1979; Leuchtenberger and Ozzello, 1983). In the scheme of Fig. 3 and in Table II, data are presented which compare the effects of vitamin C on SK-Br-3 cultures without and after exposure to smoke and without and with addition of vitamin C or L-cysteine. Figures 4–9 present the microscopical appearance observed *in vivo* and in fixed preparations of the breast cancer cultures without (Fig.

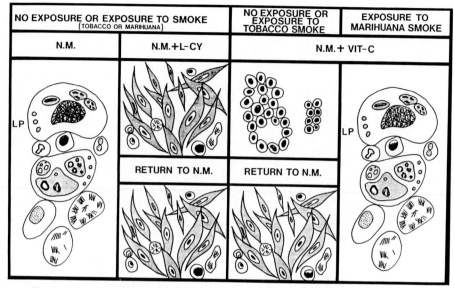

Fig. 3. Scheme of cell morphology of human breast cancer (Sk-Br-3) cultures grown in media without [normal media (N.M.)] and with addition of L-cysteine (L-CY) and vitamin C (VIT-C). LP, lipid granulas.

4a and b) and with addition of L-cysteine (Figs. 5 and 7) or vitamin C (Figs. 6, 8, and 9). As can be seen, there were significant differences between human breast cancer cultures without and with addition of vitamin C, regardless of whether the cultures were exposed or not exposed to tobacco smoke (Figs., 4, 6, and 8). Vitamin C caused in these cultures a stimulation of growth, accompanied by a marked reduction of mitotic abnormalities (Table II). Furthermore, there was an occurrence of clusters of cells in pseudoglandular arrangement suggesting differentiation (Figs. 6 and 8). All these effects of vitamin C on the breast cancer cultures were completely absent after exposure to marijuana smoke (Fig. 9). Vitamin C did not only stimulate the occurrence of abnormal proliferation, but also the dedifferentiation of the cancer cells in marijuana-exposed cultures (Fig. 9).

L-Cysteine, although it had shown previously a preventive effect similar to that of vitamin C in tobacco carcinogenesis of animal lung cultures (Leuchtenberger and Leuchtenberger, 1977a), had a very different influence on the breast cancer cultures from that of vitamin C. All the cultures became fibroblastic, whether or not exposed to tobacco or marijuana smoke in the presence of L-cysteine, and there was marked proliferation, but no decrease in mitotic abnormalities nor any sign of differentiation (Table II and Figs. 5 and 7).

TABLE II

Effects of Vitamin C or L-Cysteine on Growth and Cell Division of Human Breast Cancer SK-Br-3

Type of media	Cell type observed for			Subcultures (19–70 weeks) mean weekly increase 990[a]	Mitotic abnormalities in (%) 451[b]	Alterations and cell type after return to normal media		
	1–4 weeks	5–14 weeks	15–70 weeks			1–4 weeks	5–14 weeks	15–70 weeks
Normal medium	S + L epithelial[c]			1 ± 0.3	8.2			
Normal medium + vitamin C	S+L epithelial	S+L epithelial	S epithelial pseudo-glandular structure	14 + 2.3 PCo<0.005	2.2 PCo<0.005	Epithelial + fibro-blastlike		Fibroblastlike
Normal medium + L-cysteine	S + L epithelial	Epithelial + fibro-blastlike	Fibroblast-like	12 ± 1.5 PCo<0.005	10.5		Fibroblastlike	

[a] Number of cultures examined.
[b] Fifty fields counted at random in each culture.
[c] S, small cells; L, large cells with abnormalities.

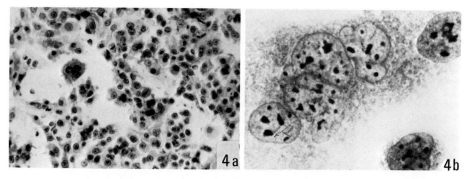

Fig. 4. (a) and (b): Light micrographs of human breast cancer culture (SK-Br-3) grown in normal media. Note: small, large atypical epithelial cells and giant multinucleated abnormal cells. Hematoxylin and eosin. (a) × 113. (b) × 600.

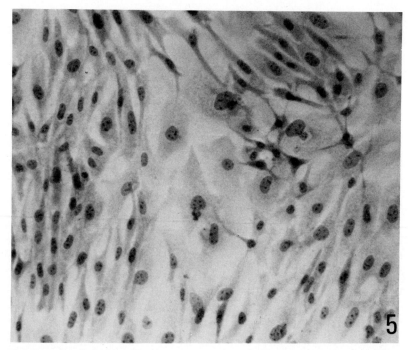

Fig. 5. Light micrograph of human breast cancer culture (SK-Br-3) grown in normal media + L-cysteine (0.05%) for 161 days. Note: fibroblastlike cells. Hematoxylin and eosin. × 188.

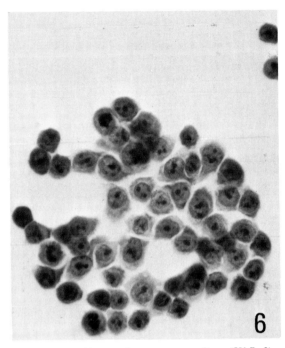

Fig. 6. Light micrograph of human breast cancer culture (SK-Br-3) grown in normal media + vitamin C (8 mg/liter) for 504 days. Note: small epithelial cells arranged as pseudoglandular structures. Hematoxylin and eosin. × 375.

It would thus appear that addition of L-cysteine to normal medium (N.M.) evoked in cultures of the human breast cancer line SK-Br-3 not only a metaplastic change from an epithelial to a fibroblastlike cell type, but also an acceleration of the growth rates of the cells. The finding that this change, observed in the presence of L-cysteine, did not regress when these fibroblastlike cultures were placed back for long periods in N.M. without L-cysteine indicates that the metaplasia caused by L-cysteine is irreversible, at least for the time examined (up to 70 weeks) and would suggest that it is accompanied by a fundamental change in cell physiology. The marked acceleration of growth rates of SK-Br-3 cultures, when grown in N.M. with L-cysteine, is in good accordance with the significant increase in growth rate of adult human lung cultures when grown with L-cysteine (Leuchtenberger and Leuchtenberger, 1977a). However, while in the breast cancer cultures exposure to L-cysteine led to fibroblastlike growth, i.e., to a marked dedifferentiation of the cells, in the adult human lung cultures it promoted the expression of epithelial features (Leuchtenberger and Leuchtenberger, 1977a). An

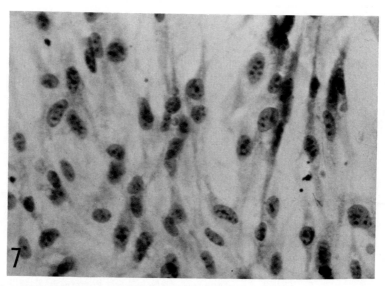

Fig. 7. Light micrograph of human breast cancer culture (SK-Br-3) seven times exposed to six puffs of fresh smoke from tobacco cigarettes and grown in normal media + L-cysteine (0.05%). Note: fibroblastlike cells resembling those in Fig. 5. Hematoxylin and eosin. × 375.

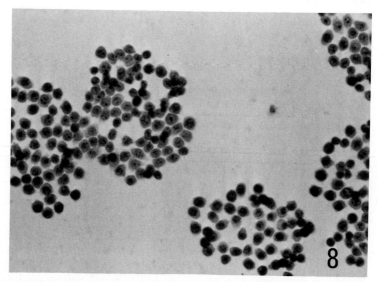

Fig. 8. Light micrograph of human breast cancer culture (SK-Br-3) seven times exposed to six puffs of fresh smoke from tobacco cigarettes and grown in normal media + vitamin C (8 mg/liter). Note: several pseudoglandular structures resembling those in Fig. 6. Hematoxylin and eosin. × 188.

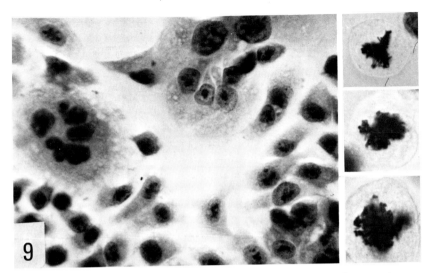

Fig. 9. Light micrograph of human breast cancer culture (SK-Br-3) seven times exposed to eight puffs of fresh smoke from marijuana cigarettes and grown in normal media + vitamin C (8 mg/liter). Note: multinucleated epithelial cells resembling those in Fig. 4 and frequent occurrence of abnormal giant mitoses. Hematoxylin and eosin. × 338. Inset × 675.

epithelial growth was also noted in normal and transformed hamster lung cultures, nonexposed or exposed to tobacco or marijuana smoke, after L-cysteine (Leuchtenberger and Leuchtenberger, 1977b). These discrepancies in results indicate that cultures prepared from animal or human tissues, as well as cultures from various human tissues, do not respond in the same manner to L-cysteine. The question of whether the difference in response of various human tissues may be due to the difference between human normal and human tumor tissues cannot be answered at present, but needs further comparative studies on cultures of normal and neoplastic tissues.

The observation that vitamin C affected SK-Br-3 cultures in a very different manner from that of L-cysteine, although the acceleration in growth was similar after exposure to either one of the metabolifes, deserves consideration. Vitamin C did not lead to overt dedifferentiation and fibroblastlike growth, but favored the expression of epithelial growth with pseudoglandular arrangement and decrease in mitotic abnormalities suggesting differentiation. These observations are in good accordance with those obtained on cultures from normal human and animal lung, and on cultures of transformed hamster lung, nonexposed or exposed to smoke from tobacco or marijuana cigarettes (Leuchtenberger and Leuchtenberger, 1977a,b). Although these studies indicate that various animal and human lung tissue cultures respond to vitamin

C in a similar manner, SK-Br-3 cultures differ in their response to vitamin C when exposed to tobacco or marijuana smoke (Leuchtenberger *et al.*, 1979). While after exposure to tobacco smoke the SK-Br-3 cultures were affected by vitamin C in a similar manner to non-smoke-exposed cultures (Figs. 6 and 8), SK-Br-3 cells exposed to marijuana smoke showed a striking dedifferentiation and no occurrence of pseudoglandular structures (Fig. 9) (Leuchtenberger *et al.*, 1979). It would thus appear that depending on environmental factors, such as type of smoke, even the same type of human cancer cultures, such as SK-Br-3, may be affected very differently by the same metabolite, such as vitamin C.

Another marked difference between the effects of L-cysteine and vitamin C on SK-Br-3 cultures is the observation that, when placed back in N.M. only, cultures previously exposed to L-cysteine did not change their fibroblastlike morphology, while cultures exposed to vitamin C lost in a relatively short period of time their striking epithelial character and pseudoglandular structures. This would indicate that the pseudoglandular arrangement of the epithelial cells, suggesting a tendency to differentiation, was dependent on the presence of vitamin C. The pathway by which vitamin C induced a tendency to differentiation is difficult to elucidate, not only because this special change took place very slowly, but also because the change to pseudoglandular structures was not observed to the same extent in all of the cultures grown in media with vitamin C. The finding that cultures showing pseudoglandular formations, when placed back in N.M. without vitamin C did not revert to the original epithelial appearance of cultures grown in N.M., but became more and more fibroblastlike, makes it even more difficult to suggest mechanisms of action of vitamin C.

Although at present nothing is known regarding the pathway of action of L-cysteine or vitamin C on SK-Br-3 cells, the marked and different effects of L-cysteine and vitamin C indicate that morphology and growth of cultured human cancer cells, such as SK-Br-3, can be altered significantly by naturally occurring metabolites.

REFERENCES

Allison, A. C. (1969). *In* "Lysosomes in Biology and Pathology" (J. T. Dingle and H. B. Fell, eds.), p. 178. North Holland Pub., Amsterdam.

Allison, A. C., and Paton, G. R. (1965). *Nature (London)* **207**, 1170.

Davies, P., Kistler, G. S., Leuchtenberger, C., and Leuchtenberger, R. (1975). *Beitr. Pathol.* **155**, 168.

Fenner, M. L., and Braven, J. (1968). *Br. J. Cancer* **22**, 474.

Fogh, J., and Trempe, G. (1975). *In* "Human Tumor Cells *in Vitro*" (J. Fogh, ed.), p. 115. Plenum, New York.

Lange, R. (1961). *Science* **134**, 52.

Leuchtenberger, C. (1947) In "Approaches to Tumor Chemotherapy" (F. R. Moulton, ed.), pp. 157–162. Science Press Printing Co., Lancaster, Pennsylvania.

Leuchtenberger, C. (1982). *ARF/WHO Sci. Meet. Adverse Health Behav. Consequences Cannabis Use* (in press).

Leuchtenberger, C., and Leuchtenberger, R. (1970a). *AEC Symp. Ser.* **21**, 329–346.

Leuchtenberger, C., and Leuchtenberger, R. (1970b). *Exp. Cell Res.* **62**, 161–172.

Leuchtenberger, C., and Leuchtenberger, R. (1974). *Soz. Praeventivmed.* **19**, 41–45.

Leuchtenberger, C., and Leuchtenberger, R. (1976). In "The Pharmacology of Marihuana" (M. C. Braude and S. Szara, eds.), pp. 595–612. Raven Press, New York.

Leuchtenberger, C., and Leuchtenberger, R. (1977a). *Cell Biol. Int. Rep.* **1**, 317–324.

Leuchtenberger, C., and Leuchtenberger, R. (1977b). *Br. J. Exp. Pathol.* **58**, 625–634.

Leuchtenberger, C., and Ozzello, L. (1983). *Prog. Surg. Pathol.* **5** (in press).

Leuchtenberger, C., Lewisohn, R., Laszlo, D., and Leuchtenberger, R. (1944). *Proc. Soc. Exp. Biol. Med.* **55**, 204–205.

Leuchtenberger, C., Leuchtenberger, R., and Schneider, A. (1973a). *Nature (London)* **241**, 137–139.

Leuchtenberger, C., Leuchtenberger, R., Ritter, U., and Inui, N. (1973b). *Nature (London)* **242**, 403–404.

Leuchtenberger, C., Leuchtenberger, R., and Zbinden, I. (1974). *Nature (London)* **247**, 565–567.

Leuchtenberger, C., Leuchtenberger, R., Zbinden, I., and Schleh E. (1976a). *Soz. Praeventivmed.* **21**, 47–50.

Leuchtenberger,C., Leuchtenberger, R., Zbinden, I., and Schleh, E. (1976b). In "Marihuana: Chemistry, Biochemistry, and Cellular Effects" (G. G. Nahas, ed.), pp. 243–256. Springer-Verlag, Berlin and New York.

Leuchtenberger, C., Leuchtenberger, R., Zbinden, I., and Schleh, E. (1976c). *Colloq.—Inst. Natl. Sante Rech. Med.* **52**, 73–80.

Leuchtenberger, C., Leuchtenberger, R., and Chapuis, L. (1979). In "Marihuana: Biological Effects" (G. G. Nahas and W. D. M. Paton, eds.), pp. 209–218. Pergamon, Oxford.

Leuchtenberger, R. (1947). In "Approaches to Tumor Chemotherapy" (R. Moulton, ed.), pp. 163–194. Science Press Printing Co., Lancaster, Pennsylvania.

Leuchtenberger, R., Leuchtenberger, C., Laszlo, D., and Lewisohn, R. (1945). *Science* **101**, 46.

Lewisohn, R. (1947). In "Approaches to Tumor Chemotherapy" (F. R. Moulton, ed.), pp 139–147. Science Press Printing Co., Lancaster, Pennsylvania.

Lewisohn, R., Leuchtenberger, C., Leuchtenberger, R., and Laszlo, D. (1941a). *Am. J. Pathol.* **17**, 251–260.

Lewisohn, R., Leuchtenberger, C., Leuchtenberger, R., Laszlo, D., and Bloch, K. (1941b). *Cancer* **1**, 799–806.

Lewisohn, R., Leuchtenberger, C., Leuchtenberger, R., and Keresztesy, J. C. (1946). *Science* **104**, 436–437.

Loo, Y. H., and Williams, R. J. (1945). *Univ. Tex. Publ.* **4507**, 123–134.

Mirvish, S. S. (1975). *Ann. N.Y. Acad. Sci.* **258**, 175.

National Research Council (1982). "Diet, Nutrition and Cancer." Natl. Acad. Press, Washington, D.C.

Pelletier, O. (1975). *Ann. N.Y. Acad. Sci.* **258**, 156.

Pollack, M. A., Taylor, A., and Williams, R. G. (1942). *Univ. Tex. Publ.* **4237**, 56–69.

Powell, G. M., and Green, G. M. (1972). *Biochem. Pharmacol.* **21**, 1785.

Styles, J. A. (1976). *Br. J. Exp. Pathol.* **57**, 286.

10

The Metabolism of Vitamin A and Its Functions

H. F. DeLuca

Department of Biochemistry
University of Wisconsin
Madison, Wisconsin

I. INTRODUCTION

Vitamin A was the first vitamin to be clearly defined on an experimental basis. In 1913, McCollum and Davis described a lipid component of the diet required for growth, which they described as "fat-soluble A." Subsequent work then provided additional evidence for a "water-soluble B" factor required for prevention of neurological symptoms in animals

149

Nutritional Factors in the Induction
and Maintenance of Malignancy

(McCollum *et al.*, 1916). This work, together with that of Osborne and Mendel (1917), firmly established the existence of the fat-soluble substance that became known as vitamin A. These initial discoveries were to usher in the era of vitamin discovery and to provide the basis for development of the new science of biochemistry.

Despite early discovery, the function of vitamin A in molecular terms remains unknown with the exception of its role in the visual cycle. On the other hand, the mechanisms of action of the B complex vitamins have been rather thoroughly described. The main reason for this obvious divergence in information is that the B complex vitamins are required by virtually all living organisms for basic metabolic reactions, such as in the transduction of energy or in the utilization of energy for the construction of macromolecules. On the other hand, the fat-soluble vitamins are not required by all organisms, but rather are required by organisms having tissues with a great division of labor. In short, they are required for the development of specialized tissues or for specialized tissues in providing specialized functions characteristic of the higher organisms. The molecular mechanisms of action, therefore, are likely to be intimately related with the process of differentiation of cells or in highly specialized processes not approachable with the use of simple microorganisms and the powerful tool of mutant forms. Vitamin A is the prime example of the fat-soluble group. Because the metabolism of vitamin A is so intimately involved with its functions, both areas will be covered and their interrelationship described.

II.   METABOLISM OF VITAMIN A

A.   Absorption of the Vitamin

The primary source of vitamin A to the animal kingdom is from plant supplies, primarily as the carotenes (Moore, 1957). In addition to these sources, vitamin A is available as the retinyl esters from animals sources. β-Carotene in the small intestine is cleaved by a dioxygenase that has an absolute requirement for molecular oxygen and a nonspecific requirement for a detergent such as bile salts (Goodman *et al.*, 1966; Olson, 1964; Olson and Hayaishi, 1965). The dioxygenase is a soluble enzyme that has been partially purified and characterized from rat, hog, and rabbit intestine (Goodman *et al.*, 1966; Fidge *et al.*, 1969; Lakshmanan *et al.*, 1972). Carotene is converted to retinal that undergoes reduction by retinyl aldehyde reductase. This enzyme has a requirement for NADH or NADPH and appears to be a nonspecific aldehyde reductase reducing retinal to retinol (Fidge and Goodman, 1968). Retinol is then esterified in the small intestine with fatty acids, usually long chain saturated fatty acids (Huang and Goodman, 1965). Retinyl esters from the diet are cleaved to form retinol in the small intestines. The retinol from either source is then, following esterification, absorbed in the chylomicrons that are then cleared into the liver where the retinol is hydrolyzed and esterified to form retinyl palmitate (DeLuca, 1979; Moore, 1957). This represents the storage form of vitamin A and can be hydrolyzed upon demand to form retinol. Retinol then is involved in the induction of formation of the transport protein, retinol binding protein, as will be described below.

B. Transport of Retinol

There is little question that the circulating form of vitamin A is retinol (DeLuca, 1979; Smith and Goodman, 1979). It circulates and binds to a transport protein known as retinol binding protein that has been isolated in pure form and quite thoroughly characterized (Goodman, 1969, 1972; Smith and Goodman, 1979). Retinol binds at a ratio of 1 mole/mole of retinol binding protein that then in turn binds to 1 mole of prealbumin that is responsible for the transport of thyroxine (Smith and Goodman, 1979). Retinol binding protein is formed in the liver, and there is an intracellular form of retinol binding protein that accumulates in vitamin A deficiency. Upon vitamin A repletion, retinol binding protein decreases in the liver and makes its appearance in the serum with bound retinol (Smith and Goodman, 1979; J. E. Smith et al., 1973). The biosynthesis of retinol binding protein is markedly limited under conditions of severe protein malnutrition, and hence therapy of subjects that have protein malnutrition in addition to vitamin A deficiency is relatively ineffective until protein repletion permits the biosynthesis of the transport protein (F. R. Smith et al., 1973). Figure 1 illustrates the nature of the transport protein in a diagrammatic sense. The mechanism whereby retinol is transferred from the transport protein to the target cells remains unknown. Nevertheless, it seems quite certain that the target cells are responsible for whatever metabolism of retinol must take place before function.

C. Target Organ Metabolism of the Retinoids

Virtually every organ possesses the ability to oxidize retinol to retinal as can be seen in Fig. 2. This reaction utilizes an NAD requiring alcohol dehydrogenase (Moore, 1957; Wald and Hubbard, 1950, 1960). Retinal in

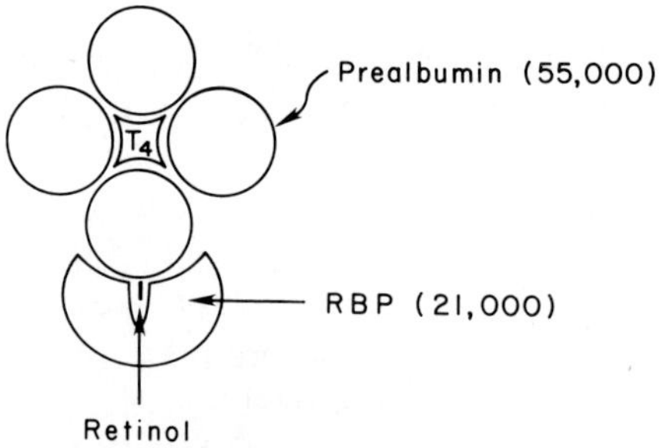

Prealbumin (55,000)

RBP (21,000)

Retinol

Fig. 1. Diagrammatic representation of retinol binding protein (RBP) in association with prealbumin as it circulates in the plasma.

the all-trans and 11-cis forms are certainly the active metabolites of vitamin A in the visual cycle as will be discussed below. Therefore, oxidation of retinol to retinal in the retina represents a target organ required modification of the vitamin A molecule (Wald and Hubbard, 1950, 1960). There is considerable question as to whether further metabolism of vitamin A is required for function in the epithelial tissue, in bone tissue, or in the reproductive organs (DeLuca, 1979; DeLuca et al., 1981). As can be seen from Fig. 2, retinol is readily oxidized to retinoic acid in a large number of tissues (Futterman, 1962; Mahadevan et al., 1962). There has been considerable question as to whether retinoic acid is a true in vivo metabolite of retinol. There is now no question that oxidation of retinol to retinoic acid occurs in vivo, with retinoic acid appearing in large amounts in many of the target tissues (Emerick et al., 1967; Ito et al.,

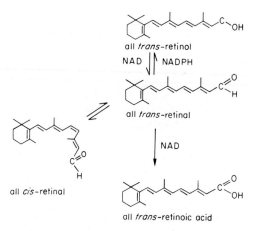

all *trans*-retinol

NAD ⇅ NADPH

all *trans*-retinal

NAD

all *cis*-retinal

all *trans*-retinoic acid

Fig. 2. The functional metabolism of retinol.

1974a; Kleiner-Bossaler and DeLuca, 1971). Retinoic acid cannot be converted back to retinal or retinol *in vivo* or *in vitro* (Arens and van Dorp, 1946; Dowling and Wald, 1958, 1960). Thus, the supply of retinoic acid or many of its analogs does not satisfy the functions that require the aldehyde or alcohol form of vitamin A. There is no question that retinoic acid is metabolized even further to a variety of products, some of which have been characterized and others which have not (Fig. 3). Some of the metabolism reported here takes place predominantly in the liver and may or may not take place in the target organs.

Work by Sporn, Roberts, and Frolik at the National Institutes of Health has demonstrated clearly that retinoic acid is oxidized to 4-hydroxyretinoic acid and subsequently to 4-ketoretinoic (Frolik *et al.*, 1978, 1979; Roberts and Frolik, 1979). The 4-hydroxylase is absent in deficient hamsters and must be induced by administration of retinoic acid (Roberts *et al.*, 1979a,b, 1980). These 4-keto and 4-hydroxyl compounds are less active than retinoic acid in the epithelial differentiating systems (Newton *et al.*, 1980). Therefore, they are regarded as primarily inactivation or degradation products. Further work by Frolik and co-workers

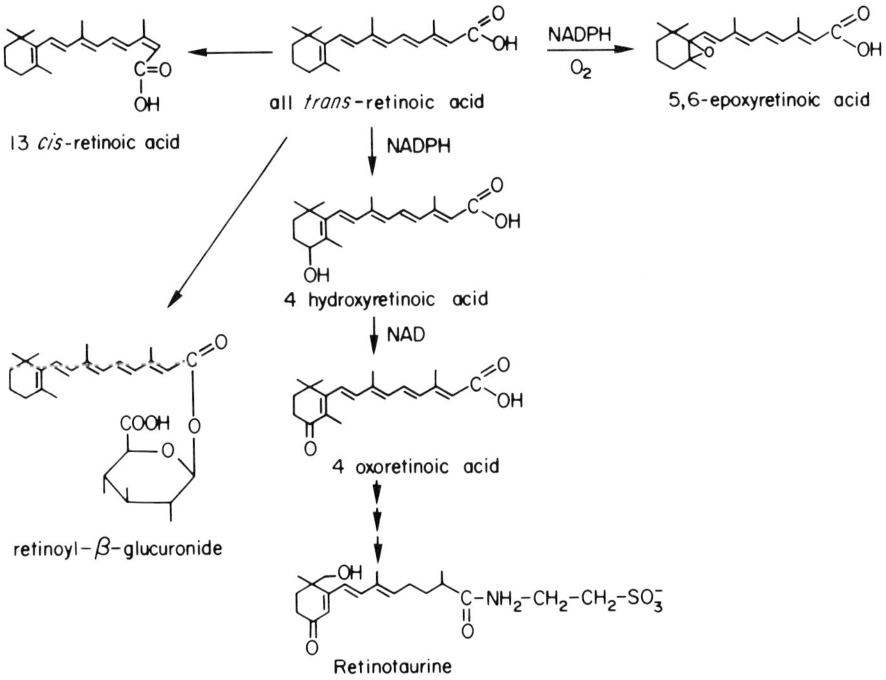

Fig. 3. Physiologic metabolism of retinoic acid as is currently understood.

(1981) has shown that these compounds can be converted to the 13-cis derivatives and subsequently can be converted to their glucuronide conjugates. Another important fact that eliminates the 4-keto- and 4-hydroxyretinoic acids for consideration as active forms is that they are not formed initially in vitamin A-deficient animals responding to retinoic acid (Roberts *et al.*, 1979b; Silva and DeLuca, 1982). The primary reason is that the 4-hydroxylase is absent and must be induced. Nevertheless, the absence of 4-hydroxy- and hence 4-ketoretinoic acid in tissues before the initial response to retinoic acid eliminates their consideration as active forms.

All-*trans*-retinoic acid is converted to 13-*cis*-retinoic acid *in vivo* (Zile *et al.*, 1967, 1982a). Although this conversion can also take place autocatalytically, it seems certain that some 13-cis isomerization is catalyzed *in vivo* (Zile *et al.*, 1982a). However, it is difficult to conclude that this is an important *in vivo* reaction. Besides these reactions, two other reactions of retinoic acid are known. One is the formation of 5,6-epoxyretinoic acid (McCormick *et al.*, 1978; Napoli *et al.*, 1978). There is no question that this epoxidation does occur *in vivo*, since the enzyme responsible for epoxidation has been clearly identified and studied (McCormick *et al.*, 1980; Sietsema and DeLuca, 1979). This enzyme forms another example of a lipid peroxidation system that is blocked by free radical inhibitors such as diphenyl-*p*-phenylenediamine (Sietsema and DeLuca, 1982b; Zile *et al.*, 1980a). The most active tissue in 5,6-epoxidation is the kidney, although a variety of other epithelial tissues will carry out the epoxidation (DeLuca, 1979). The amount of 5,6-epoxyretinoic acid found *in vivo* following an injection of radiolabeled retinoic acid is vanishingly small and can only be found 3 hours post-injection of the radiolabel. Some studies have been initiated on further metabolism of the 5,6-epoxide. The epoxide is essentially biologically inactive (Zile *et al.*, 1980a), and experiments have been carried out in which the 5,6-epoxidation can be blocked *in vivo* by the administration of diphenyl-*p*-phenylenediamine without intefering with the response of vitamin A-deficient rats to retinoic acid. These experiments eliminate 5,6-epoxyretinoic acid as a possible active form (Sietsema and DeLuca, 1982b). Other arguments include its very low concentration *in vivo* at any particular time and the fact that it certainly represents a minor pathway that is not universally demonstrable in all laboratories.

A significant metabolite of retinoic acid was isolated and identified in the laboratory of Dr. James Olson many years ago (Dunagin *et al.*, 1965, 1966). This compound is the retinoyl-β-glucuronide which was first considered as a substance involved in the enterohepatic circulation of retinoic acid (Zachman *et al.*, 1966). The retinoyl-β-glucuronide appears to be equally active if not slightly more active than retinoic acid in such epithelial differentiating systems as the vaginal smear system (Sietsema and DeLuca, 1982a; Skare *et al.*, 1982b). Of considerable importance is the fact that this metabolite is not only formed by liver but is also found in such target tissues as intestine following bile duct cannulation (Olson and Hayaishi, 1965; Zile *et al.*, 1982b). Because of its impressive biological activity in epithelial differentiating systems and because it is found in target organs following physiologic doses of retinoic acid, this compound must still be considered as a possible metabolically active form, although it is generally believed that glucuronides represent excretory products.

The complexity of retinoic acid metabolism in the target organs has recently been shown using physiologic doses of retinoic acid and high-performance liquid chromatographic separation of the metabolic products in the target organs using high specific activity radiolabeled retinoic acid (Fig. 4). There are several possible active forms of vitamin A in the sense that metabolites appear very readily in target organs prior to a measurable target organ response (Ito *et al.*, 1974b; Silva and DeLuca, 1982). In an attempt to determine whether these physiologically apparent metabolites have biological activity, we have recently administered greater than physiological levels of radiolabeled retinoic acid to vitamin A-deficient animals, removed the intestines, and extracted and chromatographed them on Sephadex LH-20 followed by high-performance liquid chromatography. All of the polar metabolite fractions have been assayed for biological activity in the vaginal smear assay (Stephens-Jarnagin *et al.*, 1983). The results have clearly shown the absence of any significant biological activity in these polar fractions. In this series of experiments the only biologically active metabolites present in significant amounts were the retinoyl-β-glucuronide and the 13-*cis*-retinoic acid. At the present time, therefore, it can be concluded that the only established metabolically active forms of vitamin A *in vivo* are retinol, retinal, and retinoic acid. Retinoyl-β-glucuronide cannot yet be excluded as a possible metabolically active form. The most definitive experiments, however, will come from a thorough investigation of the metabolism of retinoic acid in isolated cell cultures, such as the teratocarcinoma F-9 cell lines and the human myeloid leukemic cell line HL-60, that undergo differentiation in response to retinoic acid. Current results have not supported the concept that there is an active form beyond retinoic acid, however.

The major route of excretion of the retinoids is the urine and the bile (Zile *et al.*, 1980b). Three distinct pathways of retinol and retinoic acid metabolism were deduced during the 1960 era in which it was clearly

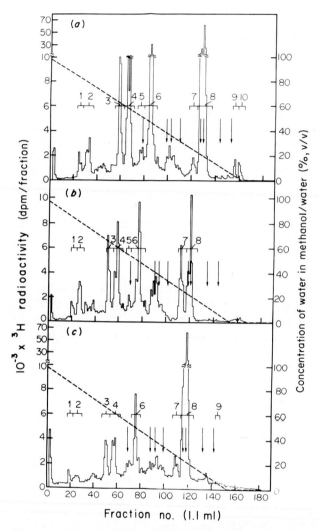

Fig. 4. High-performance liquid chromatographic profile of metabolites found in (a) blood, (b) trachea and lungs, and (c) testes of rats following a physiologic dose of [11,12-³H]retinoic acid having a specific radioactivity level of 30–40 Ci/mmole. The column is a reversed phase Zorbax ODS column (Dupont, Inc., Wilmington, Delaware) with a solvent gradient of 98% water in methanol to 100% methanol (dashed line). Standards are from left to right (arrows), 16-hydroxy-4-ketoretinoic acid, 4-ketoretinoic acid, 4-hydroxyretinoic acid, 5,6-epoxyretinoic acid, 13-*cis*-retinoic acid, all-*trans*-retinoic acid, all-*trans*-retinol, and methyl retinoate.

shown that retinoids are eliminated in urine and bile as an intact molecule, i.e., with the side chain remaining intact (60%), or without the terminal side chain carbon (20%), or without the last two carbons (Roberts and DeLuca, 1967). This resulted in the postulation of at least three pathways of retinol or retinoic acid metabolism *in vivo* (Fig. 5). So far, however, besides the 4-keto- and 4-hydroxyretinoic acid found in very small amounts as excretory products, only one major excretory form of retinoic acid has been isolated and identified in addition to retinyl-β-glucuronide if it can be assumed that that compound is a true excretory product. That product is known as retinotaurine, and the structure is shown in Fig. 3 (Skare *et al.*, 1982a). This product comprises as much as 20% of the total retinoic acid excreted (Skare *et al.*, 1982a). This interesting compound involves hydroxylation on the gem methyl, 4-keto formation, cleavage of the terminal carbon, reduction of two double bonds, and finally conjugation with taurine (Skare *et al.*, 1982a). This substance is biologically inactive in the vaginal smear assay (Skare *et al.*, 1982b).

In conclusion, the total metabolism of the retinoids is far from elucidated. However, it seems very possible that the only active forms of vitamin A are retinol, retinal, and retinoic acid. There have been claims that retinol and retinal can satisfy all of the functions of vitamin A. However, these deductions do not pay adequate attention to several important facts. First, retinoic acid is a major metabolite of retinol *in vivo* (Emerick *et al.*, 1967; Ito *et al.*, 1974a; Kleiner-Bössaler and DeLuca,

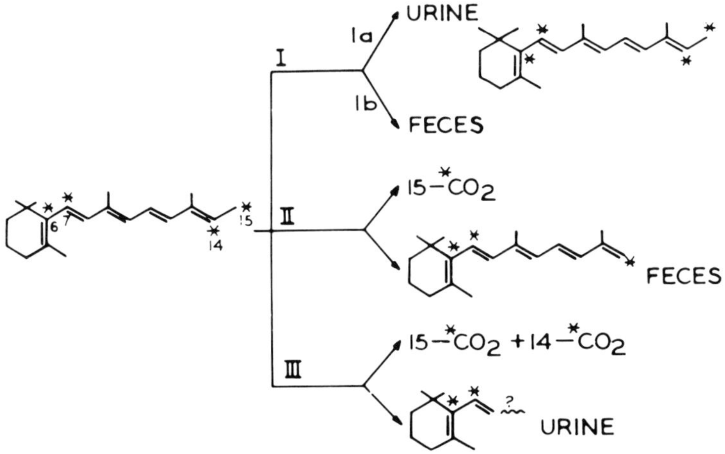

Fig. 5. *In vivo* pathways of retinoic acid metabolism. (From Roberts and DeLuca, 1967.)

1971). Second, it is extremely biologically active even in supporting growth of vitamin A-deficient rats (Dowling and Wald, 1958, 1960; Zile and DeLuca, 1968). Third, retinoic acid is more active than retinol in several epithelial differentiating systems carried out *in vitro* (Breitman *et al.*, 1980; Newton *et al.*, 1980; Strickland and Mahdovi, 1978). Since retinol is less active than retinoic acid in these cell systems and since retinoic acid cannot be converted to retinol, whereas the reverse is true, it seems very likely that retinoic acid or a further metabolite must be considered the active form in epithelial differentiation.

Besides the metabolism described above, which clearly occurs under physiologic conditions, metabolites of retinoic acid found in feces and urine have been isolated from animals given massive amounts of retinoic acid (Hänni and Bigler, 1977; Hänni *et al.*, 1976; Rietz *et al.*, 1974). Interested readers are directed elsewhere for references to this elegant chemical work. However, it must be kept in mind that these metabolic products do not necessarily occur *in vivo* when physiologic doses of retinoic acid are given, and that their appearance under the conditions used should not be regarded as a physiologic event. With this background of metabolism, the next section will be devoted to the known functions of vitamin A with comments on the possible molecular mechanism of action of the retinoids.

III. THE FUNCTIONS OF VITAMIN A

A. The Visual Cycle

Of all of the functions of vitamin A, the best characterized is its role in the visual cycle. The visual cycle in its simplistic form is illustrated in Fig. 6. All-*trans*-retinal that arises from the oxidation of retinol is converted to the 11-cis isomer by an isomerase. Alternatively, it is considered possible that the 11-cis isomerization takes place on retinyl esters (Wiggert *et al.*, 1977a,b) which then become hydrolyzed and oxidized to enter the visual cycle (for reviews, see DeLuca, 1978; Wald, 1968; Wiggert *et al.*, 1977a,b). 11-*cis*-Retinal will bind to the protein opsin to form the complex rhodopsin, which is considered to be the photoreceptor in the rods and cones. There are several types of opsins that will interact with retinal. The 11-*cis*-retinal apparently binds through a Shiff base mechanism on the ϵ-amino group of lysine available from the opsins. The rhodopsin then receives light of broad wavelength and is converted to metastable metarhodopsin and lumirhodopsin as well as other metastable forms. As these metastable forms impart electric impulses to the nerve endings, the opsin and all-*trans*-retinal dissociate. All-*trans*-retinal

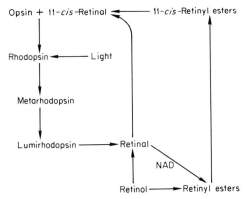

Fig. 6.   Simplistic diagrammatic representation of the visual cycle involving the vitamin A compounds.

can then be reisomerized through the 11-*cis*-isomerase or can be reduced to retinol, esterified, isomerized, and then reoxidized to the 11-*cis*-retinal to reenter the visual cycle (Fig. 6).

B.   Epithelial Differentiation

Wolboch and Howe (1925) were the first to note that in the absence of vitamin A, epithelial tissues become keratinized with the absence of mucus and ciliated cells. They correctly concluded that vitamin A is necessary for epithelial differentiation. This work was followed by a number of organ culture experiments carried out with an excess of vitamin A and later with physiologic amounts of vitamin A. Thus, Mellanby and Fell first provided *in vitro* evidence that the retinoids stimulate the differentiation of basal cells to the mucus-secreting ciliated cells. In fact, excess of vitamin A could convert in culture heavily keratinized epithelium taken from legs of embryonic chicks and cause them to differentiate into mucus-secreting tissues (Fell, 1957; Fell and Mellanby, 1953). The classic work of Lasnitzki using prostate organ culture provided strong evidence that prostate taken from vitamin A-deficient animals were heavily keratinized and could be made to differentiate into mucus-secreting tissues by the addition of retinol (Lasnitzki, 1962). Lasnitzki also carried out important experiments in which such agents as 3-methylcholanthrene that induced carcinogenesis would result in metaplastic appearance of prostate that could then be reversed by the addition of retinoids, thus highlighting the parallel between the metaplastic state of vitamin A-deficient tissues and the metaplastic state induced by chemical carcinogenesis (Lasnitzki, 1978).

Since that early work, other organ cultures, such as the tracheal organ culture system used in the laboratory of Sporn and others, have clearly demonstrated that trachea taken from vitamin A-deficient hamsters are heavily keratinized and can be made to differentiate into mucus-secreting tissues by the addition of a large number of retinoids; the most active of the natural retinoids being retinoic acid (Newton *et al.*, 1980). This epithelial differentiation of the tracheal organ cultures is illustrated in Fig. 7. Thus, *in vivo*, a large number of epithelial tissues require retinoids for differentiation. Skin, goblet cells of the intestinal epithelium, trachea, lungs, kidney, and other epithelial tissues can be shown to require vitamin A for normal differentiation. This must be regarded as a major function of vitamin A for normal differentiation and for the growth supporting activity of retinoids in vitamin A-deficient animals.

The molecular mechanism whereby the retinoids induce differentiation remains largely unknown. From the laboratory of Dingle and Lucy (1965) came the suggestion that the retinoids function in differentiation by modification of membranes, especially lysosomal membranes. However, the quantities of retinoid required to induce epithelial differentiation are so small, and the quantities required to induce membrane modification so large that this mechanism cannot be considered. Furthermore, many of the membrane changes can be induced by compounds possessing no vitamin A activity. One of the more recent suggestions has been that retinol functions as a sugar donor in the production of glycoproteins and glycolipids (Adamo *et al.*, 1979; DeLuca *et al.*, 1979). It has, therefore, been suggested that retinylphosphomannose serves as a donor of the mannose residue in the synthesis of glycolipids and glycoproteins. However, it is well known that dolichol is the accepted intermediary in this transfer reaction and is superior to retinol *in vitro* in this system (DeLuca *et al.*, 1979). Furthermore, this mechanism does not explain the fact that retinoic acid is fully effective in epithelial differentiation yet cannot participate as an acceptor for the mannosyl phosphate. It has been postulated that retinoic acid might be converted by reduction to a compound that could serve as an acceptor for mannosyl phosphate, although evidence for this is not convincing (DeLuca *et al.*, 1979). Therefore, it is not likely that this mechanism, if it occurs at all *in vivo*, plays a significant role in molecular events resulting in epithelial differentiation.

Another mechanism that has been suggested is similar to the steroid hormone mechanism in which retinol or retinoic acid interact with specific receptor molecules that then transfer to the nucleus and result in the expression of characteristic genes (Chytil and Ong, 1978, 1979; DeLuca *et al.*, 1979; Ross and Goodman, 1979; Takase *et al.*, 1979). There is no doubt in this author's mind that retinoids are involved in the ex-

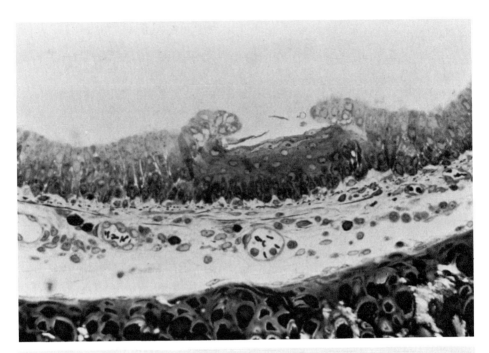

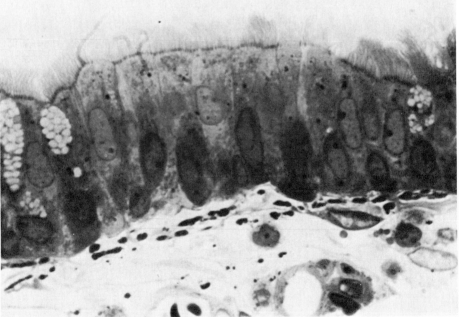

Fig. 7. Differentiation of tracheal tissues in response to retinoic acid. The tracheal tissue was removed from vitamin A-deficient hamsters (top) or from vitamin A-deficient hamsters given retinoic acid (bottom). Courtesy of Dr. Michael B. Sporn of the National Cancer Institute.

pression of a number of genes. The question of how gene expression occurs in response to retinoids, however, has not been solved. Furthermore, the molecular mechanism whereby steroid hormones induce the expression of genes remains largely unknown. There is no doubt that binding proteins have been found both for retinoic acid and retinol (Chytil and Ong, 1978, 1979; Deluca et al., 1979; Ross and Goodman, 1979; Takase et al., 1979). Some of these binding proteins have been found in some of the cell cultures that respond to the retinoids (Saari et al., 1978; Solter et al., 1979). However, there are significant cell cultures that respond to the retinoids but do not have the retinoic acid binding protein (Dover and Koeffler, 1982; Libby and Bertram, 1982). Thus, although it seems very likely that the retinoids are involved in gene expression, they probably interact with the nucleus in such a way that a large number of genes are expressed. The mechanism of this, however, remains largely unknown, and many postulates can be imagined but require experimental investigation.

C. The Function of Vitamin A in Bone

There is abundant evidence dating from the early results that both excess and deficiency of vitamin A results in changes in bone structure. There is no doubt that the pinching of the optic nerve by failure of the optic foramen to remodel is a classic example of the role of vitamin A in the function of the bone forming and regulating cells (Howell et al., 1967b; Mellanby, 1944, 1947; Moore, 1939). Unfortunately, this area has not been investigated except for the work of Mellanby (1947) in which changes of both osteoclastic and osteoblastic activity have been demonstrated in vitamin A deficiency. Although likely, it has not been clearly demonstrated that the role of vitamin A in bone is to induce differentiation of cells either into osteoblasts or into osteoclasts or both. The absence of these cells in bone results in a failure of the remodeling process to occur. Thus, normally as an animal or organism grows, bone is constantly being remodeled and shaped. In the absence of adequate induction of both bone resorption and bone-forming cells, remodeling cannot taken place and can probably account for the symptoms found in bone in vitamin A deficiency.

D. The Role of Vitamin A in Reproduction

1. Spermatogenesis

Failure of the male to reproduce is well known in vitamin D deficiency (Evans, 1928a,b). However, the most significant advance occurred with the synthesis of retinoic acid by Arens and van Dorp (1946), which permitted the use of retinoic acid in supporting some of the functions of vitamin A. Retinoic acid can clearly support growth and epithelial differentiation of whole animals and presumably can support the bone functions of vitamin A (Dowling and Wald, 1958, 1960). However, vitamin A-deficient animals supported with retinoic acid have a failure of the visual system, resulting in permanent degeneration of rods and cones causing permanent blindness (Dowling and Wald, 1958, 1960). Of considerable importance is that retinoic acid-supported animals show marked testicular degeneration and failure of spermatogenesis (Howell et al., 1963). Spermatogenesis fails at the first meiotic division in the conversion of spermatids to spermatozoa (Howell et al., 1963, 1967a; Huang and Hembree, 1979). The process of spermatogenesis is a complex one, and hence it is not possible to deduce that it is a failure of the spermatids themselves. There is evidence that both Sertoli and Leydig cells do not function adequately in vitamin A deficiency (Howell et al., 1967a; Huang and Hembree, 1979). Retinoic acid cannot satisfy the function of vitamin A in spermatogenesis, and retinol is required. A notable exception is in birds where retinoic acid can support normal spermatogenesis (Howell et al., 1969). This interesting area remains to be adequately investigated.

2.   Role of Vitamin A in the Female

In vitamin A deficiency, estrus does not occur, since the normal cycling of the epithelium of the reproductive tract of the female does not take place (Evans, 1928a). However, if the animals are supported by retinoic acid, normal estrus can be established (Thompson et al., 1964). The females under these circumstances produce eggs that can then be fertilized, and implantation occurs (Thompson et al., 1964). However, there is failure of the placenta to develop. Thus, retinoic acid cannot support the development of placental tissue. It is, therefore, apparent that retinol or some metabolite thereof is required for this differentiating system. Again, the molecular mechanism whereby retinoids are involved in placental development remains to be elucidated.

3.   Role of the Retinoids in Embryogenesis

Chick embryos fail to develop when in the vitamin A-deficient state (Thompson et al., 1969). One of the major reasons is failure of the circulatory system to develop in the embryos. Undoubtedly, other epithelial differentiation does not occur resulting in failure of embryogenesis (Thompson et al., 1969).

IV. SUMMARY OF THE ROLE OF VITAMIN A

It is clear that vitamin A satisfies many functions. There is no doubt that the aldehyde form of vitamin A is responsible for the visual cycle. It is also apparent that in its absence, the rods and cones degenerate, and thus a requirement for vitamin A in the maintenance of epithelial tissues of the eye is obvious. This is satisfied only by retinol and retinal. Vitamin A is required for growth of animals and man, and this is probably the direct result of the role of vitamin A in the differentiation of epithelial cells and cells of bone. This function is satisfied by the acid form of vitamin A, and it is likely that the acid form is the functional form, although it has not yet been deduced whether a further metabolite might be responsible for this function. The molecular mechanism of the retinoids in this system remains largely unknown and is particularly exciting in view of the possible relationship to carcinogenesis. Vitamin A is required for reproduction both in males and females and is involved in embryonic development. Retinoic acid can satisfy epithelial changes in the female urogenital track required for reproduction, but it cannot support spermatogenesis and testicular development in the male or placental development in the female. Furthermore, retinoic acid does not appear to be effective in all aspects of embryogenesis. Vitamin A, therefore, is a multifunctional vitamin in which at least two active forms are known, and several different molecular mechanisms can be anticipated for its functions. Of particular interest is the role of vitamin A in the differentiation of epithelial cells and its possible implication in the prevention and treatment of cancer. In any case, the molecular mechanism whereby retinoids support differentiation of epithelial cells, of bone cells, and the mechanism whereby spermatogenesis and placental development responds to retinoic acid will contribute valuable information required for the ultimate solution of the cancer problem.

ACKNOWLEDGMENTS

This work was supported by a Project Program Grant No. AM-14881 of the National Institutes of Health and the Harry Steenbock Research Fund of the Wisconsin Alumni Research Foundation.

REFERENCES

Adamo, S., DeLuca, L. M., Silverman-Jones, C. S., and Yuspa, S. H. (1979). *J. Biol. Chem.* **254**, 3279–3287.

Arens, J. F., and van Dorp, D. A. (1946). *Nature (London)* **158**, 622–623.
Breitman, T. R., Selonick, S. E., and Collins, S. J. (1980). *Proc. Natl. Acad. Sci. U.S.A.* **77**, 2936–2940.
Chytil, F., and Ong, D. E. (1978). *Recept. Horm. Action* **2**, 573–598.
Chytil, F., and Ong, D. E. (1979). *Fed. Prod., Fed. Am. Soc. Exp. Biol.* **38**, 2510–2514.
DeLuca, H. F. (1979). *Fed. Proc., Fed. Am. Soc. Exp. Biol.* **38**, 2519–2523.
DeLuca, H. F., Zile, M., and Sietsema, W. K. (1981). *Ann. N.Y. Acad. Sci.* **359**, 25–36.
DeLuca, L. M. (1978). *In* "Handbook of Lipid Research" (H. F. DeLuca, ed.), Vol. II, pp. 15–22. Plenum, New York.
DeLuca, L. M., Bhat, P. V., Sasak, W., and Adamo, S. (1979).*Fed. Proc., Fed. Am. Soc. Exp. Biol.* **38**, 2535–2539.
Dingle, J. T., and Lucy, J. A. (1965). *Biol. Rev. Cambridge Philos. Soc.* **40**, 422–461.
Dover, D., and Koeffler, K. P. (1982). *J. Clin. Invest.* **69**, 277–283.
Dowling, J. E., and Wald, G. (1958). *Proc. Natl. Acad. Sci. U.S.A.* **44**, 648–661.
Dowling, J. E., and Wald, G. (1960). *Proc. Natl. Acad. Sci. U.S.A.* **46**, 587–608.
Dunagin, P. E., Jr., Meadows, E. H., Jr., and Olson, J. A. (1965). *Science* **148**, 86–87.
Dunagin, P. E., Jr., Zachman, R. D., and Olson, J. A. (1966). *Biochim. Biophys. Acta* **124**, 71–85.
Emerick, R. J., Zile, M., and DeLuca, H. F. (1967). *Biochem. J.* **102**, 606–611.
Evans, H. M. (1928a). *J. Biol. Chem.* **77**, 651–656.
Evans, H. M. (1928b). *Am. J. Physiol.* **99**, 477–482.
Fell, H. B. (1957). *Proc. R. Soc. London* **146**, 242–247.
Fell, H. B., and Mellanby, E. (1953). *J. Physiol. (London)* **119**, 470–488.
Fidge, N. H., and Goodman, D. S. (1968). *J. Biol. Chem.* **243**, 4372–4379.
Fidge, N. H., Smith, F. R., and Goodman, D. S. (1969). *Biochem. J.* **114**, 689–694.
Frolik, C. A., Tavela, T. E., Newton, D. L., and Sporn, M. B. (1978). *J. Biol. Chem.* **253**, 7319–7324.
Frolik, C. A., Roberts, A. B., Tavela, T. E., Roller, P. P., Newton, D. L., and Sporn, M. B. (1979). *Biochemistry* **18**, 2092–2097.
Frolik, C. A., Swanson, B. N., Dart, L. L., and Sporn, M. B. (1981). *Arch. Biochem. Biophys.* **208**, 344–352.
Futterman, S. (1962). *J. Biol. Chem.* **237**, 677–680.
Goodman, D. S. (1969). *Am. J. Clin. Nutr.* **22**, 911–912.
Goodman, D. S. (1972). *Vitam. Horm. (N.Y.)* **32**, 1–42.
Goodman, D. S., Huang, H. S., and Shiratori, T. (1966). *J. Biol. Chem.* **241**, 1929–1932.
Hänni, R., and Bigler, F. (1977). *Helv. Chim. Acta* **60**, 881–887.
Hänni, R., Bigler, F., Meister, W., and Englert, G. (1976). *Helv. Chim. Acta* **59**, 2221–2228.
Howell, J. McC., Thompson, J. N., and Pitt, G. A. J. (1963). *J. Reprod. Fertil.* **5**, 159–167.
Howell, J. McC., Thompson, J. N., and Pitt, G. A. J. (1967a). *Br. J. Nutr.* **21**, 37–42.
Howell, J. McC., Thompson, J. N., and Pitt, G. A. J. (1967b). *Br. J. Exp. Pathol.* **48**, 450–458.
Howell, J. McC., Pitt, G. A. J., and Thompson, J. N. (1969). *Br. J. Exp. Pathol.* **50**, 181–186.
Huang, H. F. S., and Hembree, W. C. (1979). *Biol. Reprod.* **21**, 891–898.
Huang, H. N., and Goodman, D. S. (1965). *J. Biol. Chem.* **240**, 2839–2844.
Ito, Y. L., Zile, M. H., Ahrens, H., and DeLuca, H. F. (1974a). *J. Lipid Res.* **15**, 517–524.
Ito, Y. L., Zile, M., and Ahrens, H. M. (1974b). *Biochim. Biophys. Acta* **369**, 338–350.
Kleiner-Bössaler, A., and DeLuca, H. F. (1971). *Arch. Biochem. Biophys.* **142**, 371–377.
Lakshmanan, M. R., Chansang, H., and Olson, J. A. (1972). *J. Lipid Res.* **13**, 477–482.
Lasnitzki, I. (1962). *Exp. Cell Res.* **28**, 40–51.
Lasnitzki, I. (1978). *Curr. Chemother. Proc. Int. Congr. Chemother., 10th, 1977*, pp. 1292–1294.
Libby, P. R., and Bertram, J. S. (1982). *Carcinogenesis* **3**, 481–484.

McCollum, E. V., and Davis, M. (1913). *J. Biol. Chem.* **15,** 167–175.
McCollum, E. V., Simmonds, N., and Pitz, W. (1916). *J. Biol. Chem.* **27,** 33–43.
McCormick, A. M., Napoli, J. L., Schnoes, H. K., and DeLuca, H. F. (1978). *Biochemistry* **17,** 4085–4090.
McCormick, A. M., Napoli, J. L., Yoshizawa, S., and DeLuca, H. F. (1980) *Biochem. J.* **186,** 475–481.
Mahadevan, S., Murthy, S. K., and Ganguly, J. (1962). *Biochem. J.* **85,** 326–331.
Mellanby, E. (1944). *Proc. R. Soc. London* **132,** 28.
Mellanby, E. (1947). *J. Physiol. (London)* **105,** 382–399.
Moore, L. A. (1939). *J. Nutr.* **9,** 533–539.
Moore, T. (1957). "Vitamin A." Elsevier, Amsterdam.
Napoli, J. L., McCormick, A. M., Schnoes, H. K., and DeLuca, H. F. (1978). *Proc. Natl. Acad. Sci. U.S.A.* **75,** 2603–2605.
Newton, D. L., Henderson, W. R., and Sporn, M. B. (1980). *Cancer Res.* **40,** 3413–3425.
Olson, J. A. (1964). *J. Lipid Res.* **5,** 281–299.
Olson, J. A., and Hayaishi, O. (1965). *Proc. Natl. Acad. Sci. U.S.A.* **54,** 1364–1370.
Osborne, T. B., and Mendel, L. B. (1917). *J. Biol. Chem.* **31,** 149–163.
Rietz, P., Wiss, O., and Weber, F. (1974). *Vitam. Horm. (N.Y.)* **32,** 237–249.
Roberts, A. B., and DeLuca, H. F. (1967). *Biochem. J.* **102,** 600–611.
Roberts, A. B., and Frolik, C. A. (1979). *Fed. Proc., Fed. Am. Soc. Exp. Biol.* **38,** 2524–2527.
Roberts, A. B., Nichols, M. D., Newton, D. L., and Sporn, M. B. (1979a). *J. Biol. Chem.* **254,** 6296–6302.
Roberts, A. B., Frolik, C. A., Nichols, M. D., and Sporn, M. B. (1979b). *J. Biol. Chem.* **254,** 6303–6309.
Roberts, A. B., Lamb, L. C., and Sporn, M. B. (1980). *Arch. Biochem. Biophys.* **199,** 374–383.
Ross, A. C., and Goodman, D. S. (1979). *Fed. Proc., Fed. Am. Soc. Exp. Biol.* **38,** 2515–2518.
Saari, J. C., Futterman, S., Stubbs, G. W., Hefferman, J. T., Bredberg, L., Chan, K. Y., and Albert, D. M. (1978). *Invest. Ophthalmol. Visual Sci.* **17,** 988–1002.
Sietsema, W. K., and DeLuca, H. F. (1979). *Biochem. Biophys. Res. Commun.* **90,** 1091–1097.
Sietsema, W. K., and DeLuca, H. F. (1982a). *J. Nutr.* **112,** 1481–1489.
Sietsema, W. K., and DeLuca, H. F. (1982b). *J. Biol. Chem.* **257,** 4265–4270.
Silva, D. P., and DeLuca, H. F. (1982). *Biochem. J.* **206,** 33–41.
Skare, K. L., Schnoes, H. K., and DeLuca, H. F. (1982a). *Biochemistry* **21,** 3308–3317.
Skare, K. L., Sietsema, W. K., and DeLuca, H. F. (1982b). *J. Nutr.* **112,** 1626–1630.
Smith, F. R., Goodman, D. S., Zaklama, M. S., Gabr, M. K., El Maraghy, S., and Patwardhan, V. N. (1973). *Am. J. Clin. Nutr.* **26,** 973–981.
Smith, J. E., and Goodman D. S. (1979). *Fed. Proc., Fed. Am. Soc. Exp. Biol.* **38,** 2504–2509.
Smith, J. E., Muto, Y., Milch, P. O., and Goodman, D. S. (1973). *J. Biol. Chem.* **248,** 1544–1549.
Solter, D., Shevinsky, L., Knowles, B. B., and Strickland, S. (1979). *Dev. Biol.* **70,** 515–521.
Stephens-Jarnagin, A., Sietsema, W. K., Miller, D. A., and DeLuca, H. F. (1983). *Arch. Biochem. Biophys.* **220,** 502–508.
Strickland, S., and Mahdovi, V. (1978). *Cell* **15,** 393–403.
Takase, S., Ong, D. E., and Chytil, F. (1979). *Proc. Natl. Acad. Sci. U.S.A.* **76,** 2204–2208.
Thompson, J. N., Howell, J. McC., and Pitt, G. A. J. (1964). *Proc. R. Soc. London, Ser. B* **159,** 510–535.
Thompson, J. N., Howell, J. McC., Pitt, G. A. J., and McLaughlin, C. I. (1969). *Br. J. Nutr.* **23,** 471–490.
Wald, G. (1968). *Science* **162,** 230–239.
Wald, G., and Hubbard, R. (1950). *Proc. Natl. Acad. Sci. U.S.A.* **36,** 92–102.

Wald, G., and Hubbard, R. (1960). *In* "The Enzymes" (P. D. Boyer, H. Lardy, and K. Myrbäck, eds.), 2nd rev. ed., Vol. 3, pp. 369–386. Academic Press, New York.

Wiggert, B., Bergsma, D. R., Helmsen, R. J., Alligood, J., Lewis, M., and Chader, G. J. (1977a). *Biochim. Biophys. Acta* **491,** 104–113.

Wiggert, B., Bergsma, D. R., Lewis, M., Abe, T., and Chader, G. J. (1977b) *Biochim. Biphys. Acta* **498,** 366–374.

Wolbach, S. B., and Howe, P. R. (1925). *J. Exp. Med.* **42,** 753–777.

Zachman, R. D., Dunagin, P. E., Jr., and Olson, J. S. (1966). *J. Lipid Res.* **7,** 3–9.

Zile, M. H., and DeLuca, H. F. (1968). *J. Nutr.* **94,** 302–308.

Zile, M. H., Emerick, R. J., and DeLuca, H. F. (1967). *Biochim. Biophys. Acta* **141,** 639–641.

Zile, M. H., Inhorn, R. C., and DeLuca, H. F. (1980a). *J. Nutr.* **110,** 2225–2230.

Zile, M. H., Schnoes, H. K., and DeLuca, H. F. (1980b). *Proc. Natl. Acad. Sci. U.S.A.* **77,** 3230–3233.

Zile, M. H., Inhorn, R. C., and DeLuca, H. F. (1982a). *J. Biol. Chem.* **257,** 3537–3543.

Zile, M. H., Inhorn, R. C., and DeLuca, H. F. (1982b). *J. Biol. Chem.* **257,** 3544–3550.

11

Effects of Supplemental Dietary Vitamin A and β-Carotene on Experimental Tumors, Local Tumor Excision, Chemotherapy, Radiation Injury, and Radiotherapy

Stanley M. Levenson, Giuseppe Rettura,* and Eli Seifter†*

Department of Surgery*
Departments of Biochemistry and Surgery†
Albert Einstein College of Medicine and
Montefiore Hospital and Medical Center
Bronx, New York

169

Nutrition Factors in the Induction
and Maintenance of Malignancy

I. INTRODUCTION

Several years ago, we began a series of experiments dealing with the effects of supplemental vitamin A and β-carotene on neoplasia, chemotherapy, tumor surgery, radiation injury, and radiation therapy. These studies arose in part from our studies of the effects of supplemental vitamin A on wound healing, stress, and certain immunologic responses, some of which were reported briefly at the first Bristol-Myers Symposium (Levenson and Seifter, 1983; Levenson *et al.*, 1982).

We hypothesized that vitamin A and β-carotene would have beneficial effects on neoplasia because of the following experimental observations from our laboratories:

1. They are "thymotropic," that is, they lead to an increase in thymic weight and in the number of thymic small lymphocytes in normal rats and mice (Table I).

2. They increase the number of lymphocytes in the peripheral blood of thymectomized rats.

3. They mitigate various aspects of the stress response (adrenal enlargement, thymic involution, gastrointestinal ulceration) to a variety of physical and chemical stressors and toxins.

4. They accelerate skin allograft rejection.

5. Vitamin A accelerates wound healing in normal rats and rats with femoral fracture.

6. Vitamin A increases the influx of macrophages into the injured site.

Further evidence in support of the hypothesis may be seen in the observations of Cohen and associates:

1. There is an increase in the number of splenic antibody producing cells in vitamin A supplemented mice inoculated with sheep red blood cells (Cohen and Cohen, 1973).

2. Supplemental vitamin A increases resistance of mice to certain bacterial infections (Cohen and Elin, 1974).

3. It has been shown in humans that elective operation under general anesthesia induces relative lymphopenia and diminished lymphocyte responsiveness to mitogens *in vitro* (Cohen *et al.*, 1979); these were prevented when dietary supplements of vitamin A were fed to patients, and are thus closely related to the findings in rodents.

It was our hypothesis then that supplemental vitamin A and β-carotene would increase the defense mechanisms of the host, thereby enabling the host to combat neoplasms more effectively. Also, it had been shown in preliminary studies in the mid-1960s that supplemental vitamin A had some mitigating effects in mice with experimental C3HBA and BW10232 breast tumors (Seifter and Norris, 1965).

In addition, we had shown that supplemental vitamin A obviates the impaired wound healing and thymic involution of streptozotocin diabetic rats, without affecting the hyperglycemia, polydipsia, glycosuria, and polyuria (Seifter et al., 1981b). Since streptozotocin is an alkylating agent, we thought it likely that supplemental vitamin A and β-carotene would ameliorate the toxicity of other therapeutic alkylating agents without impairing their antineoplastic effects.

Further, because there are many similarities in the actions and responses of animals and patients to alkylating agents and radiation injury, we thought it likely that supplemental vitamin A and β-carotene would ameliorate many of the adverse effects of radiation without interfering with its antitumor action.

The effects of supplemental β-carotene were studied as well as those of supplemental vitamin A based on the view that β-carotene would have effects similar to those of vitamin A, but would have the added virtue of less potential toxicity; our initial studies with β-carotene were the first experiments of their types.

II. EXPERIMENTAL FINDINGS

This chapter will describe our findings of the effects of supplemental vitamin A and β-carotene in five areas: (1) experimental neoplasms, (2) chemotherapy, (3) limited local excision of tumors, (4) radiation injury, and (5) radiotherapy. No attempt is made in this chapter to present a comprehensive review of these matters; rather a summary of our studies will be presented, along with a discussion of some possible mechanisms underlying our findings.

In a typical experiment, commercial rat feed [Purina Chow (Ralston Purina Co., St. Louis, Missouri) or Teklad (Taklad, Inc., Monmouth, Illinois)], containing 15,000 units of vitamin A palmitate and 6.5 mg β-carotene per kilogram of diet or 6190 I.U. of vitamin A and 4.3 mg β-carotene/kg diet, respectively, (about 2–3 times the National Research Council recommended daily allowance for vitamin A for healthy rodents) was fed as the control or basal ration after grinding to a coarse powder in our laboratory. Supplemented diets were made as follows: Vitamin A-supplemented diet was made by dissolving 90 mg of vitamin A palmitate (1000 I.U./mg, ICN Pharmaceuticals, Cleveland, Ohio) in 30 ml of absolute ethanol. While the powdered feed was being mixed, the 30 ml of vitamin A solution was treated with 200 ml of tap water, causing

TABLE I

Effects of Supplemental Vitamin A and C3HBA Tumor on Thymus and Adrenal Glands, Thymocytes, and Peripheral White Blood Cell Counts in Mice

Group	Inoculum C3HBA cells	Vitamin A	Sacrifice day post-inoculum	Thymus (mg)	Adrenals (mg)	Thymocytes (10^6)	Peripheral white blood cell count		
							Total ($10^3/mm^3$)	Lymphocytes (%)	Neutrophils (%)
II	—	—	5	28.5±1.4	4.3±0.4	19.5±0.8	10.3±0.3	76.6±0.9	19.2±0.9
III	—	—	5	38.4±2.2	4.3±0.3	31.1±2.1	11.9±0.4	77.0±1.4	19.0±1.1
IV	—	—	5	23.9±2.3	5.7±0.4	9.1±0.7	19.4±0.9	61.6±1.1	35.6±1.2
V	—	—	5	30.9±1.2	4.9±0.9	16.0±0.9	16.3±0.3	71.2±1.5	24.6±1.3
VI	—	—	10	28.4±1.1	4.3±0.3	17.4±1.0	10.8±0.5	73.6±1.2	22.2±1.2
VII	—	—	10	35.6±1.0	4.1±0.2	27.2±1.3	11.4±0.3	73.8±1.3	22.0±1.2
VIII	—	—	10	20.1±0.3	5.8±0.2	7.3±0.5	28.7±1.6	40.4±1.5	56.8±1.9
IX	—	—	10	28.9±0.4	4.8±0.2	22.0±0.1	22.2±0.9	59.0±1.3	36.0±1.4
X	—	—	13	25.3±1.6[a]	19.7±1.6	4.3±0.2	13.2±0.5	72.6±1.1	24.2±1.0
XI	—	—	13	35.0±0.9	36.2±1.4	4.3±0.3	12.6±0.4	73.8±1.0	22.9±1.1
XII	—	—	13	18.1±1.2	7.8±1.1	5.8±0.4	37.9±2.6	28.8±0.9	66.0±2.5
XIII	—	—	13	34.0±2.0	27.2±2.1	5.0±0.2	22.1±1.7	49.8±1.2	46.4±1.4
XVII	—	—	17	25.5±1.6[a]	14.9±1.7	4.4±0.2	11.9±1.3	71.4±0.9	25.4±0.7
XVIII	—	—	17	33.9±2.2	27.6±1.4	4.3±0.3	11.8±1.0	72.8±1.3	23.7±0.9

XIX	17	—	16.9±1.0	5.5±0.4	7.2±0.4	48.0±1.9	21.4±1.0	75.4±0.8
XX	17	—	25.1±1.1	16.3±0.9	6.5±0.4	27.9±1.0	47.8±1.8	48.0±0.8
XXIV	20	—	27.4±1.0[a]	19.6±1.2	4.4±0.2	10.7±1.0	68.2±1.8	28.4±0.9
XXV	20	—	34.3±1.2	32.3±1.0	4.3±0.3	10.9±1.1	71.8±1.5	25.9±1.1
XXVI	20	—	11.4±0.3	2.9±0.2	7.0±0.4	74.7±2.3	25.0±1.1	72.4±1.0
XXVII	20	—	23.4±1.0	12.0±0.9	5.5±0.3	40.5±1.9	39.0±1.1	58.0±1.7
p value[b]								
II versus III			<0.01	NS	<0.001	NS	NS	NS
IV versus V			<0.02	NS	<0.001	<0.01	<0.001	<0.001
VI versus VII			<0.001	NS	<0.001	NS	NS	NS
VIII versus IX			<0.001	<0.01	<0.001	<0.01	<0.001	<0.001
X versus XI			<0.001	<0.001	NS	NS	NS	NS
XII versus XIII			<0.001	<0.001	<0.1	<0.001	<0.001	<0.001
XVII versus XVIII			<0.02	<0.001	NS	NS	NS	NS
XIX versus XX			<0.001	<0.001	NS	<0.001	<0.001	<0.001
XXIV versus XXV			<0.001	<0.001	NS	NS	NS	NS
XXVI versus XXVII			<0.001	<0.001	<0.005	<0.001	<0.001	<0.001

[a] Mean ± standard error of the mean.
[b] Analyzed by the Student's t test for small unpaired samples; NS, not significant.

a fine insoluble film precipitate of vitamin A. The suspension was added to 6 kg of powdered chow in small portions with constant mixing. Finally, 15 ml of absolute alcohol were used to wash the residue of vitamin A into the mixture. The diets were mixed for 2 or more hours. To prepare β-carotene-supplemented diets, 540 mg of β-carotene (Eastman Kodak, Rochester, New York) were used in place of vitamin A. Control diets were made from the ground feed similarly treated with alcohol and water.

It should be emphasized that the control basal feeds are not deficient in vitamin A or β-carotene. They support normal growth, reproduction, lactation, and longevity of normal mice and rats. All rats and mice ate and drank (tap water) *ad libitum*.

For the experiments with C3HBA tumors, the C3HBA adenocarcinoma was obtained from The Jackson Laboratory as a transplant in young C3H/HeJ female mice. The inocula were prepared from solid tumors 1.2 cm in diameter. The tumor tissue was gently minced in a cold phosphate-buffered saline solution containing penicillin and streptomycin and filtered through a wire screen. The residue was discarded, and the filtrate was centrifuged for 10 minutes at $1800 \times g$. The supernatant was discarded and the precipitate was suspended in cold buffer. To count the viable cells, an aliquot of the suspension was stained with 0.4% trypan blue. The concentration of cells was adjusted with buffer so that a 0.1 ml suspension contained 1×10^6 viable cells. Mice received tumor cells subcutaneously in an area of the nipple line, approximately 1.3 cm above the right inguinal lymph node.

Inocula for these experiments were prepared by passing the C3HBA tumor through CBA hosts, harvesting the tumors, and then preparing the inocula as described above. Although C3HBA cells are immunogenic in C3H, CBA, and C57 mice, significant immunity develops only in C57 mice, which reject C3HBA tumors.

In all cases inoculum sites were gently palpated daily to determine the date of tumor appearance. After a tumor appeared, its size was estimated daily with the use of a caliper with millimeter divisions. Tumor size was recorded as the average of the major and minor diameters of the generally ovate tumor. Latency was recorded as the number of days required for the development of a palpable tumor.

For the experiments with the Moloney sarcoma virus tumors, the virus (MuSV-M) used in these experiments was originally obtained from Dr. J. B. Moloney, National Cancer Institute, and was designated as lot No. 206. For use as an inoculum, the virus was passed through CBA/J mice from which the tumors were harvested and treated for extraction of the virus. The virus was reconstituted with a phosphate–saline buffer so that virus recovered from 1 gm of tumor was present in 1 ml of suspension, yielding 1 gm-eq/ml. In the reported experiments, the virus was used in tenfold (10^{-1} gm-eq/ml) or hundredfold (10^{-2} gm-eq/ml) dilutions. Inoculations consisted of intramuscular (im) injection of 0.1 ml of virus suspension in the inner aspect of the left thigh. Tumors were graded on a scale of 1 to 4, as described by Blumenschein and Moloney (1969).

A.   Transplanted Tumors

Neoplasms induce various responses that are unfavorable for survival; these are mitigated both by supplemental vitamin A and supplemental β-carotene. For examples, (a) neoplasms are immunosuppressive. C3H mice with C3HBA tumors did not readily reject C57 skin allografts; supplemental vitamin A increased their ability to reject the allografts. (b) There is a decrease in thymic lymphocytes, thymic weight, peripheral blood lymphocytes and an increase in adrenal weights in rodents subjected to experimental neoplasms; supplemental vitamin A and supplemental β-carotene each largely prevented these changes (Table I). (c) Neoplasms cause loss of nontumor body weight; this was reduced by supplemental vitamin A.

Supplemental vitamin A altered the "critical tumor mass" required for tumor development in mice inoculated with C3HBA cells. The TD_{50} (and, therefore, its LD_{50}) in normal C3H mice was an inoculum of 1×10^4 C3HBA cells. When the vitamin A-supplemented diet was begun 3 days prior to or just after C3HBA inoculation, 1×10^4 cells was the TD_{10} and the TD_{50} was 1×10^5 cells. In mice subjected to a variety of stressors, the TD_{100} was 1×10^4 cells; supplemental vitamin A altered this so that 1×10^4 cells was the TD_{50}. Comparable findings were observed in other tumor systems, e.g., the MuSV-M.

Supplemental vitamin A given to young C3H/HeJ female, C3H/He female or CBA male mice inoculated with C3HBA tumor cells reduced tumor incidence, prolonged the latency period, slowed tumor growth, and prolonged survival of those mice that developed tumors. In these experiments, the supplemental vitamin A was begun 3–4 days prior to tumor inoculation and continued thereafter. Supplemental β-carotene had similar effects. Also, importantly, supplemental vitamin A and supplemental β-carotene each begun immediately after tumor inoculation or later after tumors developed slowed tumor growth and increased survival time (Figs. 1 and 2).

This work is believed to be the first demonstration of the antitumor action of β-carotene in animals with a transplanted tumor.

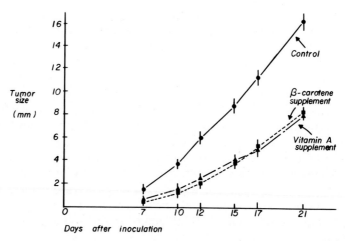

Fig. 1.   Female C3H/HeJ mice were inoculated with 2×10^5 syngeneic C3HBA cells. Feeding of supplemented diets was started several hours after inoculation. (From Rettura *et al.*, 1982.)

We found that C3H/HeHa mice were less resistant to tumor development and growth than C3H/HeJ mice as judged by tumor incidence, latent period, tumor size (growth rate), and survival time. Resistance to disease and death following inoculation with tumor cells was related to thymus status in the following way: thymic involution was associated

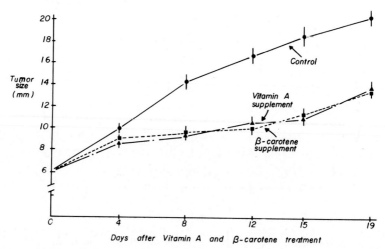

Fig. 2.   Male CBA/J mice were inoculated with 2×10^5 C3HBA tumor cells. Treatments were begun when tumor diameters were 6.2 ± 0.3 mm (mean $\pm$ SEM, range = 5.5–7.0 mm). (From Rettura *et al.*, 1982.)

with decreased resistance of the mice to tumor development. When C3H/HeHa mice were fed supplemental vitamin A, a treatment that increases their thymus size and number of thymic small lymphocytes, their resistance to the C3HBA tumor was markedly increased (Fig. 3) (Seifter *et al.*, 1981a).

Marked neutrophilia occurred in C3H/HeJ mice inoculated with C3HBA mammary adenocarcinoma (Fig. 4). The rise in neutrophil count correlated with increasing tumor size, strongly indicating a causal relationship. This was further supported by the fall in neutrophil count after tumor excision and the persistent low levels after administration of supplemental vitamin A which inhibited tumor regrowth (Fig. 5). The mechanism of the neutrophilia is strongly suggested by the demonstration by Lan *et al.* (1981) of marked granulopoietic stimulating activity *in vitro* by media conditioned with tumor cells and by serum of tumor-bearing mice.

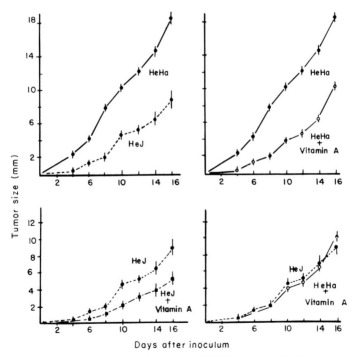

Fig. 3.   Mice were inoculated with 1×10^6 C3HBA tumor cells. Tumors grew more rapidly in C3H/HeHa mice (upper left). Supplemental vitamin A slowed growth in both C3H/HeHa and C3H/HeJ mice (upper right and lower left). Supplemental vitamin A increased resistance of C3H/HeHa mice to equality with that of unsupplemented C3H/HeJ mice (lower right). (From Seifter *et al.*, 1981a.)

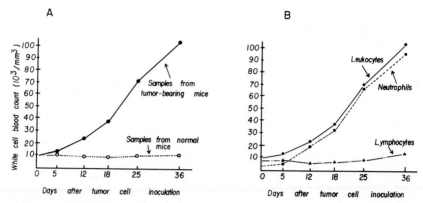

Fig. 4. (A) White blood cell counts after inoculation with 10⁵ cells on day 0 (●——●), control (○- - -○). (B) White blood cell counts after inoculation with 10⁵ cells on day 0 (●——●), neutrophil count after inoculation (■- - -■), lymphocyte count after inoculation (▲- - -▲). Each point represents the mean of 10 mice. (From Lan *et al.*, 1981.)

Supplemental vitamin A also slowed the growth of BW10232 breast tumors. Seven-week-old C57B1 mice were inoculated subcutaneously with one of three doses of BW10232 tumor cells (10⁴, 10⁵, 10⁶) 3 days after half the mice had been started randomly on the vitamin A-supplemented chow while the other half were continued on the control chow. The supplemental vitamin A reduced tumor incidence when the inocu-

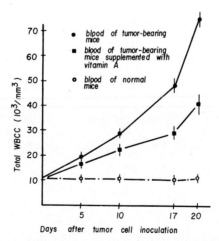

Fig. 5. Effect of supplemental vitamin A on peripheral WBC count in mice inoculated with C3HBA tumor cells. Vertical markings indicate standard errors of the mean.

lum was 10^4 ($p<0.001$), and prolonged the latency period ($p<0.01$) and increased survival time ($p<0.05$) when the inoculum was 10^5.

Citral, a vitamin A antagonist, decreased thymic weight and number of small lymphocytes, increased adrenal weight, and decreased the resistance of C57/B1 mice to BW10232 tumor; supplemental vitamin A partially overcame these effects of citral (Seifter *et al.*, 1979).

B. Virus-Induced Tumor (Moloney Sarcoma)

Supplemental vitamin A and β-carotene each increased the resistance of mice to Moloney sarcoma tumor virus (MuSV-M), an RNA virus (Seifter *et al.*, 1982a). Our experiments showed a decreased tumor frequency, increased latent period, slowed rate of tumor growth, and an increased rate of tumor regression in young male inbred CBA/J mice fed supplemental vitamin A or β-carotene continuously beginning 2–3 days before they were inoculated with the Moloney sarcoma virus (Table II). Mean tumor size was reduced by β-carotene supplementation, which had an effect similar to that of reducing the inoculum size by 1 log unit. When these supplements were begun after tumors were already present (mean tumor score, grade 2), the rate of tumor regression was increased markedly and mortality decreased (Fig . 6).

This is believed to be the first demonstration of the antitumor action of β-carotene in mice inoculated with an oncogenic virus.

TABLE II

Supplemental β-Carotene and Latent Period of MuSV-M Tumors in CBA/J Mice[a]

MuSV-M inoculum (gm-eq/ml)	Diet	Experiment 1			Experiment 2		
		Latent period[b] (days)	No. of mice with tumor/ No. inoculated	p^c	Latent period[b] (days)	No. of mice with tumor/ No. inoculated	p^c
10^{-1}	Control	5.8±0.3	10/10	<0.005	6.1±0.2	10/10	<0.01
	β-Carotene supplemented	8.3±0.6	8/10		7.1±0.2	5/10	
10^{-2}	Control	7.1±0.4	9/10	<0.008	7.9±0.3	8/10	<0.05
	β-Carotene supplemented	10.5±0.8	4/10		9.8±1.0	4/10	

[a] From Seifter *et al.* (1982a).
[b] Mean ± SEM.
[c] Analyzed by Student's *t* test for small samples.

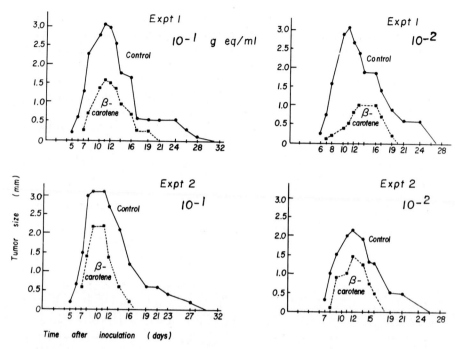

Fig. 6. All mice received 0.1 ml of MuSV-M inoculum. Control mice were fed a chow containing 6190 IU vitamin A palmitate/kg and 4.3 mg β-carotene/kg, while the others were fed the same chow supplemented with 90 mg β-carotene/kg in Expt. 1 and 120 mg β-carotene/kg in Expt. 2. (From Seifter *et al.*, 1982a.)

The vitamin A and β-carotene supplements each minimized the virus-induced thymus gland involution that accompanied tumor growth. For example, after 3 days of β-carotene supplementation, the size of the thymus glands increased and the numbers of small lymphocytes in the gland increased by more than 50%. Inoculation with MuSV-M caused a rapid and progressive loss in thymus mass due to the decrease in the numbers of small thymic lymphocytes. Supplemental β-carotene largely prevented this (Table III).

Supplemental vitamin A protected rodents inoculated with pox virus (DNA), an indication of its broad spectrum immunostimulatory actions (Seifter *et al.*, 1976).

C. Tumors Induced by a Chemical Carcinogen

Supplemental vitamin A and supplemental β-carotene each significantly decreased tumor incidence, adrenal and ovarian enlargement, thymic involution, and death following a single dose of 20 mg 7,12-dimethylbenz[a]anthracene (DMBA) given to young female Sprague-Dawley rats by gastric intubation without prior food deprivation. This occurred when the supplements were begun either 2 days before or as long as 2 weeks after DMBA administration. When supplements of β-carotene were begun 3, 5, 7, or 9 weeks after DMBA administration, an ameliorating effect was seen for the 3 and 5 week groups, but little or no effect was seen for the 7 or 9 week groups (Tables IV and V) (Seifter et al., 1982b).

TABLE III

Supplemental β-Carotene and Thymus Gland Effects on MuSV-M Inoculated CBA/J Mice[a]

| | Days on diet/days postinoculation | | | | | |
| | 3/0 | | 6/3 | | 10/7 | |
Treatment groups	Thymus weight[b] (mg)	TTL[c] (10^{-6})	Thymus weight[b] (mg)	TTL[c] (10^{-6})	Thymus weight[b] (mg)	TTL[c] (10^{-6})
A. Control diet	46.8±1.0	33.3±0.9	45.5±1.0	35.0±1.1	45.8±1.3	31.3±1.2
B. Control diet and MuSV-M inoculated	47.5±1.1	32.4±1.0	31.5±1.4	15.0±1.2	25.0±1.3	11.5±1.2
C. β-Carotene-supplemented diet	56.0±1.6	55.8±2.0	53.9±1.9	54.1±0.9	54.7±2.1	52.6±1.5
D. β-Carotene-supplemented diet and MuSV-M inoculated	55.2±0.8	54.9±2.4	40.3±1.0	24.9±1.2	40.2±2.2	38.3±1.5
p values[d]						
A versus B	NS	NS	<0.005	<0.001	<0.001	<0.001
A versus C	<0.001	<0.001	<0.002	<0.001	<0.005	<0.001
A versus D	<0.001	<0.001	<0.05	<0.01	NS	<0.01
B versus D	<0.001	<0.001	<0.005	<0.001	<0.001	<0.001
C versus D	NS	NS	<0.005	<0.001	<0.001	<0.001

[a] From Seifter et al. (1982a).
[b] Values are means ± SEM.
[c] TTL, total thymic lymphocytes. Values are means ± SE.
[d] Determined by the variance analysis and the Newman-Keuls test; NS, not significant.

TABLE IV

Effect of Supplemental Vitamin A and β-Carotene on the Thymus and Adrenal of Mice Given DMBA

	1 Week after DMBA		4 Weeks after DMBA	
Dietary supplement	Thymus (mg)	Adrenal (mg)	Thymus (mg)	Adrenal (mg)
None (1)	270±17	116 ±1.8	269±25	69.4±1.2
Vitamin A (2)	494±23[a]	83.4±1.0[a]	361±32	48.8±0.8[a]
β-Carotene (3)	440±22[a]	83.8±1.1[a]	405±24[a]	49.6±0.8[a]
Control (no DMBA, no supplement) (4)	508±30[a]	68.2±1.3[a]	451±19[a]	64.8±3.1[a]

[a] p value <0.001 compared with group (1).

D. Interaction of Vitamin A and β-Carotene with Therapy

1. Chemotherapy

Alkylating chemotherapeutic agents have a number of adverse effects. For example, cyclophosphamide (24 mg/kg weight) given by gastric intubation to Sprague-Dawley male rats (about 450 gm in weight) on the day of operation and for the next 4 days and again on the eighth postoperative day, led to thymic involution, lymphopenia, increased adrenal weight, bleeding, weight loss, and impaired wound healing; the rats were killed on the fourteenth postoperative day. We found that supplemental vitamin A begun immediately after operation alleviated these adverse effects of cyclophosphamide without interfering with its antitumor action (Tables VI and VII and Figs. 7 and 8) (Stratford *et al.*, 1980). In fact, supplemental vitamin A, itself effective as an antitumor agent, added significantly to the antitumor effect of cyclophosphamide in C57B1 mice with the breast tumor BW10232 and in C3H mice with C3HBA breast adenocarcinoma (Fig. 9). Thus, supplemental vitamin A and β-carotene given to CBA mice when their C3HBA tumors were 6.2 mm mean tumor size, each slowed tumor growth and increased survival time to the same extent as cyclophosphamide alone (begun at the same time) (Table VIII). The antitumor action of the supplemental vitamin A and β-carotene were additive to that of cyclophosphamide. In another experiment, cyclophosphamide, by itself, caused slight tumor regression, but 30% of the mice died of drug toxicity; in contrast, cyclophos-

TABLE V

Effect of Supplemental Vitamin A and β-Carotene on DMBA Carcinogenesis[a]

	Experiment 1			Experiment 2				
	No supple-ment	Vitamin A[b]	β-Carotene[b]	No supple-ment	Vitamin A[c]	β-Carotene[c]	Vitamin A[d]	β-Carotene[d]
Rats with tumors	18	7	3	15	3	4	3	4
Tumor deaths	10	0	0	4	0	0	0	0
Non-tumor deaths	2	0	0	1	0	0	0	0
Total tu-mors/ group	59	15	5	40	3	4	4	5

[a] Tumor incidence and mortality using 20 rats/group.
[b] Supplements started 2 days before DMBA administered.
[c] Supplements started 1 week after DMBA administered.
[d] Supplements started 2 weeks after DMBA administered.

TABLE VI

Effect of Supplemental Vitamin A on Thymus and Adrenal Glands in Rats and Mice Injected with Cyclophosphamide[a]

		Rats		Mice	
Group	Treatment	Thymus (mg)	Adrenals (mg)	Thymus (mg)	Adrenals (mg)
a	None	345±18	65.3±1.2	59±3	5.6±0.3
b	CY[b]	64±4	81.4±3.2	20±2	10.2±0.2
c	CY + vitamin A	232±9	67.0±0.8	38±3	6.7±0.2
p value[c]					
a versus b		<0.001	<0.001	<0.001	<0.01
a versus c		<0.001	NS	<0.001	NS
b versus c		<0.001	<0.001	<0.001	<0.01

[a] Cyclophosphamide (24 mg/kg body weight) was given by gavage for 6 days (rats), for 10 days (mice). Rats were killed 14 days later than the first gavage; mice 35 days later.
[b] CY, cyclophosphamide.
[c] NS, not significant.

TABLE VII

Effect of Supplemental Vitamin A on Breaking Strength of Cyclophosphamide (CY) Treated Rats

Group	Breaking strength (gm)		Hydroxyproline (mg/100 mg dry sponge)
	Fresh	Fixed	
1 Normal	491±39	2167±114	1.55±0.07
2 CY	302±41	1115±65	0.09±0.04
3 CY + vitamin A	495±49	1899±112	1.39±0.05
p value[a]			
1 versus 2	0.01	0.001	0.001
2 versus 3	0.01	0.001	0.001
1 versus 3	NS	NS	NS

[a] NS, not significant.

phamide plus the vitamin A or β-carotene supplementation caused marked tumor regression without any deaths.

Furthermore, supplemental vitamin A diminished the lethality of cyclophosphamide for rats subjected to wounding. For example, in Fischer male rats, neither wounding (simple skin incision) nor cyclophosphamide was separately lethal; the combination, however, killed more than 75% of the rats. Vitamin A supplementation prevented this completely.

2. Limited Local Excision of Tumors

Supplemental vitamin A lessens some of the metabolic sequelae of anesthesia and surgery, i.e., weight loss, adrenal enlargement, thymic involution, and lymphopenia. Importantly, supplemental vitamin A, begun at the time of tumor inoculation (C3HBA tumor; young female C3H/HeJ mice) and continued after limited local excision of the tumor or begun later at the time of the tumor excision, increased the time for tumor reappearance, slowed the rate of tumor growth of the tumors that reappeared, and increased survival time. The operation consisted of removing all macroscopically visible tumor nodule(s) without attempting to excise healthy surrounding tissue under pentobarbital anesthesia. If the tumor was fixed to the abdominal muscles, the tumor excision included a limited *en bloc* resection of the immediately underlying muscle wall. The operation, then, was in no sense intended as a "curative" procedure, but survival time was increased by operation, and this was increased still further by supplemental vitamin A. For example, in one

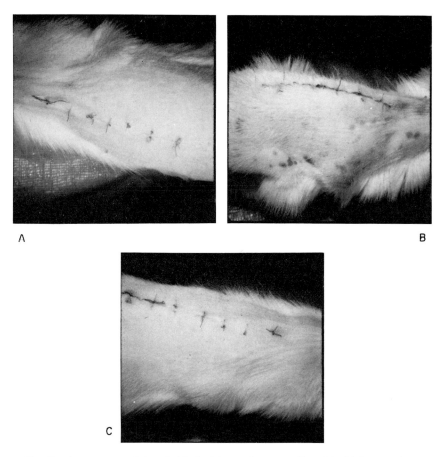

A   B

C

Fig. 7.   Appearance of dorsal skin incision and surrounding skin 14 days postopera-tively. (A) Normal control rat. (B) Cyclophosphamide-treated rat. (C) Cyclophosphamide-treated rat given supplemental vitamin A starting right after operation.

experiment, eight groups of ten mice each were inoculated with 7.5 × 10^5 C3HBA cells. Two groups served as unoperated controls; one of these was started on supplemental vitamin A feeding immediately after inoculation. Of the remaining six groups, on days 9, 13, and 16 after inoculation, two groups of mice each underwent limited local tumor excision. At these times, tumor scores were 4.6, 7.2, and 9.4 mm, respec-tively, and the average weights of the excised tumors were 7.7, 64.3, and 187 mg, respectively. After excision, one of each pair of groups was started on the vitamin A supplement, while the other continued eating the control chow.

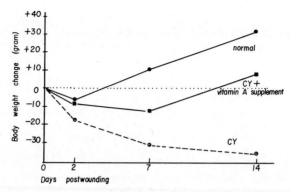

Fig. 8. Effect of supplemental vitamin A on body weight in wounded Sprague-Dawley rats treated with cyclophosphamide (CY).

Among unoperated mice, those given supplemental vitamin A starting the day of inoculation survived significantly longer than unsupplemented animals (76.1 ± 13.3 days versus 32.2 ± 1.7 days, $p<0.005$). Among mice not given supplemental vitamin A, those that had local tumor excision survived significantly longer than unoperated mice (43.9 ± 3.8 days for mice operated on day 9 after inoculation, $p<0.01$; 45.6 ± 4.6 days for mice operated on day 13, $p<0.01$; and 48.7 ± 3.9 days for mice operated on day 16, $p<0.001$). The combination of operation plus supplemental vitamin A starting immediately after excision prolonged survival significantly over operation alone (63.2 ± 5.6 days versus 43.9 ± 3.8 days for mice operated on day 9 after inoculation, $p<0.01$; 58.2 ± 2.2 days versus 45.6 ± 4.6 days for mice operated on day

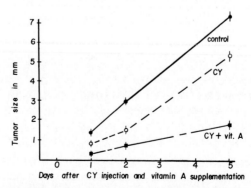

Fig. 9. Effect of supplemental vitamin A on BW10232 tumor growth in C57B1 mice treated with cyclophosphamide.

TABLE VIII

Antitumor Effects of Supplemental Vitamin A, β-Carotene, and Cyclophosphamide

| | Survival time (days) | | | | | |
| | Expt. 1 | | Expt. 2 | | Expt. 3 | |
Dietary supplement	No CY	With CY[a]	No CY	With CY[a]	No CY	With CY[b]
None	41 ± 2[c]	62 ± 2	46 ± 2	56 ± 3	40 ± 1	65 ± 3
Vitamin A	57 ± 3	78 ± 6	59 ± 3	72 ± 5	64 ± 2	85 ± 5
β-Carotene	58 ± 4	77 ± 4	—	—	63 ± 2	83 ± 2

[a] Cyclophosphamide (CY), 24 mg/kg body weight.
[b] Cyclophosphamide, 36 mg/kg body weight.
[c] Mean ± SEM.

13, $p<0.02$; and 75.4 ± 12.4 days versus 48.7 ± 3.9 days for mice operated on day 16, $p<0.05$).

In one experiment, supplemental vitamin A begun at the time of limited local tumor excision (day 10 after tumor inoculation) decreased the incidence of tumor recurrence during the 75 day postoperative observation period. In this experiment, the limited local tumor excision again increased survival time (52 ± 4 versus 32 ± 3 days, $p<0.001$) as did the supplemental vitamin A (without excision) (53 ± 2 versus 32 ± 3 days, $p<0.001$). When both limited local excision and ingestion of supplemental vitamin A were carried out, tumors failed to recur in 4/20 mice during the 75 day postoperative study period, while tumors recurred in all other mice. Also, the latency period for tumor recurrence was prolonged for those mice following local excision and supplemental vitamin A (13 ± 1 versus 7 ± 1 days, $p<0.001$) as was the survival time for the 16/20 mice in which tumors recurred (72 ± 6 versus 53 ± 2 days, $p<0.001$).

3. Radiation Injury: Local and Whole Body

We hypothesized that supplemental vitamin A and β-carotene would mitigate radiation injury because of our findings that such supplements alleviated many of the adverse effects of streptozotocin and cyclophosphamide, two drugs with radiomimetic actions. To test our hypothesis, experiments were carried out using both local and whole-body irradiation.

a. Local Radiation.   We were interested in local radiation not only as a way of testing the above-mentioned hypothesis, but also as a preliminary to testing in later experiments another of our hypotheses, namely, that supplemental vitamin A and β-carotene would add substantially to the antitumor action of local radiation.

A series of experiments was carried out using young C3H/HeJ female mice subjected to 3000 R irradiation of one hindlimb. For the radiation, the mice were anesthetized lightly with sodium pentobarbital (1 mg/20 gm body weight intraperitoneally) and irradiated using a Picker-Vanguard 280 KVp X-ray therapy unit, half-value layer (HVL)—0.5 mm copper. The unit was calibrated to deliver 450 R/minute and was timed to deliver a single dose of 3000 R to a hindleg. The dimensions of the port were 9.5×7.3 cm, giving a port area of 60.4 cm^2. The entire body of each mouse, except one hindlimb, was shielded from the radiation by a 0.2 cm thick rectangular lead shield 27.3×11.3 cm.

All mice ingested the control chow diet during their adaptation period. The supplemental vitamin A feeding was begun for some mice selected at random either 3 days before radiation, immediately after radiation, or 3 days after radiation and continued during the postirradiation period; the remaining mice continued to eat the control feed pre- and postirradiation. All mice ate and drank (tap water) *ad libitum.*

Weight loss, thymic involution (decrease in thymic weight and number of thymic small lymphocytes), adrenal enlargement, and lymphopenia due to local X irradiation was lessened by supplemental vitamin A, whether it was begun 3 days before, immediately after, or 3 days after radiation (Tables IX and X) (Seifter *et al.*, 1981c).

b. Whole-Body Radiation. Supplemental vitamin A and β-carotene each increased significantly the resistance of male CBA mice to whole-body irradiation. Weight loss, thymic involution, renal enlargement, and lymphopenia were lessened; survival time was increased; and the $LD_{50/30}$ was shifted from 560 to 630 R and the $LD_{100/30}$ from 630 to 730 R (Tables XI and XII and Fig. 10). In these experiments the mice received whole-body irradiation in a ^{137}Cs small animal irradiator (Gamma-cell-40). This unit contains two ^{137}Cs sources, approximately 1800 Ci each, positioned above and below the exposure cavity so as to produce a uniformity of $+5\%$ for the 0.66 MeV gamma radiation within the sample chamber (diameter 30 cm, height 10 cm). Dose rate within the chamber, calibrated with thermoluminescent dosimeters, was 137 rads/minute. Whole-body doses of 450 to 750 rads thus were delivered in 3.3 to 5.5 minutes. Forced ventilation was maintained within the exposure cavity during irradiation.

The mice were maintained on the control chow (Purina) during their adaptation period. The ameliorating effects of supplemental vitamin A

TABLE IX

Influence of Local Radiation and Supplemental Vitamin A on Changes in Body Weight, Weights of the Adrenal and Thymus Glands, and Small Lymphocyte Content of the Thymus[a]

Expt.	Days after radiation	Group	Treatment	Changes in body weights (gm)	Adrenal weights (mg)	Thymic weights (mg)	Numbers of lymphocytes per thymus (10⁶)
2	12	I	None	+2.3±0.4[b]	4.6±0.2	30.8±1.3	21.3±0.8
		II	Sham	+2.2±0.6	4.7±0.3	29.9±0.9	20.9±0.9
		III	3000 R	+1.3±0.2	5.4±0.2	25.8±0.7	18.6±0.5
		IV	3000 R + vitamin A	+1.7±0.2	4.8±0.2	31.3±0.7	24.5±0.5
3	3	I	None	0.0±0.0	5.0±0.3	36.0±2.7	26.9±1.0
		II	3000 R	−2.3±0.7	7.5±0.4	17.8±1.9	9.0±0.2
		III	Vitamin A, then 3000 R	−0.5±0.3	5.7±0.7	33.7±2.5	30.3±2.1
		IV	3000 R, then vitamin A	−0.8±0.3	6.0±0.3	32.0±1.2	27.4±7.0
3	8	V	None	0.0±0.0	4.3±0.2	29.7±0.9	25.4±1.5
		VI	3000 R	−3.0±0.4	6.3±0.2	17.3±0.2	10.7±0.7
		VII	Vitamin A, then 3000 R	−0.7±0.3	5.0±0.2	29.3±0.9	26.8±7.0
		VIII	3000 R, then vitamin A	−0.9±0.3	5.0±0.2	29.7±0.6	24.2±0.6

Expt.	Days after radiation	Comparison			p values[c]		
2	12	I versus II	NS	NS	NS	NS
		I versus III	<0.05	<0.01	<0.005	<0.01
		III versus IV	NS	<0.05	<0.001	<0.001
		I versus IV	NS	NS	NS	<0.005
3	3	I versus II	<0.01	<0.001	<0.001	<0.001
		II versus III	<0.01	<0.05	<0.001	<0.001
		II versus IV	<0.01	<0.001	<0.001	<0.001
		III versus IV	NS	NS	NS	NS
3	8	V versus VI	<0.001	<0.001	<0.001	<0.001
		VI versus VII	<0.001	<0.002	<0.001	<0.001
		VI versus VIII	<0.001	<0.004	<0.001	<0.001
		VII versus VIII	NS	NS	NS	NS

[a] From Seifter et al. (1981c).
[b] Weights are expressed as mean ± SEM.
[c] p values, ANOVA-Newman-Keuls test; NS, not significant ($p > 0.05$).

TABLE X

Influence of Local Radiation and Supplemental Vitamin A on the Numbers of Circulating WBC in Experiment 3[a]

Group	Treatment	Days postradiation			
		1	2	3	8
I	None	13,700±580[b]	14,380±410	13,700±210	14,550±215
II	3000 R	8,300±770	7,400±800	4,740±410	6,260±260
III	Vitamin A, then 3000 R	10,740±390	12,480±481	9,730±470	9,340±220
IV	3000 R, then vitamin A	9,980±360	9,160±310	8,720±900	9,070±230

Comparison	p values[c]			
I versus II	<0.001	<0.001	<0.001	<0.001
II versus III	<0.02	<0.001	<0.001	<0.001
II versus IV	<0.08	<0.05	<0.001	<0.001
III versus IV	NS	<0.001	NS	NS

[a] From Seifter *et al.* (1981c).

[b] Mean ± SEM in leukocytes/mm^3 of blood.

[c] *p* values, ANOVA-Newman-Keuls test; NS, not significant ($p > 0.05$).

and β-carotene were greatest when the supplements were begun 3 days before, the day before, or promptly after irradiation, although the mice probably did not eat until several hours after radiation.

Supplemental vitamin A was also significantly effective, although somewhat less so, when begun 2 or 3 days after irradiation. Survival time was prolonged, but survival rate was not, when supplemental vitamin A was begun 6 days after radiation (Seifter *et al.*, 1981b).

4. Antitumor Effects of Supplemental Vitamin A, β-Carotene, and Local Radiation

To test our hypothesis that supplemental vitamin A and β-carotene would add to the therapeutic effectiveness of local tumor irradiation, two similarly designed experiments separated by a 9-week interval were conducted. The first experiment began in November 1980 and the second in March 1981. In each experiment young male CBA/J mice were inoculated in the right hind leg with 2×10^5 tumor cells. On the thirteenth postinoculation day, when tumors had a mean diameter of 6.2

TABLE XI

Effect of Supplemental Vitamin A and β-Carotene on Survival of Mice following Whole-Body Irradiation[a]

Dietary supplement	Experiment 2					Experiment 3				Experiment 4				
	Number of mice surviving					Number of mice surviving				Number of mice surviving				
	450 R	550 R	650 R	750 R	LD_{50}	450 R	550 R	650 R	LD_{50}	550 R	600 R	650 R	700 R	LD_{50}
None	12	6	1	0	550 R	12	4	0	505 R	7	5	4	0	495 R
Vitamin A	13	14	5	4	620 R	15	11	6	620 R	—	—	—	—	—
β-Carotene	—	—	—	—	—	—	—	—	—	15	13	9	1	660 R
p values[b]	NS	<0.001	<0.01	<0.001		NS	<0.001	<0.001		<0.001	<0.001	<0.05	NS	

[a] Male CBA mice, 15 in each group.
[b] NS, not significant.

TABLE XII

Effect of Supplemental Vitamin A on the Thymus and Adrenals of CBA Male Mice
following Whole-Body Irradiation[a]

	450 R		550 R	
	No supplement	Vitamin A supplement	No supplement	Vitamin A supplement
Thymus (mg)	27.2±2.0	39.0±1.0 ($p<0.001$)	23.0±1.9	34.8±2.0 ($p<0.001$)
Adrenals (mg)	5.5±0.3	4.7±0.3 ($p<0.01$)	5.9±0.2	5.2±0.2 ($p<0.01$)

[a] Dual-beam cesium source (0.662 MeV, γ radiation).
[b] 150,000 I.U. vitamin A per kilogram of diet, started a few hours after radiation.

mm in experiment No. 1 and 5.6 mm in experiment No. 2, the mice in each experiment were separately divided randomly into two major groups, one of which received 3000 R local radiation to the tumor-bearing limb (the rest of the mouse was shielded) while the other group was not radiated. In turn, each of these two groups was divided into three subgroups, one of which continued on the control chow (Purina) while the other two subgroups were started on the chow supplemented with either vitamin A or β-carotene (Seifter *et al.*, 1981d).

The local tumor radiation was delivered as described earlier in Section II,D,3,a.

We are aware that such single dose local radiotherapy is not used in clinical radiotherapy, but we have used it in these studies as an experi-

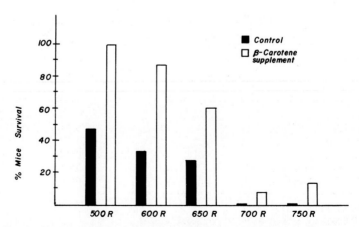

Fig. 10. Effect of β-carotene supplement on percent survival of whole-body irradiated CBA mice. β-Carotene supplement begun right after irradiation.

mental tool. We found that the supplemental vitamin A and β-carotene each added remarkably to the antitumor effect of the local X-irradiation therapy. In the unsupplemented mice given the local X irradiation, the tumor regressed temporarily, but regrew in several weeks, and all mice died of the tumors in 2–3 months; their mean survival time was twice as long as that of the unsupplemented mice not radiated. Supplemental vitamin A and β-carotene, each by itself without radiation, had antitumor effects similar to, but less than, that of local radiation alone; they slowed tumor growth, but led to tumor regression uncommonly, and all such mice died. However, their survival time was greater (one and one-half times) than that of unsupplemented nonirradiated mice, but less than that of unsupplemented radiated mice. When tumor-bearing locally irradiated mice were given supplemental vitamin A or supplemental β-carotene starting immediately after radiation, the tumor regressed "completely" in all mice and reappeared in less than 10% of these mice after several months. These latter mice survived 50–60 days longer than those receiving the control chow after radiation. Ninety percent (22/24) of the mice were living and well with no evident tumor at the end of 1 year in experiment 1 and at the end of $13\frac{1}{2}$ months in experiment 2 (Table XIII and Figs. 11 and 12).

To determine whether the tumors had been eradicated or rather held in "complete" check by the combined single dose local radiation and the

TABLE XIII

Antitumor Effects of Supplemental Vitamin A, β-Carotene, and Local Radiation[a]

Treatment	No. of mice with complete tumor regression		No. of mice surviving 1 year		Mean survival time of nonsurviving mice (days)	
	Expt. 1	Expt. 2	Expt. 1	Expt. 2	Expt. 1	Expt. 2
None	0	0	0	0	41.2±2.5	43.3±0.8
3000 rads	0	0	0	0	84.4±5.4[c,d]	99.1±5.9[c,d]
β-Carotene	0	0	0	0	61.2±2.1[c]	63.3±1.8[c]
Vitamin A	0	0	0	0	60.2±3.0[c]	64.2±1.9[c]
3000 rads + β-carotene	12[b]	12[b]	11[b]	11[b]	136[b]	128[b]
3000 rads + vitamin A	12[b]	12[b]	11[b]	11[b]	142[b]	131[b]

[a] C3HBA tumors, CBA/J male mice.
[b] $p < 0.0001$, compared with all other groups.
[c] $p < 0.001$, compared with group receiving no treatment.
[d] $p < 0.001$, compared with groups receiving either vitamin A or β-carotene alone.

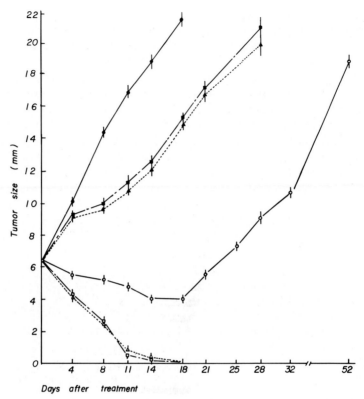

Fig. 11. Results obtained in experiment 1. Tumors averaged 6.2 ± 0.3 mm in diameter when treatments were begun. Mean tumor diameters ± SEM for mice not treated (●——●), treated with supplemental vitamin A (■– - –■), treated with supplemental β-carotene (▲- - -▲), 3000 rads X irradiation (○——○), 3000 rads and supplemental vitamin A (□– · –□), 3000 rads and supplemental β-carotene (△- - -△).

dietary supplements, at the end of 12 months in experiment 1 and $13\frac{1}{3}$ months in experiment 2, half the mice in the vitamin A- and β-carotene-supplemented groups were maintained on their respective supplements, while the other half were switched to the control chow (Table XIV). As of December 1, 1982, none of the mice that continued to receive supplemental vitamin A or supplemental β-carotene redeveloped tumors during the next 12 months in experiment 1 (24 months after the local irradiation and dietary supplements) or during the next 9 months in experiment 2 ($22\frac{1}{2}$ months after the local radiation and start of the dietary supplements). Eighteen percent of those kept on β-carotene (2/11) and 60% (6/10) of those kept on vitamin A died without evidence of tumor at autopsy (gross), 19–23 months after the local radiation and start of the supplements.

Of the mice that had been on supplemental vitamin A for 12–13½ months and then switched to the control chow, 67% (8/12) redeveloped tumors at 2–2½ months and died 2–3 months later; 17% (2/12) died without evidence of tumor at autopsy (gross) 15–18 months after tumor inoculation. Eighteen percent (2/11) of the mice that continued on the β-carotene supplement died without evidence of tumor at autopsy (gross) 20–22 months after tumor inoculation. Among the mice that had been on the supplemental β-carotene and switched to the basal diet, 20% (2/10) redeveloped a tumor; this occurred 4½–6 months after stopping

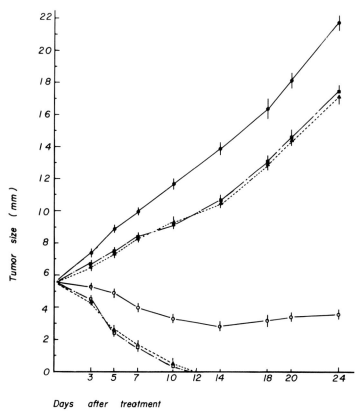

Fig. 12.   Results obtained in experiment 2. Tumors averaged 5.6 ± 0.2 mm in diameter when treatments were begun. Mean tumor diameters ± SEM for mice not treated (●——●), treated with supplemental vitamin A (■- - -■), treated with supplemental β-carotene (▲- - -▲), 3000 rads X irradiation (○——○), 3000 rads and supplemental vitamin A (□- · -□), 3000 rads and supplemental β carotene (△- - -△).

TABLE XIV

Influence of Continuing or Discontinuing Vitamin A and β-Carotene Supplements on Tumor Regrowth

	Vitamin A supplemented		β-Carotene supplemented	
	Kept on vitamin A	Switched to control chow[a]	Kept on β-carotene	Switched to control chow[a]
No. mice/group	10	12	11	10
No. mice with tumor reappearance	0	8	0	2
Time of tumor reappearance (days after diet switch)	—	58–75	—	(133, 175)
Time of death following tumor reappearance (days)	—	47–105	—	52
No. mice dying without evidence of tumor at autopsy (gross) (days after irradiation)	6 (589–697)	2 (463–559)	2 (619–677)	5 (557–669)
No. mice surviving (as of December 1, 1982)	4[b]	2[b]	9[b]	3[b]

[a] Diet switches: 1 year after irradiation and start of supplements in first experiment, 13½ months after irradiation and start of supplements in second experiment.

[b] >754 days in experiment 1, >683 days in experiment 2.

the β-carotene supplement; 50% (5/10) of this group of mice died without evidence of tumor at autopsy (gross) 19–22 months after tumor
inoculation.

As of December 1, 1982, 24 months after the start of experiment 1 and
$22\frac{1}{2}$ months after the start of experiment 2, 40% (4/10) of the locally
radiated mice continued on the vitamin A supplement and 82% (9/11) of
those continuing on the β-carotene are alive without evidence of tumor
recurrence. It is noteworthy that mice bearing C3HBA transplants and
receiving vitamin A or β-carotene supplements continuously are surviving more than $1\frac{1}{2}$ years and some more than 2 years after inoculation;
they are behaving in terms of weight and longevity as a nontumor
population of this strain surviving to old age, indicating not only
therapeutic effectiveness but also lack of toxicity of the supplements.

These data indicate that, in the 90% of mice receiving vitamin A or β-
carotene supplementation that were alive 4–5 months after the start of
the experiment, while vitamin A or β-carotene supplementation was
continued the tumor was kept in "complete" check, but not eradicated.
The duration of the antitumor effect of the β-carotene supplementation
appears to be greater than that of the vitamin A supplementation after
the supplements were discontinued.

III. SUMMATION OF EXPERIMENTAL DATA

These experiments demonstrate the salutary actions of supplemental
vitamin A and supplemental β-carotene on (1) the prevention and treatment of various experimental neoplasms [viral (MuSV-M), nonviral
transplantable (C3HBA and BW10232), and chemically induced
(DMBA)]; (2) the mitigation of many adverse effects of an alkylating agent
chemotherapeutic drug (cyclophosphamide) not only without interfering
with its antitumor action but, in fact, adding substantially to it; (3) the
addition to the antitumor benefits of limited local excision of tumors
(C3HBA breast adenocarcinoma); (4) the mitigation of adverse effects of
local and whole-body radiation; and (5) the dramatic additional benefit to
the antitumor action of local radiation.

IV. DISCUSSION

What is the basis for these effects? It is our view that multiple actions
of supplemental vitamin A and β-carotene are involved. A comprehensive discussion of these actions is beyond the scope of this chapter.

Some of the actions have been of special interest to us and have been addressed in our experiments. This is not to be interpreted as our minimizing other important actions of vitamin A and β-carotene, such as the effect of vitamin A on epithelial cell differentiation; the reader is referred elsewhere for a discussion of these effects (Bollag and Matter, 1981).

We consider the action of vitamin A and β-carotene in increasing host resistance to be very important. Supplemental vitamin A and β-carotene are each thymotropic in normal mice and rats; they minimize thymic involution in injured and in tumor-bearing mice and rats, increase peripheral blood lymphocytes, increase the *in vitro* mitogenic activity of lymphocytes, accelerate skin allograft rejection, increase the influx of macrophages into the site of injury (Barbul *et al.*, 1978), and lessen adrenal enlargement.

In this regard, spontaneous resistance of inoculated MuSV-M in syngeneic BALB/c mice is strongly dependent on lymphocytes, particularly on T lymphocyte activity. Similarly, resistance to MuSV-M tumor in CBA/J mice is strongly decreased by agents or conditions that inhibit lymphocyte activity, such as anti-lymphocytic serum, thymectomy, cortisone or ACTH administration, or burns or other physical stress, whereas resistance is increased greatly by thymic hormones, supplemental vitamin A, or other agents that induce lymphopoiesis or prevent injury-induced lymphopenia.

In this same vein, resistance to experimental C3HBA tumors is decreased by stress and is lower in C3H/HeHa mice (with small thymuses and enlarged adrenals) than in C3H/HeJ mice (with larger thymuses and smaller adrenals). Correlated with the increased resistance to the C3HBA tumor in both strains as a result of supplemental vitamin A and β-carotene is a thymotropic effect in normal mice of both strains, a decrease in the adrenal weight of normal C3H/HeHa mice, and a lessening of the thymic involution and adrenal weight increase in C3HBA tumor inoculated mice of both strains.

We believe the route by which we have given the supplemental vitamin A and β-carotene is important in these actions. In our experiments, these supplements have been incorporated in the diet. When given via the gastrointestinal tract, dietary vitamin A and that originating in the gut mucosa from β-carotene is absorbed and transported in the lymph. In addition thereby to generating lymph high in vitamin A, the lamina propria and Peyer's patches provide the lymph with high concentrations of B lymphocytes and monocytes. We believe that the interactions between vitamin A and these cells in the lymph may lead to activation of these two cell types. The lymph containing the activated cells and the vitamin A then enters the peripheral circulation via the subclavian vein.

Medawar and Hunt (1981) have pointed out that the immunity-promoting action of vitamin A is probably through its actions on the cellularity of thymus glands and that this action is probably critical for the antitumor action of the vitamin. This view is similar to the one we had expressed earlier (Seifter *et al.*, 1978). Similarly, Lotan and Dennert (1979) and Lotan (1980) have related the thymic effects of vitamin A to the enhancement of the tumor immunity by vitamin A. The role of vitamin A in the promotion of epithelial differentiation can be fulfilled by certain chemicals lacking other vitamin A activity, such as reproduction or sense perception. However, the role of vitamin A (and of β-carotene) in tumor prevention and therapy, which involves lymphopoiesis and immune mechanisms, in our experience is not fulfilled by compounds such as retinoic acid that are not convertible to retinol *in vivo*.

The amounts of supplemental vitamin A that we have added (two to three times the NRC recommended daily allowance for normal rodents) to the basal control diets did not lead to vitamin A toxicity when ingested daily for over 1 year by mice. This, too, we think may be associated with the route by which the supplemental vitamin A was given, namely, with the diet. At the doses we have used, vitamin A is not cytotoxic nor does it labilize lysosomal membranes.

The action of supplemental vitamin A and β-carotene on ameliorating many of the adverse effects of cyclophosphamide while at the same time adding to its antitumor activity we believe is due, in part, to minimizing the stress and immunosuppressant effects of cyclophosphamide and the bleeding. Supplemental vitamin A also mitigates the effects of cyclophosphamide on wound neovascularization, fibroblast multiplication, and reparative collagen accumulation. It is not clear that these latter activities of supplemental vitamin A are related to the antitumor action of cyclophosphamide, but they are important in terms of wound healing and in minimizing the decreased resistance to infection caused by cyclophosphamide in the early postoperative period. Since these salutary effects of vitamin A occur without inhibiting, but in fact adding to, the antitumor action of cyclophosphamide, this may permit its use clinically immediately after surgery, a time when tumor load is at a nadir, rather than waiting about 2 weeks as is current clinical practice. Also, supplemental vitamin A and β-carotene permitted the use of higher levels of cyclophosphamide when used for tumor therapy in laboratory animals, and this may be clinically important.

Our findings that the adverse effects, notably mortality, of whole-body radiation are mitigated to a substantial degree by supplemental vitamin A and β-carotene show that (1) they have prophylactic action when begun prior to radiation, as do other radio-protective agents; (2)

they have therapeutic action when given up to several days after radiation, an action which differentiates them from other radio-protective agents; (3) even when radiation dosage was so high that neither supplemental vitamin A nor β-carotene decreased mortality, each prolonged survival significantly. This last finding would furnish additional time for other therapeutic measures to be beneficial, e.g., antimicrobial agents, transfusions of blood, platelets, white blood cells, or marrow cells. This contrasts with the effects of most other radio-protective agents, such as sulfhydryl compounds, which must be given prior to or during radiation to be protective. These data suggest that therapeutic supplemental vitamin A and β-carotene may reduce morbidity and mortality in humans following accidental or purposeful radiation exposure.

Local radiation of normal C3H/HeJ mice produced systemic responses that were all moderated significantly by supplemental vitamin A. Since the adrenal and thymus glands were shielded from radiation, the changes in these organs were not due primarily to direct radiation effects per se. Our data suggest that a major protective action of the supplemental vitamin A is due to prevention of the sequelae of radiation injury rather than an immediate direct radio-protective action. This is supported by our observation that supplemental vitamin A offered several hours after radiation also moderated the weight loss, adrenal hypertrophy, thymic involution, and leukopenia. Support for this view is also given by our finding that supplemental vitamin A and β-carotene begun 1–3 days after whole-body radiation shifted the $LD_{50/30}$ and $LD_{50/100}$ to the right.

However, this in no way rules out the concept that supplemental vitamin A and β-carotene may also have direct radio-protective action and a role in the repair of radiation damage. β-Carotene and other terpenes related to vitamin A (but not retinoic acid) exert protection against ultraviolet phototoxicity; this suggests that vitamin A could elicit radio-protective action against ionizing radiation. However, because of the very high energy content of X radiation, β-carotene and vitamin A cannot act as barriers to the radiation. This is in contrast to the way in which β-carotene and vitamin A prevent the primary event damage in ultraviolet radiolysis.

Although vitamin A and β-carotene cannot prevent the primary radiolytic reactions of X radiation, they could prevent damage to cell constituents by products of X radiolysis of the solvent. For example, X radiation promotes the following reaction

$$
\begin{array}{ll}
H_2O \rightarrow H_2O^+ + e^- & \text{(ionization of water)} \\
H_2O^+ + H_2O \rightarrow H_3O^+ \ (H^+ + H_2O) + OH \\
\hline
2H_2O \rightarrow H_3O^+ + OH^- + e^-
\end{array}
$$

The OH free radical or its dimer H_2O_2 are responsible for some of the radiation-induced cell damage. Enzymes, such as peroxidases and catalase, can decompose the H_2O_2 into $H_2O + \frac{1}{2}O_2$. The hydrated electron produced by radiolysis of water is sufficiently energized to cause radical formation in nucleic acids and thereby favor cross-linking of nucleic acids or cleavage of the link between the base and the deoxysugar. Detoxication of the hydrated electron can occur by metabolic utilization of the electron by enzymes involved in superoxide (O_2^-) metabolism. Theoretically, vitamin A could protect cells against the radiolytic products of water, OH^- and e^-, because vitamin A has a very high degree of conjugation of single and double bonds. The highly conjugated double bond system of vitamin A makes it possible for these molecules to "buffer" hydrated electrons until these are disposed of by chemical interactions with electrophilic agents or by metabolic utilization of hydrated electrons attached to oxygen (superoxide, O_2^-). In this regard, β-carotene may be even more effective than vitamin A.

In this connection, the earlier work of Lucy and Lichti (1969) shows that retinol (but not retinoic acid) reacts with electron acceptors such as iodine and can donate or share electrons with quinones. Also, the double bond of the B-ionine ring of vitamin A or retinoic acid is readily oxidized by OH^- or H_2O_2 to the epoxy derivatives as shown by DeLuca (1979). Oxidation of retinoic acid to the epoxy or hydroxyl derivatives may be a part of a natural mechanism for enzymatic and chemical detoxication of peroxides and hydroxyl free radicals.

High doses of vitamin A and vitamin A acid have been used in some patients undergoing radiotherapy (Kleibel and Huelswitt, 1975). Tannock and associates (1972) used loosely defined doses of vitamin A in conjunction with radiation of tumor-bearing rodents and reported that the combination of vitamin A with radiation was an effective treatment against the experimental tumor in mice. In those publications, there was no discussion of possible vitamin A–radiation interactions leading to decreased radiation injury. In cell culture, added retinol sensitized murine L1210 leukemic cells to X irradiation (Brandes et al., 1974). Similarly, an aromatized analog of vitamin A acid inhibited radiation-induced oncogenic transformation of C3H mouse embryonic fibroblasts in vitro (Harisiadis et al., 1978).

The possible direct radio-protective effects of supplemental vitamin A (in doses used in our experiments, which are considerably lower than those used by Tannock) and β-carotene do not interfere with the antitumor action of local tumor X irradiation, but, in fact, we found that each adds substantially to the antitumor action. We think that this added antitumor action is largely the result of the indirect radio-protective effects of the supplemental vitamin A and β-carotene, as a result of which host resistance to neoplasms is increased by the mechanisms already discussed. We have speculated also that tumor destruction by radiation gives rise to antigens and the development of antitumor immune reactions to these tumor antigens is stimulated by vitamin A and β-carotene supplementation. We have speculated also that supplemental vitamin A may modify systemic radiation-induced disease in part by inhibiting the release of white cells into the circulation following radiation and thus lessening their rapid early destruction.

V. CONCLUSION

These findings and those of others suggest strongly that supplemental vitamin A and β-carotene will be useful in the management of patients with malignant tumors, including those undergoing operation, chemotherapy, and radiation injury. Our findings lead us to believe also that supplemental vitamin A and β-carotene will lessen the immune suppression which follows radiation and thereby decrease the risk of radiation-induced tumorigenesis and the increased susceptibility of radiated individuals to infection. Although we have not addressed in any detail the subject of cancer prevention, we think it likely that supplemental vitamin A and/or β-carotene will be shown to play an important role(s) in the prevention of certain cancers.

β-Carotene, because of its lesser toxicity and more prolonged effect in restraining tumor growth after discontinuation in mice with experimental C3HBA leg tumors receiving single-dose local X radiation (3000 R) and prolonged (1 year) supplementation with β-carotene or vitamin A may have an advantage over vitamin A. We believe that the more diffuse storage of β-carotene as compared with vitamin A may be a factor. It is possible that β-carotene may have some additional antitumor effects both quantitatively and qualitatively different from those which result purely from its conversion to vitamin A, as suggested also by Peto and associates (1981). Our experiments were not designed to determine this. Also, others have suggested that the conversion of β-carotene to vitamin A at sites other than the gut may be important in β-carotene's antitumor effect; this seems reasonable but, as far as we know, experimental data to establish this have not been published.

ACKNOWLEDGMENTS

Supported in part by NIH Grant 5K06 GM14208, Research Career Award (S.M.L.) and Research Funds of the Combined Department of Surgery, Albert Einstein College of Medicine, Yeshiva University, and Montefiore Hospital and Medical Center.

REFERENCES

Barbul, A., Thysen, B., Rettura, G., Levenson, S. M., and Seifter, E. (1978). *JPEN, J. Parenter. Enteral Nutr.* **2,** 129–140.

Blumenschein, G. R., and Moloney, J. B. (1969). *JNCI, J. Natl. Cancer Inst.* **42,** 123–133.

Bollag, W., and Matter, A. (1981). *In* "Modulation of Cellular Interactions by Vitamin A and Derivatives (Retinoids)" (L. DeLuca and S. S. Shapiro, eds.), pp. 9–23. N.Y. Acad. Sci., New York.

Brandes, D., Rundell, J. O., and Ueda, H. (1974). *JNCI, J. Natl. Cancer Inst.* **52,** 945–949.

Cohen, B. E., and Cohen, I. K. (1973). *J. Immunol.* **111,** 1376–1380.

Cohen, B. E., and Elin, R. J. (1974). *J. Infect. Dis.* **129,** 597–600.

Cohen, B. E., Gill, G., Cullen, P. R., and Morris, P. J. (1979). *Surg., Gynecol. Obstet.* **149,** 658–662.

DeLuca, H. F. (1979). *Fed. Proc., Fed. Am. Soc. Exp. Biol.* **38,** 2519–2523.

Harisiadis, L., Miller, R. C., Hall, E. J., and Borek, C. (1978). *Nature (London)* **274,** 486–487.

Kleibel, F., and Huelswitt, I. (1975). *Therapiewoche* **25,** 3388–3392.

Lan, S., Rettura, G., Levenson, S. M., and Seifter, E. (1981). *JNCI, J. Natl. Cancer Inst.* **67,** 1135–1138.

Levenson, S. M., and Seifter, E. (1983). *In* "Nutritional Support of the Seriously Ill Patient" (W. Winters and H. L. Greene, eds.), Vol. 1, pp. 53–62. Academic Press, New York.

Levenson, S. M., Hopkins, B. S., Waldron, M. M. A., and Seifter, E. (1982). *In* "Relevance of Nutrition to Sepsis" (J. E. Fischer, ed.), pp. 111–116. Ross Laboratories, Columbus, Ohio.

Lotan, R. (1980). *Biochim. Biophys. Acta* **605,** 33–91.

Lotan, R., and Dennert, G. (1979). *Cancer Res.* **39,** 55–58.

Lucy, J. A., and Lichti, F. U. (1969). *Biochem. J.* **112,** 231–241.

Medawar, P. B., and Hunt, R. (1981). *Immunology* **42,** 349–353.

Peto, R., Doll, R., Buckley, J. D., and Sporn, M. B. (1981). *Nature (London)* **290,** 201–208.

Rettura, G., Stratford, F., Levenson, S. M., and Seifter, E. (1982). *JNCI, J. Natl. Cancer Inst.* **69,** 73–77.

Seifter, E., and Norris, H. (1965). "Progress Report to the National Science Foundation." SSTP Loomis Institute, University of Hartford, Connecticut.

Seifter, E., Rettura, G., Padawer, J., Demetriou, A. A., and Levenson, S. M. (1976). *JNCI, J. Natl. Cancer Inst.* **57,** 355–359.

Seifter, E., Rettura, G., Levenson, S. M., and Critselis, A. (1978). *Curr. Chemother., Proc. Int. Congr. Chemother., 10th, 1977* Vol. II, pp. 1290–1291.

Seifter, E., Rettura, G., Liu, S., and Levenson, S. M. (1979). *Fed. Proc.* **38,** 714.

Seifter, E., Rettura, G., and Levenson, S. M. (1981a). *JNCI, J. Natl. Cancer Inst.* **67,** 467–472.

Seifter, E., Rettura, G., Padawer, J., Stratford, F., Kambosos, D., and Levenson, S. M. (1981b). *Ann. Surg.* **194,** 42–50.

Seifter, E., Rettura, G., Stratford, F., Yee, C., Weinzweig, J., Jacobson, N. L., and Levenson, S. M. (1981c). *JPEN, J. Parenter. Enteral Nutr.* **5,** 288, 294.

Seifter, E., Rettura, G., Stratford, F., Goodwin, P., and Levenson, S. M. (1981d). *Int. Symp. Carotenoids, 1981* Abstract.

Seifter, E., Rettura, G., Padawer, J., and Levenson, S. M. (1982a). *JNCI, J. Natl. Cancer Inst.* **68,** 835–840.

Seifter, E., Rettura, G., and Levenson, S. M. (1982b). *Proc. Conf. Radioprot. Anticarcinogens, 1st, 1982* pp. 14–15. Abstract.

Stratford, F., Rettura, G., Babyatsky, M., Levenson, S. M., and Seifter, E. (1980). *Surg. Forum* **31,** 224–225.

Tannock, I. F., Suit, H. D., and Marshall, N. (1972). *JNCI, J. Natl. Cancer Inst.* **48,** 731–741.

12

Vitamin A and Synthetic Derivatives (Retinoids) in the Prevention and Treatment of Human Cancer

Frank L. Meyskens, Jr.
Department of Internal Medicine
and Cancer Center Division
University of Arizona Health Sciences Center
Tucson, Arizona

Nutrition Factors in the Induction
and Maintenance of Malignancy

I. BACKGROUND

A.   Laboratory Studies

Epidemiological observations of malnourished humans led to the observation that epithelial dysplasias could be reversed by dietary supplementation with dark-colored vegetables, particularly carrots (Steenbock, 1919). This information provided the necessary clue from which von Euler *et al.* (1929) and Moore (1929) were able to isolate a vitamin A precursor (β-carotene) and vitamin A. In early animal trials, vitamin A produced substantial hepatotoxicity at high doses, and interest in these groups of compounds as preventive or anticancer compounds waned. In the late 1950s synthetic derivatives were developed. Subsequently, a large number of *in vitro* and *in vivo* investigations have demonstrated that the phenotypic expression of malignancy, whether initiated by chemical, physical, or viral carcinogens, can be suppressed (and in some cases ablated) by vitamin A and the synthetic retinoids (for reviews, see Sporn, 1977; Meyskens, 1981). The biology and biochemistry of many of these model systems have been extensively studied and provide a convincing rationale for clinical studies.

B.   Epidemiological Investigations

Prospective and retrospective dietary and retinol level studies implicate β-carotene and/or vitamin A as natural inhibitors of cancer development in humans and are summarized by Peto *et al.* (1981). Overall, these investigations support two major conclusions. A diet impoverished in β-carotene, and perhaps in vitamin A, produced a higher risk for several different types of cancers, particularly of the epithelial histological subtype. Also, minor decreases in serum vitamin A levels, even within the "normal range," placed individuals at substantial risk for the subsequent development of cancer. These observations strongly support intervention trials in groups of individuals at high risk for a malignancy, selected because of an intrinsic (genetic or familial) or extrinsic (carcinogen exposure) risk factor.

C.   Clinical Trials

Vitamin A has long been known to have a salutory effect on some forms of acne and dyskeratoses. In the late 1960s and early 1970s β-*trans*-retinoic acid (RA), a natural derivative of vitamin A, was shown by

Bollag (1970) to inhibit the growth of benign and malignant skin lesions. Additionally, beneficial effects of retinoids on actinic keratoses (Moriarity *et al.,* 1982), leukoplakia (Koch, 1978), and other premalignant conditions have been demonstrated. Recently, other investigators have shown that retinoids may also modulate hematopoietic progenitor cell function *in vitro* (Douer and Koeffler, 1982).

II. CLINICAL STUDIES AT THE UNIVERSITY OF ARIZONA

A. Prevention of Cervical Cancer with β-*trans*-Retinoic Acid (RA)

Systemic vitamin A clearly can reverse certain dysplastic lesions of the skin and mucosa. Topical application of RA can inhibit or suppress the growth of a variety of skin lesions (Bollag, 1970), and recently derivatives of RA have been shown to suppress actinic keratoses (Moriarity *et al,* 1982) and leukoplakia (Koch, 1978). Elsewhere, we have discussed extensively the advantages of locoregional chemoprevention (Dorr and Meyskens, 1983; Meyskens, 1981). Briefly, these features include the lack of systemic toxicities and site-specific application. A number of premalignancies could serve as useful models for locoregional chemoprevention in humans; the well-characterized natural history and easy accessibility of the involved site for serial observations makes cervical intraepithelial neoplasia particularly attractive. Although a number of retinoid preparations could have been used for the initial study, we chose RA for a number of clinical and practical reasons. These include the known toxicity and side effects of this agent on skin and mucosal surfaces, the availability of several different carrying vehicles, and the accessibility of this retinoid for such an investigation.

Our initial attempts at locoregional delivery of retinoic acid to the dysplastic cervix are described in Surwit *et al.* (1982). Our first prototype delivery device consisted of a simple diaphragm within which was a collagen sponge insert saturated with RA in an inert carrying vehicle. These initial studies indicated that the cream base was the best vehicle. However, the diaphragm leaked, producing unpredictable non-dose-related vaginal toxicity. No undesirable cervical side effects were noted, even at very high concentrations of RA, and preliminary evidence for reversal of some dysplastic lesions was obtained. Subsequently, we have developed an improved delivery system in the form of a cervical cap which has the desirable features of a molded rim (for individual fit) and self-adherence by differential osmotic pressure. This device also is amenable to the attachment of a positioning applicator which will allow self-treatment.

We have conducted a phase I dose-escalation study of RA using the cervical cap/collagen sponge insert for mild and moderate cervical dysplasia (Meyskens *et al.*, 1983b). Thirty-five patients were treated for a total of 4 days with daily changing of the cap, sponge, and RA. No limiting cervical or systemic side effects were noted at concentrations lower than 0.484% RA. Dose-limiting vaginal toxicity developed at a concentration of 0.484% RA following the 4-day application. We speculate that the cervix was oversaturated at this concentration, and vaginal side effects were secondary to leaching of the RA after the 4-day period. These results suggested that a concentration of RA of 0.372% would be a safe dose for investigations of efficacy. We plan to conduct a randomized trial of RA versus placebo in cervical intraepithelial neoplasia II (moderate dysplasia). Patients will be treated for an initial 4-day period. In the maintenance phase treatment will be done for 2 days every 3 months for 1 year. Patients will be followed indefinitely for disease progression and regression. The data from this trial should provide a definitive answer regarding the efficacy of RA for the suppression of moderate cervical dysplasia and establish a *modus operandi* for other studies of preneoplasia.

B. Adjuvant Treatment of Surgically Resected High-Risk Relapse Malignant Melanoma

A number of laboratory studies have shown that vitamin A and the retinoids (Lotan and Dennert, 1979; Sidell, 1983) improve certain immune parameters. In animal models vitamin A has inhibited the development of several transplantable tumors, an effect which was enhanced when the retinoid was combined with BCG (Felix *et al.*, 1975). Additionally, retinoids have inhibited the proliferation of both murine and human melanoma cells, an event frequently accompanied by differentiation, as measured by increased melanogenesis (Lotan and Lotan, 1980; Meyskens and Fuller, 1980). We have also demonstrated that retinoids, including vitamin A, can inhibit the clonogenic growth of some cells obtained from biopsies of melanoma tissue (Meyskens and Salmon, 1979).

Based on these laboratory observations and the absence of useful treatment for malignant melanoma in the adjuvant setting, we initiated a stratified randomized trial of BCG (by scarification) versus BCG + oral vitamin A (100,000 units/day) for surgically resected stage I (>1.0 mm thickness) and stage II malignant melanoma in April of 1978. This study was first analyzed in the spring of 1981 (Meyskens *et al.*, 1981) and updated in February of 1982 (Meyskens *et al.*, 1983a). At the last analysis, 98 patients had been registered on study, of whom 75 were fully eligible and evaluable. The key results from this preliminary evaluation are summarized in Table I. Side effects and toxicity were acceptable, as only two patients had therapy discontinued secondary to problems from vitamin A. These results demonstrated that most patients could tolerate 18 months of vitamin A at 100,000 units/day. Analysis of the data showed that there were fewer relapses of patients on the BCG + vitamin A arm, but this result was only significant at the level of $p = 0.20$. Nevertheless, these results were encouraging, inasmuch as an initial criticism of this trial was that vitamin A, acting as a hormone or growth factor, would produce a higher relapse rate. This does not appear to be so. However, a longer duration of follow-up will be needed to determine whether vitamin A is indeed useful as an adjuvant treatment for malignant melanoma.

C. Activity of Retinoids against Established Malignancies

1. In Vitro *Studies*

A number of investigators have demonstrated that RA, 13-*cis*-retinoic acid, retinyl palmitate (and retinol), an aromatic ethyl ester derivative of retinoic acid (RO-10-9359), and other retinoids can inhibit the growth of cultured malignant animal and human cells *in vitro* (review, Lotan, 1980). Experience with human cell lines is more limited, but inhibition of proliferation of several malignant cell types has been demonstrated, an event frequently accompanied by evidence for differentiation or matura-

TABLE I

Adjuvant Treatment of Stage I and Stage II Malignant Melanoma

	Treatment[a]	
	BCG	BCG + vitamin A
No. patients	33	42
No. relapses	7	4
Relapse free survival	$p = 0.20$	

[a] Patients were treated weekly (as tolerated) with Connaught BCG by scarification with or without vitamin A (retinol, 100,000 units) orally per day.

tion. Most notably these tumors include malignant melanoma (Meyskens and Fuller, 1980), neuroblastoma (Sidell, 1983), and leukemic cells (Breitman *et al.*, 1980). We and others have also shown that retinoids can reduce the colony-forming ability of clonogenic cells obtained from fresh biopsies of malignant tissue (Meyskens and Salmon, 1979). Our preliminary *in vitro/in vivo* correlative studies also indicate that activity of retinoids against clonogenic cells may be an accurate reflection of clinical potency.

2. Clinical Studies

a. Advanced Cancers. A number of investigators have used RA to treat premalignant and malignant skin conditions (Bollag, 1970; Meyskens *et al.*, 1982), most notably basal cell carcinomas (Peck *et al.*, 1978). Additionally, the activity of retinoids (particularly RO-10-9359) against psoriasis (Tsambaos and Orfancos, 1981) suggested that the antiproliferative response to these compounds might be more general than originally suspected. We, therefore, conducted a broad phase II anticancer trial of 13-*cis*-retinoic acid. This study has been previously reported (Meyskens *et al.*, 1982), and the key data from our initial experience with 105 patients are reproduced here (Table II). No responses were seen in 21 patients with nonepithelial malignancies. One of 13 patients with malignant melanoma and 1 of 45 patients with nonsquamous epithelial malignancies responded. The most encouraging results were with patients with squamous epithelial cell cancers, in whom a 25% response rate was obtained. Although the activity of 13-*cis*-retinoic acid was essentially limited to skin and subcutaneous disease sites, these results demonstrated that this noncytotoxic compound could act on human malignant cells *in vivo*. A remarkable feature of this drug was that no bone marrow toxicity was noted, thereby suggesting that combination therapy with conventional cytotoxic agents would be a useful approach.

b. Preneoplastic Conditions. A number of studies have demonstrated clinical activity of retinoids against preneoplastic or low-grade tumors, including cutaneous squamous (Bollag, 1970) and basal (Peck *et al.*, 1978) cell carcinomas, keratoacanthomas (Haydey *et al.*, 1980), leukoplakia (Koch, 1978), and epidermal dysplasia verucciformis (Lutzner and Blanchet-Bordon, 1980). In our initial experience with 13-*cis*-retinoic acid against neoplastic disorders, we also treated several patients with severe preneoplastic conditions, and substantial clinical responses were noted in 3 of 5 patients (Table III), including patients with keratoacanthomas,

TABLE II

Patient Distribution and Response Rate of Eligible and Evaluable Patients Treated with Isotretinoin[a]

Histologic class	No. of patients	No. of responses[b]	
		Including mixed responses	Excluding mixed responses
Epithelial[c]			
Squamous cell			
Advanced	24	6 (25%)	2 (8%)
Low grade (preneoplastic)	5	3 (60%)	3 (60%)
Nonsquamous cell	45	1 (2%)	1 (2%)
Malignant melanoma	13	1 (7%)	1 (7%)
Nonepithelial[c]	21	0	0

[a] Reproduced with permission from Meyskens *et al.* (1982).

[b] Responses include only mixed, partial, and complete; improvements are not included.

[c] Tumor types included: epithelial squamous cell, high-grade (8 lung, 10 head and neck, and 6 other); epithelial squamous cell, low-grade (3 multiple basal cell, 1 keratoacanthoma, and 1 epidermal dysplasia verruciformis); epithelial nonsquamous cell (8 breast, 12 ovarian, 12 colon, 4 bladder, and 9 miscellaneous); and nonepithelial (3 choriocarcinoma, 5 lymphoma, 4 leukemia, and 9 miscellaneous).

multiple basal cell carcinoma, and epidermal dysplasia verruciformis (Meyskens *et al.*, 1982). Subsequently, we have treated several additional patients with other malignant conditions, and our experience is summarized in Table III. We have treated 4 patients with severe laryngeal papillomatosis, a hyperproliferative, viral-induced condition which is frequently lethal (Zur Haussen and Gissman, 1980). One adult failed a course of therapy and one has been stable for 6 months. Two children with this disease have responded, one with a partial response lasting more than 8 months and a second patient who has had a complete response lasting greater than 18 months.

We have also recently treated two patients with mycosis fungoides (Kessler *et al.*, 1983), a T cell lymphoma of the skin which appears to be the consequence of RNA tumor virus infection (Popovic *et al.*, 1982). Both patients were drug refractory, and have responded dramatically to oral 13-*cis*-retinoic acid. The first patient has had nearly complete clearing of large whole body tumorous skin plaques. The effect has occurred slowly over 13 months, but no new lesions have been recorded during this duration. The second patient, who also had far advanced and exten-

TABLE III

Details of Responses of Patients with Preneoplastic Cell Disorders to 13-*cis*-Retinoic Acid

Disease	Prior treatment	Response description	Response[a]	Response duration (months)	Virus-associated[b]
Keratoacanthomas	Multiple surgery	Disappearance of 24 of 25 lesions (0.5–2.0 cm), one resected	CR	+24	HPV
Multiple basal cell carcinomas	Concurrent radiation to 2 large face lesions	Complete response of several unirradiated areas; partial response of additional areas	PR	+25	No
Epidermal dysplasia erruciformis	None	Resolution of 50% of total mass of multiple lesions	PR	2[c]	HPV
Laryngeal papillomatosis	Extensive surgery	Partial resolution	PR	+6	HPV
Laryngeal papillomatosis	Extensive surgery	Complete resolution of life-threatening disease	CR	+12	HPV
Mycosis fungoides	Extensive chemotherapy	Nearly complete clearing of massive disease	PR+	+10	HTLV
Mycosis fungoides	Extensive chemotherapy	Initial rapid clearing	—	+1	HTLV

[a] CR, complete response; PR, partial response.
[b] Virus-associated: HPV, human papilloma viruses; HTLV, human T cell leukemia virus.
[c] Discontinued due to skin toxicity, prompt relapse followed.

sive disease has only received the retinoid for 4 months, and substantial clearing of lesions has occurred.

These preliminary results with 13-*cis*-retinoic acid in patients with a diversity of conditions are very encouraging and suggest that further exploration of the clinical activity of this retinoid in premalignant and malignant conditions may lead to other surprising responses.

III. FUTURE DIRECTIONS

A. High-Risk Individuals

A large number of situations have been identified for which individuals are put at high risk for the development of cancer. Some of the more common conditions include exposure to smoking, asbestos, and aniline dyes. Another large group of high-risk individuals are patients who have had a nonmelanoma skin cancer resected, as they have a 5% reoccurrence rate per year. A substantial number of epidemiological studies suggest that patients who develop epithelial cancers have low β-carotene ingestion and decreased vitamin A levels (for review, see Peto *et al.*, 1981). The design and implementation of large-scale intervention trials, whether by dietary replacement or pharmacological treatment, will be difficult. The ethical issues as well as the problems of adherence and compliance are formidable and require careful planning and monitoring.

B. Premalignant Conditions

Laboratory, epidemiological, and clinical data strongly suggest that a number of preneoplastic conditions may be altered by retinoids. In terms of practical considerations for chemoprevention in humans, two major forms of preneoplasias exist—those which can be treated by locoregional application and those which require systemic therapy. We have discussed the strengths and problems of locoregional chemoprevention in detail elsewhere, and a few of the conditions most amenable to this approach are listed in Table IV as well as some conditions which should be considered for systemic chemoprevention therapy.

The nature of the preneoplastic conditions which have responded to the retinoids to date is of considerable interest. Epidermal dysplasia verruciformis, keratoacanthomas, and laryngeal papillomas are all caused by papillomas viruses (Zur Hausen and Gissman, 1980), and mycosis fungoides is clearly associated, if not caused, by a unique

TABLE IV

Some Candidate Preneoplasia for Chemoprevention

Locoregional
  Cervical dysplasias
  Oral leukoplakias
  Bladder papillomas
Systemic
  Preleukemias/dysplastic marrow syndromes
  Preneoplastic bowel syndromes
  Squamous dysplasias of lung

human retrovirus (Popovic *et al.*, 1982). Other neoplasms which have been associated with viruses, such as Burkitt's lymphoma, nasopharyngeal carcinoma, and hepatocellular carcinoma, should be considered as prime malignancies for experimental treatment with retinoids.

C. Malignant Diseases

Two major directions for the use of retinoids against established cancers seem likely: the development of new retinoids and combination therapy. A large number of retinoids have been synthesized (Sporn *et al.*, 1976), and clinical experience with these agents are now being obtained in premalignant and malignant conditions. To date, the major activity of retinoids is confined to cutaneous conditions or lesions located in the skin. A key question that has not yet been answered is whether these responses occur because of the intrinsic nature of the diseases localized to the skin or whether they respond because retinoids concentrate in the skin with high local concentrations of the compound being obtained. The distinction is important (but little considered), and if the latter is the case, a redirection of synthesis efforts from improving therapeutic/toxicity ratios (a maximum appears to have been reached) to the design of retinoids with different tissue specificity seems warranted.

In the future combination therapy may be considered either with conventional cytotoxic agents or other biological modifiers. The toxicity of retinoids is clearly different from most cytotoxic compounds, making combination therapy very attractive. Additionally, a large number of noncytotoxic biological modifiers have been developed in the past several years, many of which have promise as differentiating and maturation agents (Fidler *et al.*, 1982). Combinations of these and other agents may eventually allow the development of effective nontoxic regimens.

Overall, extensive laboratory data, numerous epidemiological investigations, and clinical studies suggest an important role for retinoids in the prevention and treatment of cancer in humans.

ACKNOWLEDGMENTS

The author thanks his numerous colleagues for their contributions to these studies, particularly E. Surwit, D. Alberts, V. Graham, L. Loescher, N. Levine, and S. Jones and also R. Collie and L. Kimball for secretarial assistance. Supported in part by Grant CA27502 and Contract CM17500 from the National Institutes of Health and a grant from Hoffmann-LaRoche, Inc., Nutley, New Jersey.

REFERENCES

Bollag, W. (1970). *Int. J. Vitam. Nutr. Res.* **3**, 299 311.
Breitman, T. R., Selonick, S. E., and Collins, S. J. (1980). *Proc. Natl. Acad. Sci. U.S.A.* **77**, 2936–2940.
Douer, D. and Koeffler, H. P. (1982). *J. Clin. Invest.* **69**, 277–283.
Dorr, R. and Meyskens, F. L., Jr. (1983). *J. Natl. Cancer Inst.* (in press).
Felix, E. L., Lloyd, B., and Cohen, M. H. (1975). *Science.* **189**, 886–888.
Fidler, I. J., Berendt, M., and Oldham, R. K. (1982). *J. Biol. Respir. Mod.* **1**, 15–26.
Haydey, R. P., Reed, M. L., and Dzubow, L. M. (1980). *N. Engl J. Med.* **303**, 560–562.
Kessler, J., Meyskens, F. L., Jr., Levine, N., and Jones, S. E. (1983). *Lancet* **1**, 1345–1347.
Koch, H. F. (1978). *J. Max. Fac. Surg.* **6**, 59–63.
Lotan, R. (1980). *Biochim. Biophys. Acta* **605**, 33–91.
Lotan, R., and Dennert, G. (1979). *Cancer Res.* **39**, 55–58.
Lotan, R. and Lotan, D. (1980). *Cancer Res.* **40**, 3345–3350.
Lutzner, M. and Blanchet-Bordon, C. (1980). *N. Engl. J. Med.* **302**, 1091–1093.
Meyskens, F. L., Jr. (1981). *Life Sci.* **28**, 2323–2327.
Meyskens, F. L., Jr., and Fuller, B. B. (1980). *Cancer Res.* **40**, 2194–2916.
Meyskens, F. L., Jr., and Salmon, S. E. (1979). *Cancer Res.* **39**, 4055–4057.
Meyskens, F. L., Jr., Aapro, M. S., Voakes, J. B., Moon, T. E., and Martin, E. (1981). *In* "Adjuvant Therapy of Cancer III" (S. E. Salmon and S. E. Jones, eds.), pp. 217–224. Grune & Stratton, New York.
Meyskens, F. L., Jr., Gilmartin, E., Alberts, D. S., Levine, N. S., Brooks, R., Salmon, S. E., and Surwit, E. A. (1982). *Cancer Treat. Rep.* **66**, 1315–1319.
Meyskens, F. L., Jr., Alberts, D. S., Aapro, M. S., and Surwit, E. A. (1983a). *In* "Proceedings of the First International Conference on the Modulation and Mediation of Cancer by Vitamins" (F. L. Meyskens, Jr., and K. N. Prasad, eds.). Karger, Basel (in press).
Meyskens, F. L., Jr., Graham, V., Chvapil, M., Dorr, R. T., Alberts, D. S., and Surwit, E. A. (1983b). *J. Natl. Cancer Inst* (in press).
Moore, T. (1929). *Lancet* **2**, 380–381.
Moriarity, M., Dunn, D., Oawagh, A., Lambe, R., and Buick, I. (1982). *Lancet* **1**, 364–365.
Peck, G. L., Olsen, T. G., Yoker, F. W. (1978). *Dermatologica* **157**, Suppl. 1, 11–12.
Peto, R., Doll, R., Buckler, J. D., and Sporn, M. B. (1981). *Nature (London)* **290**, 201–208.
Popovic, M., Reitz, M. S., Jr., Sarngadharan, M. G., Robert-Guroff, M., Kalyanaramin, V. S., Nakoo, Y., Miyoshi, I., Minowada, J., Yoshida, M., Ito, Y., and Gallo, R. C. (1982). *Nature (London)* **300**, 63–66.

Sidell, N. (1983). *JNCI J. Natl. Cancer Inst.* (in press).

Sporn, M. B. (1977). *Nutr. Rev.* **35,** 59–65.

Sporn, M. B., Dunlop, N. M., Newton, D. L., and Henderson, W. R. (1976). *Nature (London)* **263,** 110–113.

Steenbock, H. (1919). *Science* **57,** 289–291.

Surwit, E., Graham, V., Droegemueller, W., Alberts, D., Chvapil, M., Dorr, R. T., Davis, J. R., and Meyskens, F. L., Jr. (1982). *Am. J. Obstet. Gynecol.* **143,** 821–823.

Tsambaos, D., and Orfancos, C. E. (1981). *Pharmacol. Ther.* **14,** 355–374.

von Euler, B., von Euler, H., and Karrer, P. (1929). *Helv. Clin. Acta* **12,** 278–285.

Zur Hausen, H., and Gissman, L. (1980). *In* "Viral Oncology" (G. Klein, ed.), pp. 433–445. Raven Press, New York.

13

Vitamins C and E (or Fruits and Vegetables) and the Prevention of Human Cancer

Elizabeth Bright-See

Ludwig Institute for Cancer Research
Toronto Branch for Human Cancer Prevention
Toronto, Ontario, Canada

I. INTRODUCTION

The way people eat is associated with what types of cancer they may develop (Peto and Doll, 1981; National Research Council, 1982). Whether the differences in dietary patterns are responsible for the different cancer rates is not yet known. However, much research recently has been dedicated to trying to identify which factors in a particular food supply that might be potentially harmful and, conversely, which factors might be protective.

Vitamins C and E are two nutrients being considered as potentially protective food components. Much of the research has centered on the ability of vitamins C and E to block the formation of nitrosamines both *in vitro* (Tannenbaum and

Nutrition Factors in the Induction
and Maintenance of Malignancy

Mergens, 1980; Newmark and Mergens, 1981a) and *in vivo* (Oshima and Bartsch, 1981; Oshima *et al.*, 1982; Lintas *et al.*, 1982). Many nitrosamines are potent carcinogens in animal models, but their relationship to any human cancer has not been confirmed, and they will not be considered further here.

Epidemiological studies have often been used to support the theory that vitamin C plays a role in preventing human cancer. (Studies of human populations have not attempted to estimate vitamin E intakes.) This chapter will review the findings and the methods of measuring or estimating vitamin C of these studies as well as some more recent studies that may influence their interpretation.

II. MEASUREMENT OF VITAMIN C INTAKE

The results of several studies have been used to implicate vitamin C in the prevention of carcinogenesis. Some of these are shown in Table I along with the types of food–nutrient measurements made. In only one study, that of the Institute for Cancer Research, Chinese Academy of Medical Sciences (1979), was an actual marker of vitamin C intake measured. The daily urinary output of inhabitants of a region with a high esophageal cancer rate (Linhsien) was only one-eighth to one-ninth of that among the residents of a low-risk area (Hsinyaghsian). Low vitamin C availability is being considered as one of several possible factors, including low levels of molybdenum in the soil, high nitrates and nitrites in foods, and the use of fermented and moldy foods (Yang, 1980).

Vitamin C intake can also be calculated using food intake data and food composition tables. Kolonel *et al.* (1981) calculated vitamin C intakes from reported weekly intakes of about 80 food items of four groups at different risks for stomach cancer in Hawaii. They found a negative association of vitamin C intakes with risk for male subjects; however the difference between the lowest and highest risk groups was only 29 mg/day, and the level of significance was not reported. In one recent case control study of cervical dysplasia (Wassertheil-Smoller *et al.*, 1981), vitamin C intakes were calculated from 24 recall or 3 day food records. Subjects had lower intakes than did controls.

Such calculations may only represent indices, as accurate estimates of current intakes may require records of up to 21 days in length (James *et al.*, 1981). Because of the instability of vitamin C in foods, calculations from even these extensive records may not represent true intakes.

Other indices of intakes of vitamin C have also been used. In the case of Graham *et al.* (1981) and Marshall *et al.* (1982), these were based on the

TABLE I

Studies of Diet and Several Types of Cancer and the Methods Used to Assess "Vitamin C" Foods or Vitamin C

Cancer	Reference	"Measurement" of vitamin C			
		Direct measures	Calculated intake	Index of intakes	Foods presumed to correlate with intake
Stomach	Meinsma (1964)				+
	Higginson (1966)				+
	Graham et al. (1967)				+
	Graham et al. (1972)				+
	Haenszel et al. (1972)				+
	Kolonol et al. (1981)		+		
Lung	Hirayama (1977)				+
	Bjelke et al. (1982)			+	
	Kvale and Bjelke (1982)			+	
Esophagus	Institute for Cancer Research, Chinese Academy of Medical Sciences (1979)	+			
	Aoki et al. (1982)				+
Mouth	Marshall et al. (1982)			+	
Larynx	Graham et al. (1981)			+	+
Cervical dysplasia	Wassertheil-Smoller et al. (1981)		+		

frequency of use of 27 food items, and a standard serving size (100 gm) was assumed for all foods.

The majority of the studies have not attempted to assess nutrient intakes, either as calculations or indices, but rather have dealt with the frequency of use of different foods or groups of foods. Fruits and/or vegetables were among the foods found to be associated with cancer in case-control studies and with the risk of cancer in surveys.

In the case of stomach cancer, individuals with cancer were found to have lower intakes of fruits (Meinsma, 1964), lettuce (Graham et al.,

1967), total raw vegetables (Graham *et al.*, 1972), or fresh fruits and vegetables (Higginson, 1966) than did control subjects. Hirayama (1977) reported that Japanese who ate yellow and green vegetables daily had a lower risk of lung cancer; this was true for both smokers and non-smokers. Fruit and vegetable intake was also negatively associated with a lower risk of lung cancer in Norway (Bjelke *et al.*, 1982). Cases with esophageal cancer had low intakes of a series of "Western" fruits and vegetables (Aoki *et al.*, 1982) and low total vegetable consumption was as strongly associated with laryngeal cancer as was the "vitamin C index" (Graham *et al.*, 1981).

III. THE IMPORTANT FACTORS IN FRUITS AND VEGETABLES

The data on fruit and vegetable consumption is often used as indirect evidence that vitamin C is a protective agent (National Research Council, 1982). Is this justified, and are there other possible explanations for the associations between risks for certain types of cancer and fruit and vegetable consumption?

In most studies fruits and vegetables were simply identified as classes of foods. Where associations have been found in particular vegetables and fruits (Haenszel *et al.*, 1972; Aoki *et al.*, 1982), these food items are not all high in vitamin C and may in fact rather be good sources of vitamin A (in the form of carotene) and dietary fiber (Table II).

Foods that are sources of vitamin C supply other important nutrients and food factors. Pennington (1976) found that the vitamin C content of foods in a food composition table was correlated with the content of total vitamin A ($r=0.290$), folic acid ($r=0.276$), and fiber ($r=0.315$). In our own studies of international data (G. Eyssen and E. Bright-See, unpublished data) the daily average availability of vitamin C (Food and Agriculture Organization, United Nations, 1977) is associated with the availability of total vegetables ($r=0.69$) and fruit ($r=0.41$), but also with carotene ($r=0.62$), fruit fiber ($r=0.56$), vegetable fiber ($r=0.78$), and fruit and vegetable fiber ($r=0.84$).

As Marshall *et al.* (1982) aptly pointed out, vitamins C and A may be important in the etiology of oral cancer or neither may be relevant but "instead be markers for the presence in the diet of other substances." The same may be true for other types of cancer.

Thus far, the "other substances" receiving the most attention are the known nutrients. However, recent studies on some nonnutrients indicate that it would perhaps be unwise to take a limited view of dietary factors that may be important in preventing human cancers.

TABLE II

Composition of Some Foods Negatively Associated with Risk of Cancer

Reference	Cancer	Food	Vitamin C[a] per 100 gm wet weight (mg)	Vitamin A[a] per 100 gm wet weight (IU)	Fiber[b] per 100 gm wet weight (gm)
Haenszel et al. (1972)	Stomach cancer	Tomato	23	900	1.5
		Celery	9	240	1.8
		Corn	7	400	—
Aoki et al. (1982)	Esophageal cancer	Cabbage	47	130	3.4
		Tomato	23	900	1.5
		Cucumber	11	250	0.4
		Carrot	8	11,000	2.9
		Egg Plant	3	10	—
		Lettuce	18	1,900	—
		Plum	4	300	2.1
		Strawberry	59	60	2.2
		Peach	7	1,330	1.4

[a] U.S. Department of Agriculture.
[b] Paul and Southgate (1978).

The nonnutrient compounds of interest are the plant phenols. The presence of these substances in plants (and human foods from plants) have been known for many years. Newmark and Mergens (1981b) reported that two of these, caffeic acid and ferulic acid, are more potent blockers of nitrosamine formation than either vitamin C or vitamin E. Wattenberg et al. (1980) found that caffeic acid and ferulic acid decreased the incidence of forestomach tumors in mice treated with carcinogen benzo[a]pyrene. Recently, series of phenolic compounds were tested for their ability to block the mutagenicity of the ultimate carcinogen form of benzo[a]pyrene, benzo[a]pyrene-7,8-diol-9,10-expoxide-2 (Wood et al., 1982). Ferulic, caffeic, and chlorogenic acids were all effective, but the polyphenol, ellagic acid, was 80–300 times more effective than the other compounds. All of these phenolic compounds occur naturally in many plant materials, are normally ingested by humans, and may act to inhibit carcinogenicity of the polycyclic aromatic hydrocarbons and the formation of nitrosamines.

Foods contain more nonnutrient than nutrient chemicals, so it can be expected that other nonnutrients may be identified that may offer protection against specific types of cancer. That will only be done by taking a broad view of foods and dietary patterns without any bias about which of the many food components, nutrient and nonnutrient, may be identified as important.

The evidence shows that the consumption of fruits and vegetables is associated with a low risk for a number of types of cancer. Whether this is primarily due to vitamin C, other nutrients, or nonnutrient compounds in these foods has yet to be determined. Nutrients, such as vitamin C, vitamin A, and folate, are worthy of continued study but not to the exclusion of other materials. In studies of these nutrients, intakes will need to be assessed accurately by comprehensive dietary data or by markers of intake, such as blood or urine values (Sauberlich *et al.*, 1973).

For sometime, we may be stuck with the intellectually unsatisfying situation that specific foods or types of foods or dietary patterns are found to be either harmful or protective without knowing why. Medical and nutritional history is full of examples of cures or preventions being found and effectively applied before the rationale, mechanism, or individual active agent was known. If we are truly interested in preventing cancer, rather than just studying it, we must be able to accept that prevention may be achieved without a full understanding of the biological mechanism.

REFERENCES

Aoki, K., Okada, H., Takeda, S., Segi, M., Ohno, Y., Sasaki, R., and Tominaga, S. (1982). *Proc. Int. Cancer Congr. 13th, 1982*, p. 175. Abstract.

Bjelke, E., Schuman, L. M., Gart, J. J., and Heuch, I. (1982). *Proc. Int. Cancer Congr., 13th, 1982*, p. 175.

Food and Agriculture Organization, United Nations (1977). "Provisional Food Balance Sheets, 1972–74 Average." FAO/UN, Rome.

Graham, S., Lilienfold, A. M., and Tidings, J. E. (1967). *Cancer* **20**, 2224–2234.

Graham, S., Schotz, W., and Martino, P. (1972). *Cancer* **30**, 927–938.

Graham, S., Mettlin, C., Marshall, J., Priore, R., Rzepka, T., and Shedd, D. (1981). *Am. J. Epidemiol.* **113**, 675–680.

Haenszel, W., Kurihara, M., Segi, M., and Lee, R. K. C. (1972). *JNCI, J. Natl. Cancer Inst.* **49**, 969–988.

Higginson, J. (1966). *JNCI, J. Natl. Cancer Inst.* **37**, 527–545.

Hirayama, T. (1977). *In* "Naturally Occurring Carcinogens—Mutagens and Modulators of Carcinogenesis" (E. C. Miller *et al.*, eds.), pp. 359–380. University Press, Baltimore, Maryland.

Institute for Cancer Research, Chinese Academy of Medical Sciences (1979). *Adv. Med. Oncol., Res. Educ., Proc. Int. Cancer Congr., 12th, 1978*, Vol. 3, pp. 39–44.

James, W. P. T., Bingham, S. A., and Cole, T. J. (1981). *Nutr. Cancer* **2**, 203–212.

Kolonel, L. N., Nomura, A. M. Y., Hirohata, T., Hankin, J. H., and Hinds, M. W. (1981). *Am. J. Clin. Nutr.* **34**, 2478–2485.

Kvale, G., and Bjelke, E. (1982). *Proc. Int. Cancer Congr. 13th, 1982*, p. 175. Abstract.

Lintas, C., Clark, A., Fox, J., Tannenbaum, S. R., and Newberne, P. M. (1982). *Carcinogenesis* **3**, 161–165.

Marshall, J., Graham, S., Mattlin, C., Shedd, D., and Swanson, M. (1982). *Nutr. Cancer* **3**, 145–149.

Meinsma, L. (1964). *Voeding* **25**, 357–365.

National Research Council (1982). "Diet, Nutrition and Cancer." Natl. Acad. Press, Washington, D.C.

Newmark, H. L., and Mergens, W. J. (1981a). *In* "Criteria of Food Acceptance" (J. Solms and R. L. Hall, eds.), pp. 379–390. Forster Publ. Ltd., Zurich.

Newmark, H. L., and Mergens, W. J. (1981b). *In* "Inhibition of Tumor Induction and Development" (M. S. Zedeck and M. Lipkin, eds.), pp. 127–168. Plenum, New York.

Oshima, H., and Bartsch, H. (1981). *Cancer Res.* **41**, 3658–3662.

Oshima, H., Bereziat, J. C., and Bartsch, H. (1982). *Carcinogenesis* **3**, 115–120.

Paul, A. A., and Southgate, D. A. T. (1978). "McCance and Widdowson's The Composition of Foods," 4th ed. Elsevier North-Holland Biomedical Press, New York.

Pennington, J. A. (1976). "Dietary Nutrient Guide." AVI Publ. Co., Westport, Connecticut.

Peto, R., and Doll, R. (1981). *JNCI, J. Natl. Cancer Inst.* **66**, 1194–1265.

Sauberlich, H. E., Dowdy, R. P., and Skala, J. H. (1973). *CRC Crit. Rev. Clin. Lab. Sci.* **4**, 215–227, 228–235, 263–274.

Tannenbaum, S. R., and Mergens, W. (1980). *Ann. N.Y. Acad. Sci.* **355**, 267–277.

U.S. Department of Agriculture (1975). *U.S., Dep. Agric., Agric. Handb.* **456.**

Wassertheil-Smoller, S., Romney, S. L., Wylie-Rosett, J., Slagle, S., Miller, G., Lucide, D., Duttagupta, C., and Polan, P. R. (1981). *Am. J. Epidemiol.* **114**, 714–724.

Wattenberg, L. W., Coccia, J. B., and Lam, L. K. T. (1980). *Cancer Res.* **40**, 2820–2823.

Wood, A. W., Huang, M. T., Chang, R. L., Newmark, H. L., Lehr, R. E., Nagi, H., Sayer, J. M., Jerina, D. M., and Conney, A. H. (1982). *Proc. Natl. Acad. Sci. U.S.A.* **79**, 5513–5517.

Yang, C. S. (1980). *Cancer Res.* **40**, 2633–2644.

14

Role of Folate Deficiency in Carcinogenesis

Carlos L. Krumdieck

Department of Nutrition Sciences
University of Alabama in Birmingham
Birmingham, Alabama

I. INTRODUCTION

The use of antagonists of folic acid, the antimetabolites aminopterin and methotrexate (MTX), resulted in the first production by therapeutic means of temporary remissions in acute leukemia in children (Farber *et al.*, 1948) and permanent cures of advanced choriocarcinoma of the uterus (Hertz *et al.*, 1963; Hertz, 1963). Since both of these drugs exert their anti-

225

Nutrition Factors in the Induction
and Maintenance of Malignancy

tumor effect by producing a severe deficiency of the biologically active tetrahydrofolates, it seemed logical to assume that folate deficiency, of whatever origin, ought to be associated with a decreased risk of cancer development. This untested notion is presently being challenged by a significant body of experimental evidence supporting the contrary hypothesis: that folate deficiency renders normal cells more susceptible to neoplastic transformation. It is the purpose of this chapter to present and discuss some of this evidence and to propose several nonmutually exclusive mechanisms to explain the postulated cocarcinogenic role of folate deficiency.

Considering that folate deficiency is one of the most common vitamin deficiencies in this country (Bailey *et al.*, 1979, 1980) and in the world (Colman, 1977), and that hidden "localized deficiencies" affecting one or a few tissues in the presence of normal systemic levels of the vitamin are now believed to occur (Whitehead *et al.*, 1973; Branda *et al.*, 1978), a very large number of persons may, if our hypothesis is validated, face an increased risk of developing cancer. Furthermore, preliminary results indicate that progression of preneoplastic lesions may in some cases be arrested or reversed by folate supplementation (Butterworth *et al.*, 1982).

II. SUPPORTIVE EVIDENCE

A. Chromosomal Damage and Neoplastic Transformation

Chromosomal damage to human cells *in vivo* as a result of folate or B_{12} deficiency is extensive and very commonly observed. Table I summarizes the morphological abnormalities described by Menzies *et al.* (1966) in the chromosomes of bone marrow cells of patients with megaloblastic anemia. Chromatid breaks, thin elongated chromosomes, despiralization, and marked accumulation of mitosis in prophase were their most

TABLE I

Chromosome Aberrations in Megaloblastic Anemia Bone Marrow Cells[a,b]

Prominent centrometric constrictions
Prominent satellites
Chromatid breakages (5–33%)
Mitosis arrested in prophase (52%)
Reduced contraction—despiralization

[a] Menzies *et al.* (1966).
[b] Morphologic chromosome abnormalities found in *all* cases examined.

prominent findings. Similar chromosomal damage in lymphocytes, persisting long after correction of the folate deficiency, has been reported by Das and Herbert (1978), and many workers, referred to by Sieber and Adamson (1975), have demonstrated the production of chromosomal damage *in vivo* by the administration of MTX (Table II). Chromatid breaks and gaps, fragmented chromosomes, and chromatid exchanges have been reported in peripheral white cells and in some marrow cells of patients treated with MTX for malignant or nonmalignant disease (Sieber and Adamson, 1975; Voorhees *et al.*, 1969).

In vitro work has also demonstrated the susceptibility of the chromosome to folate deprivation or to the inclusion of folate antagonists in the culture medium. Recent studies, beginning with Sutherland's pioneering observation that culturing lymphocytes from a group of mentally retarded patients in a folate-deficient medium resulted in the expression of a characteristic abnormality of the X chromosome (Sutherland, 1977), have led to the recognition of several heritable folate-sensitive fragile sites in the human karyotype. A number of culture variables capable of inducing or inhibiting expression of the folic acid-sensitive fragile sites have been identified. It is thus well established that the antifolates, MTX and aminopterin, induce expression (Sutherland, 1979; Fonatsch, 1981; Mattei *et al.*, 1981) as does the thymidylate synthetase inhibitor 5-fluorodeoxyuridine (FUdR) (Glover, 1981; Hecht *et al.*, 1982). Conversely, addition of a folate, thymidine, or bromodeoxyuridine (BrUdR) to the medium inhibits expression of folate-sensitive fragile sites (Sutherland, 1977). This is in keeping with prior *in vitro* work demonstrating that 24-hour exposure of hamster cells to MTX at concentrations similar to those obtained during cancer chemotherapy produced a very high number of chromosomal aberrations (Benedict *et al.*, 1977) (Table III). Ninety to

TABLE II

In Vivo **Human Chromosomal Damage Induced by Methotrexate**[a]

		Aberrations	
Cell type	Dose	Percent	Types[b]
Leukocyte	25 mg t.d.	10.6	GaT; BrT; ExT
Lymphocyte	50 mg t.d.	16	BrT; GaT; BrS; GaS
Leukocyte	—	1.3	BrS; TrS; Fr
Marrow	25–50 mg	10–22	BrT; BrS; Fr
Marrow	20–35 mg/week	15	GaT; BrT

[a] Sieber and Adamson (1975).
[b] T, chromatid; S, chromosome; Fr, fragment; Ga, gap; Br, break; Ex, exchange.

TABLE III

Chromosomal Aberrations Produced in A(T₁) C1-3 Cells by Methotrexate (MTX)[a]

MTX (μg/ml)	Percent of cells with aberrations	x̄ chromatid breaks/cell	Chromatid exchanges
100	100	12.8	36
10	98	10.5	30
1	90	9.5	30

[a] Benedict *et al.* (1977).

100% of the exposed cells showed chromosomal changes ranging from chromatid breaks and chromatid exchanges to the appearance of dicentric chromosomes. The significance of the chromosome-damaging effect of folate deficiency or of folate antagonists resides in the fact, pointed out by Benedict *et al.* (1977), that all agents capable of producing malignant transformation *in vitro* or cancer *in vivo* produce chromosomal changes similar to those described above. That these cytogenetic aberrations indeed represent an increased risk of neoplastic transformation has been demonstrated by *in vitro* and *in vivo* studies. Neoplastic transformation of a mouse cell line (C3H/10T1/2CL8) with low incidence of spontaneous transformation by 24-hour exposure to MTX has been shown by Benedict *et al.* (1977). Using the same system, Jones *et al.* (1976) obtained a high yield of transformed cells using the thymidylate synthetase inhibitor FUdR and, most importantly, were able to show that the transformation frequency produced by FUdR was markedly decreased by simultaneous treatment with a 10-fold excess of thymidine (TdR) (Table IV).

In vivo studies using hamsters receiving MTX by injection and simul-

TABLE IV

Transformation of C3H/10T1/2CL8 Cells by MTX and FUdR

Drug	Concentration (μg/ml)	Type III foci/ total dishes	Transformation frequency (%)
MTX[a]	100	7/25	0.16
	10	3/50	0.03
	1	0/33	0.0
FUdR[b]	0.1	13/30	3.5
	0.01	18/43	0.55
FUdR + TdR	0.1 + 1.0	1/7	0.13

[a] Benedict *et al.* (1977).
[b] Jones *et al.* (1976).

taneous topical applications of 9,10-dimethyl-1,2-benzanthracene (DMBA) to their buccal pouches developed epidermoid carcinomas much earlier than controls that did not receive MTX (Shklar et al., 1966). Their tumors were larger and much more malignant than those produced by DMBA alone (Table V). In these experiments, control animals receiving only the MTX injections did not develop tumors. A cocarcinogenic role of MTX is clearly indicated by these studies. The ability of MTX to retard and occasionally abolish the growth of established tumors is, paradoxically, replaced in experimental carcinogenesis by a facilitation of neoplastic transformation. To this author's knowledge, similar experiments designed to test directly the possible cocarcinogenic role of folate deficiency have not been conducted.

In humans, the administration of MTX for nonmalignant disease, most often for the treatment of psoriasis or for the purpose of immunosuppression (Calabresi and Parks, 1980), has been associated occasionally with the development of lymphomas, leukemia, carcinomas of various sites, and Kaposi's sarcoma (Table VI) (Sieber and Adamson, 1975; Herman et al., 1980). Similarly, secondary neoplasms have been shown to develop in a significant number of patients following MTX therapy for a primary tumor (Sieber and Adamson, 1975; Chung et al., 1981; Ruyman et al., 1977) (Table VII). In all the latter cases other potentially carcinogenic chemotherapeutic agents and/or radiation were also utilized. The appearance of a second neoplasm cannot therefore be attributed to MTX alone. Rather, as in the experiments with the hamsters, MTX or, more properly, the deficiency of the biologically active tetrahydrofolates that it produces, seems to exert a cocarcinogenic effect facilitating the action of complete or incomplete carcinogens to which the host is simultaneously exposed.

TABLE V

Effect of MTX upon Chemical Carcinogenesis in the Hamster Buccal Pouch[a]

Treatment	Tumor size (mm)	Microscopy
Control	—	Normal mucosa
MTX	—	"Collagen degeneration"
DMBA	1–3	Well-differentiated carcinoma (6/6)
DMBA + MTX	10–15	Anaplastic carcinoma (5/6)

[a] Shklar et al. (1966).

[b] Treatments were given for 12 weeks. One group received MTX, one group received DMBA, and one group received DMBA and MTX. MTX and DMBA were administered subcutaneously and topically, respectively, three times per week.

TABLE VI

Neoplasms Developing in Patients Treated with MTX for Nonmalignant Disease

Disease	Neoplasm	Comments	Reference
Psoriasis	Lymphosarcoma	Regressed, similar to phenytoin	Sieber and Adamson (1975)
	Pharynx carcinoma		
	Skin cancer		
	Renal carcinoma (2)[a]		
	Mammary cancer		
	Basal epithelioma (2)		
	Lymphoma		
	Leukemia		
	Cervix carcinoma		
	Rectal cancer		
	Kaposi's sarcoma		
	Keratoacanthomas (6)		
Sarcoidosis	Leukemia		Herman et al. (1980)

[a] Number of cases.

B. Lipotrope Deficiency

Although no attempt to correlate pure folate deficiency with carcinogenesis has been published, a number of important papers dealing with lipotrope deficiency and neoplastic transformation support our hypothesis. Copeland and Salmon (1946) demonstrated that 58% of rats fed a diet deficient in choline and methionine (and, unknown to them, also devoid of vitamin B_{12} and folic acid) developed various types of neoplasms. Adenocarcinomas of the liver were found in 30%, lung carcinomas in 38%, and hemangioepitheliomas and sarcomas in 10 and 6%, respectively, of the animals. The increased susceptibility to neoplastic transformation brought about by "lipotrope" deficiency has been subsequently confirmed by the work of Newberne, Rogers, and collaborators. A diet marginal in methionine and choline and devoid of vitamin B_{12} and folic acid was shown to increase the susceptibility to aflatoxin tumorigenesis in rats (Newberne et al., 1968). Later, Rogers and Newberne (1973a) reported a new diet marginal in methionine and choline with adequate vitamin B_{12} but no folic acid which rendered rats more susceptible to tumor induction by the carcinogens, dimethylhydrazine (Rogers and Newberne, 1973b) N-2-fluorenylacetamide, 3,3-diphenyl-3-dimethylcarbamoyl-1-propyne, aflaxatoxin B_1 (Rogers, 1975), N-nitrosodiethylamine and N-nitrosodibutylamine (Rogers *et al.*, 1974; Rogers and Newberne, 1975). The cocarcinogenic effect of "lipotrope" deficiency was thus shown not to be limited to aflatoxin-induced tumorigenesis. The importance of folate deficiency as a factor aggravating a methionine–choline deficiency has been clearly demonstrated by Tuma *et al.* (1975). These authors showed that a folate deficiency, produced by MTX administration, markedly worsened the manifestations of choline–methionine deficiency and blocked the lipotropic effect of vitamin B_{12}. It is not surprising, therefore, that the cocarcinogenic effect of lipotrope deficiency should be enhanced by a superimposed folate lack. In this regard, it is important to note that most of the lipotrope-deficient diets, capable of increasing the susceptibility to carcinogenic agents, contained no folic acid. It is also important to emphasize that rats fed a folate-free diet (even if devoid of sulfa drugs intended to sterilize the gut) will develop a state of marginal folate deficiency that is easily demonstrated (Thenen, 1979). Furthermore, a superimposed deficiency of

TABLE VII

Second Neoplasms after MTX Therapy

Tumor		Other therapy[a]	Reference
Primary	Secondary		
ALL[b]	Carcinoma of pancreas	VCR; Cyt; 6MP Rad.	Sieber and Adamson (1975)
Lymphoepithelioma	AML[c]	Rad.	
Ovarian adenomas	AML	S-TEPA; 5FU	
Ovarian carcinoma	AML	S-TEPA	
Ovarian + mammary carcinoma	AML	S-TEPA; Cyt; S	
Mammary carcinoma	AML (monocytic?)	Cyt; S; VCR; 5FU	
Mammary carcinoma	AML	Cyt; 5FU; VCR; CMBL	
ALL	Glioblastoma	Rad (brain) MTX (intrathecal) VCR; S; 6MP; Cyt	Chung *et al.* (1981)
ALL	Hepatoma	VCR; S	Ruyman *et al.* (1977)

[a] VCR, vincristine; Cyt, cytoxan; 6MP, 6-mercaptopurine; Rad., radiation therapy; S-TEPA, triethylenethiophosphoramide; 5FU, 5-fluorouracil; S, steroids; CMBL, chlorambucil; MTX, methotrexate.

[b] ALL, acute lymphocytic leukemia.

[c] AML, acute myelogenous leukemia.

methionine, choline, or vitamin B_{12} will shift the bulk of available folates toward the pathway of homocysteine remethylation depriving the pathways of nucleotide biosynthesis of folate coenzymes (Thenen and Stokstad, 1973) (see Section III below). It is therefore clear that a folate deficiency of ill-defined severity has been imposed in most experiments on the cocarcinogenicity of lipotrope-deficient diets. Evidence for this comes from experiments showing that incorporation of exogenous [³H]thymine by the nuclei of renal tubule cells *in vivo* of the "lipotrope"-deficient animals was more than seven times greater than in the sufficient controls (Newberne *et al.*, 1968). These results, which clearly indicate impairment of the folate-requiring pathway of *de novo* thymidylate biosynthesis, were not interpreted in this light.

We believe that the folate deficiency, worsened by the superimposed deficiencies of methionine and choline, played a major role in rendering the lipotrope-deficient animals more susceptible to carcinogen-induced tumor development. For instance, while supplementation of a lipotrope-deficient diet with choline alone had no effect on diethylnitrosamine tumor induction, the addition of methionine, choline, and folic acid essentially eliminated the cocarcinogenic effect of the lipotrope-deficient diet (Rogers, 1977). The author attributes most of the protective effect to the addition of methionine, dismissing the role of the folic acid supplement on the arguable grounds (Thenen, 1979) that folate deficiency cannot be produced in rats in the absence of antibiotic therapy. Not only would a deficiency have occurred in the rats deprived of dietary folate, but it would have been markedly aggravated by the administration of diethylnitrosamine, which itself causes a folate deficiency in the rat (Buehring *et al.*, 1976). We believe that the folate supplement in the above studies (Rogers, 1977) must have played an important part in the elimination of the cocarcinogenic effect of the lipotrope deficiency. It is unfortunate that in none of these important studies was the severity of the imposed folate deficiency assessed in any way.

Although considerable effort has gone into determining which components of the lipotrope-deficient diets are primarily responsible for altering the susceptibility of rats to chemical carcinogenesis (Rogers *et al.*, 1980) a clear picture has not yet emerged. It is, however, well established that combined deficiencies of choline, methionine, vitamin B_{12}, and folic acid, compounds all involved in the *de novo* synthesis and transfer of methyl groups, enhance the induction of tumors in various organs by a variety of chemical carcinogens.

As concluded by Rogers *et al.* (1980), it seems that specific interactions between carcinogens and lipotropes vary with the carcinogens in question. Furthermore, as pointed out by Shinozuka *et al.* (1978), lipotrope deficiency can change the organ susceptibility to a given carcinogen. In their words, "extrapolation from one organ to another of findings concerning effects of [lipotrope] nutrition in the causation of cancer should be made with caution."

C. Localized Folate Deficiency Associated with Neoplastic Transformation of Affected Tissues

That localized folate deficiencies affecting one or a few tissues in the presence of normal systemic levels of the vitamin can occur was first indicated by the work of Whitehead *et al.* (1973), who showed megaloblastic changes in the cervico-vaginal epithelium of oral contraceptive users in which no other sign of deficiency could be demonstrated. Upon oral supplementation with folic acid, however, the megaloblastic changes reverted to normal.

The existence of these localized deficiencies offers an interesting way of challenging the validity of our hypothesis, since it would require the deficient tissues, and only those tissues, to be more susceptible to neoplastic transformation.

One notable example of such a disorder was reported by Branda *et al.* (1978). These authors described a familial abnormality of folate uptake by bone marrow cells and by phytohemagglutinin-stimulated lymphocytes. In this family, the intracellular folate levels of erythrocytes and bone marrow cells are very low, even during folate supplementation. In support of our hypothesis is the fact that this unfortunate family shows an extremely high incidence of neoplastic transformation affecting only the blood-forming organs. Of 34 members with some form of hematologic disease, there were 5 confirmed cases of acute leukemia, with 12 more who died in infancy or early childhood of infections associated with severe leukopenia, a history suggestive of more cases of acute leukemia.

Another example of localized folate deficiency associated with neoplastic transformation of the affected tissue is provided by the anticonvulsant drugs. Phenytoin and phenobarbital are known to produce a significant lowering of the folate content of the brain (Smith and Obbens, 1979), and their administration during pregnancy has been associated repeatedly (Ehrenbard and Chaganti, 1981; Pendergrass and Hanson, 1976) with the development of neuroblastoma in the offspring. The association of neoplasia and a number of birth defects (motor and developmental delays, mental retardation, etc.) occurring in the fetal hydantoin syndrome may well be due to the known interference with folate metabolism produced by the anticonvulsant drugs. It should be remembered that antifolates administered during brief critical periods during pregnancy result in the production of severe brain malformations in the rat (Nelson *et al.*, 1955).

Although it seems clear that the risk of brain tumor development following anticonvulsant administration is much higher during embryogenesis or early childhood (Gold *et al.*, 1978), there is evidence that adult patients treated with phenobarbital, phenytoin, or primidone also show a significantly increased incidence of cancers of the brain and nervous system (Clemmesen *et al.*, 1974). Tumors of other organs showed no, or marginally significant, increases over expected incidence. These results are summarized in Table VIII. Phenobarbital has been shown to enhance spontaneous hepatic tumorigenesis in mice (Peraino *et al.*, 1973) and is a promoting agent in hepatocarcinogenesis (Pitot and Sirica, 1980). To our knowledge no experiments have been conducted attempting to reverse the promoting effect of phenobarbital by folate supplementation.

D. Reversal of Preneoplastic Lesions by Folate Supplementation

The morphological similarity of folate-deficient epithelial cells and the cells observed in cervical dysplasia led Butterworth *et al.* (1982) to postulate that the two processes might be related and that supplementation with folate might correct the dysplastic lesion. In a double-blind study of oral contraceptive users with cervical dysplasia, folate supplementation resulted in significant improvement of cytology scores. No changes were observed in the patients receiving the placebo. Furthermore, the

TABLE VIII

Localized Folate Deficiency Associated with Neoplastic Transformation in Humans

Cause	Deficient tissue	Tumor	Frequency odds	Reference[a]
Defective folate uptake (familial)	Bone marrow, lymphocytes	Leukemia	5/34 confirmed 17/34 suspected	1
Fetal hydantoin syndrome	Offspring's CNS	Neuroblastoma		2–5
Barbiturates (children)	CNS	Brain tumors	8% of brain tumors in children	6
Anticonvulsants (adults) (?)	Brain and nervous system	Brain tumors	36/2.3; 32/1.8[b]	7

[a] Key to references: 1, Branda *et al.* (1978); 2, Ehrenbard and Chaganti (1981); 3, Pendergrass and Hanson (1976); 4, Sherman and Roizen (1976); 5, Allen *et al.* (1980); 6, Gold *et al.* (1978); 7, Clemmesen *et al.* (1974).

[b] Ratios of observed–expected cases in males and females, respectively.

biopsy scores in the folate-supplemented subjects were significantly better than in the unsupplemented controls (Fig. 1). The possibility that the dysplastic lesion may be arrested, and occasionally reversed, by oral folic acid supplements is indicated by these studies. It is worth noting that the natural course of dysplasia, as documented by Richart and Barron (1969), is toward progression to carcinoma. The rate of spontaneous regression from moderate dysplasia given by these authors is zero, compared to a regression of 4 out of 22 patients with moderate dysplasia who received the folate supplements in the study of Butterworth *et al.* (1982).

It is noteworthy that the average red cell folate level among the oral contraceptive users with dysplasia was at the lowest limit of normal, significantly below that of a control population not receiving oral contraceptions.

The impact of the contraceptive steroids upon the folate metabolism of its target tissues in humans remains unknown, but we have demonstrated profound changes in the folate content and in the activity of the

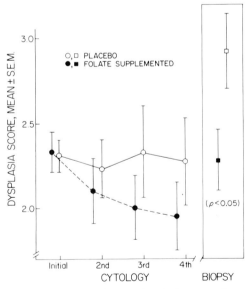

Fig. 1. Mean ± SEM cytology and biopsy dysplasia scores (1, negative; 2, mild dysplasia; 3, moderate dysplasia; 4, severe dysplasia; 5, carcinoma *in situ*) of oral contraceptive users with dysplasia of the uterine cervix receiving oral supplements of 10 mg folic acid or a placebo (10 mg ascorbic acid) daily for 3 months under double-blind conditions. Successive changes from the first visit at which time the protocol was initiated are shown. Follow-up smears for cytologic examination were obtained at monthly intervals. Biopsies were obtained at the end of the study. (From Butterworth *et al.,* 1982. © *Am. J. Clin. Nutr.* American Society for Clinical Nutrition.)

polyglutamate cleavage enzyme pteroylpoly-γ-glutamyl hydrolase of rat uterus during the normal estrous cycle (Krumdieck et al., 1976). Furthermore, similar changes could be elicited in ovariectomized rats by the administration of physiologic doses of estradiol-17β (Krumdieck et al., 1975).

E. Epidemiological Correlates

Epidemiologically, several disorders that lead to folate deficiency have been associated with increased cancer incidence. Thus, the incidence of carcinoma of the stomach in patients with pernicious anemia is about three times that found in the general population. Conversely, as many as 40% of patients with gastric carcinoma were found to have pernicious anemia when first diagnosed (Chanarin, 1979). Chronic and acute lymphocytic leukemia and myelocytic leukemia also occur with higher than expected frequency in pernicious anemia patients as do a variety of myeloproliferative disorders, primarily erythremia (Chanarin, 1979). Celiac disease, in which folate deficiency is almost always present (Dormandy et al., 1963; Grasbeck et al., 1961), is accompanied by the development of malignancy in 9 to 11% of cases (Holmes et al., 1976; Selby and Gallagher, 1979). Interestingly, esophageal carcinoma is often observed, as is the case among alcoholic and cirrhotic (Martinez, 1969; Steiner et al., 1959) patients in whom a history of folate deficiency is the rule (Blakley, 1969, p. 412). A remarkable overlap exists between the geographical distribution of Burkitt's lymphoma and malaria (Kafuko and Burkitt, 1970; Ziegler, 1981) which, perhaps more than any other hemolytic process, leads to folate deficiency (Blakley, 1969, p. 425; Strickland and Kostinas, 1970).

Furthermore, these same populations are often afflicted with high incidence of iron deficiency (due to intestinal parasitism and poor diets) which can cause a secondary folate deficiency (Velez et al., 1966) and mask its effects with a resultant underestimation of its prevalence (World Health Organization, 1972).

III. POSTULATED MECHANISMS BY WHICH FOLATE DEFICIENCY MAY FACILITATE NEOPLASTIC TRANSFORMATION

Folate coenzymes are required for two fundamental groups of reactions: (1) those involved in the remethylation of homocysteine to methionine and (2) those participating in the biosynthesis of the purine nucleotides and thymidylate. The former constitutes the sole source of *de novo* synthesis of methyl groups necessary to regenerate S-adenosylmethionine (SAM) to satisfy the constant demand for this very important coenzyme. The second group of folate-requiring reactions is essential for cell replication and DNA repair. As shown schematically in Fig. 2, these two groups of reactions can be seen as competing for the available folates of the cell. In folate deficiency, when the available folate cofactors do not satisfy the requirements of both groups of reactions, those reactions whose interruption poses a more immediate threat to the survival of the cell must be satisfied first. It now seems clear that maintenance of a normal rate of synthesis of SAM is given first priority in this metabolic competition. The supply of this coenzyme, required for more than 100 transmethylation reactions, is jealously protected. Its vital metabolic importance is obvious when considering only its role in the methylation of membrane phospholipids, required for the transmission of biological signals, as demonstrated by Hirata and Axelrod (1980). Inadequate biosynthesis of SAM should thus lead (among other things!) to severe malfunction of most, if not all, cellular membranes, posing an immediate threat to the survival of the organism. On the other hand, the

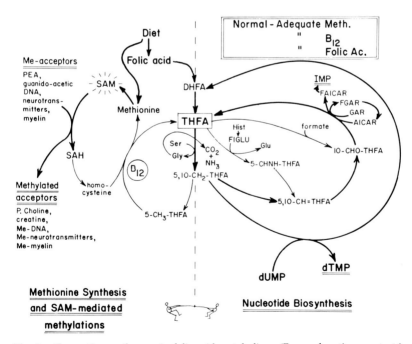

Fig. 2. Competing pathways in folic acid metabolism. (For explanation see text.)

interruption of nucleotide biosynthesis pathways does not pose an immediate threat to cell survival. Growth, and the replacement of rapidly turning over tissues would be delayed, but these are consequences that can be tolerated for considerable periods of time. Safeguarding the biosynthesis of SAM implies ensuring the supply of methionine. In the presence of an inadequate dietary supply of methionine, the levels of SAM drop (Scott and Weir, 1981), the enzyme 5,10-methylenetetrahydrofolate (5,10-CH_2-THFA) reductase, which is inhibited by SAM, is released from inhibition diverting the key folate intermediate 5,10-CH_2-THFA to the formation of 5-methyl tetrahydrofolate (5-CH_3-THFA) needed for the vitamin B_{12}-requiring methionine synthetase reaction. Essentially the same sequence of events occurs in response to choline and vitamin B_{12} deficiency, with the aggravating consequence in the latter case, that the folates accumulate in a form (5-CH_3-THFA) which cannot be utilized in the absence of vitamin B_{12}—the well-established folate trap of Herbert and Zalusky (1962) and Noronha and Silverman (1962). The shift in available folate coenzymes away from the pathways of nucleotide biosynthesis occurring in folate deficiency, vitamin B_{12} deficiency, or inadequate intake of methionine and/or choline, interferes primarily with the 5,10-CH_2-THFA-requiring conversion of deoxyuridylate (dUMP) to thymidylate (dTMP). It is known that the resulting "thymine starvation" produces DNA damage (Brozmanova and Sedliakova, 1980), affecting the regions with high AT base pair concentrations, and stalls its replication with the formation of partially single-stranded DNA (Andersen and Keiding, 1977). The genetic damage caused by thymine starvation leads to cell death, if extremely severe, and to the induction of mutations if the cell survives (Barclay and Little, 1978; Aizenberg et al., 1981).

A characteristic consequence of inhibition of dTMP synthesis is a very pronounced change in the relative pool sizes of intracellular deoxyuridine triphosphate (dUTP) and thymidine triphosphate (dTTP). The level of dTTP decreases to about 2% of the original amount, while the pool of dUTP expands by three orders of magnitude or more (Goulian et al., 1980). Under these circumstances, the mechanisms that normally prevent incorporation into DNA of dUMP in place of dTTP are overwhelmed, and uracil appears as a DNA component (Goulian et al., 1980; Sedwick et al., 1981; Luzzatto et al., 1981). We believe that the misincorporation of uracil in place of thymine in DNA is a molecular event closely related to the development of chromosomal aberrations, to the expression of folate-sensitive fragile sites, and to neoplastic transformation.

Replacement of thymine by uracil, although not interfering with the base pairing restrictions of DNA (Tye *et al.*, 1978), results in the loss of a methyl group (at position 5 of thymine) which normally appears in an exposed position in the major groove of the DNA double helix (Razin and Riggs, 1980). The methyl group of 5-methylcytosine (5-mCyt) also appears exposed in the major groove. It is now well established that loss of methyl groups in this key region, be it by conversion of 5-mCyt to cytosine or thymine to uracil, interferes with the binding of regulator proteins to DNA. Thus, it is known that changing only one nucleotide, the thymidylate at position 13 in the *lac* operator, to uracil or cytosine greatly decreases the affinity of the repressor protein for the operator (Fisher and Caruthers, 1979). Introduction of a 5-mCyt in place of the original thymine at position 13, although a mispairing, restores the missing methyl group, and with it, the affinity of the repressor for the operator gene.

The role of protein–DNA interactions in establishing the high degree of coiling and folding necessary to condense the extremely long DNA molecule to the small dimensions of a chromosome is well recognized (Razin and Riggs, 1980; Comings and Riggs, 1971). Allosteric proteins, which on binding to specific DNA sites undergo conformational changes that enable them to bind to each other to form loops of chromatin, were postulated as early as 1971 (Comings and Riggs, 1971). The role played by the 5-methyl group of thymine residues in determining both site recognition and binding of these chromosome "folding" proteins to certain DNA regions is unknown, but given the demonstrated role of the thymine methyl group in binding the *lac* repressor protein, it is reasonable to hypothesize that they, together with the methyl groups of 5-mCyt, play a very important role in the interaction of chromosome structural proteins with specific DNA sequences. Failure of these DNA–protein interactions could therefore result in both structural chromosomal damage and abnormal regulation of gene expression (Felsenfeld and McGhee, 1982; Johnson, 1982; Mohandas *et al.*, 1981).

If *vis-à-vis* cytosine and 5-mCyt, we think of thymine as 5-methyluracil (5-mUra), we can, instead of considering 5-mCyt as the only methylated base in DNA, state that all the uracil residues of DNA are methylated at the 5 position. The DNA–protein interactions that these methyl groups would make possible may well represent the *raison d'être* for the exclusive presence of thymine in DNA. The spacing of the methyl groups of 5-mCyt and 5-mUra (thymine) exposed along the major groove may constitute a binary code whose function would be to specify protein–DNA interactions while participating at the same time in protein–DNA binding. The DNA molecule would thus be seen as containing a double code, the familiar nucleotide triplet-based genetic code stipulating the nucleotide sequences of messenger RNA, and a binary methyl–nonmethyl code required for directing interactions with specific regulatory and structural proteins.

In all of the above, a crucial role is assigned to the methyl groups of thymine in the stabilization of chromosomal structure; this view is supported by the fact that thymidine supplementation inhibits fragile X expression promoted either by 5-FUdR or by folate deficiency. Also, the fact that the halogenated analog 5-bromodeoxyuridine (5-BUdR) inhibits expression of the fragile X points to the importance of the methyl group for thymine. The 5-BUdR with its bulky bromine atom (van der Waals radius 1.95 Å), closely approaching the dimensions of the methyl group of thymine (2.00 Å), is known to be incorporated into DNA mimicking the natural thymine. It is therefore extremely interesting to note that the same factors that induce and prevent expression of folate-sensitive fragile chromosomal sites also induce and prevent neoplastic transformation of C3H/10T1/2CL8 cells *in vitro* (Table IX). A conspicuous gap in the table is the effect of folic acid deficiency on transformation, which to this author's knowledge has never been investigated. The data in Table IX, in particular the protective effects of thymidine and 5-BUdR, strongly support the idea that damage to the proposed methyl-based binary second coding system of DNA may be a significant factor in carcinogenesis. We believe that the expression of fragile chromosomal sites elicited by folate deprivation represents an easily demonstrable example of a general mechanism of DNA damage of far reaching biological significance.

One of the better documented consequences of folic acid deficiency is prolongation of the cell cycle, affecting primarily the S phase and accumulating cells in prophase. These should result in an increased subpopulation of cells that should be more susceptible to the attack of tumor

TABLE IX

Factors Affecting the Expression of Fragile Chromosomal Sites and Neoplastic Transformation of C3H/10T1/2CL8 Cells

Factor[a]	Fragile site expression[b]	Transformation
FA⁻	↑	?
MTX	↑	↑
FUdR	↑	↑
Thymidine	↓	↓
BUdR	↓	↓

[a] FA⁻, folic acid deficiency; MTX, methotrexate; FUdR, 5-fluorodeoxyuridine; BUdR, 5-bromodeoxyuridine.
[b] ↑, increased; ↓, decreased.

initiating agents. This notion is strongly supported by the experiments of Berenblum and Armuth (1977) using colchicine as a means of causing accumulation of cells in metaphase prior to the administration of a single initiating dose of urethane. Mice injected with colchicine 5 and 9 hours before urethane initiation showed a significant increase ($P<0.001$) in skin tumor incidence in the 9-hour group, and an increase in percentage malignancy in both the 5-hour ($P<0.001$) and the 9-hour groups. These two time periods corresponded to the approximate peak of metaphase arrest. The concept that susceptibility to initiation is augmented by stimulation of cell division is well established (Pound and Withers, 1963; Scherer and Emmelot, 1975a,b, 1976) and implicitly carries the notion that initiation itself occurs either during a mitotic cycle or during preparation for it. There is at present no agreement about the exact phase of the cell cycle when initiation takes place, and it is indeed likely that different carcinogens may exert their effects at different stages of the cycle. In support of our hypothesis are the works of Frei and Ritchie (1964), Marquardt (1974), and Jones et al. (1976), who believe that it is during the S phase, i.e., the time of DNA replication prolonged by folate deficiency, that initiation occurs.

Figure 3 presents schematically the proposed increased susceptibility

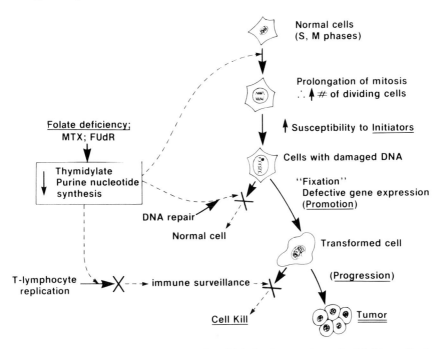

Fig. 3. Three proposed mechanisms by which the decrease in nucleotide biosynthesis resulting from folate deficiency may facilitate neoplastic transformation (see text).

to initiation brought about by folate deficiency. It also shows two additional mechanisms which may facilitate neoplastic transformation in folate deficiency. The first is by impeding normal DNA repair and the second by interfering with the normal processes of immune surveillance. The effects of folate deficiency on DNA repair have not been described. It stands to reason, however, that, in the presence of defective synthesis of purine nucleotides and thymidylate, DNA repair mechanisms requiring the reconstruction of long DNA segments should malfunction. The extent of DNA damage inflicted by initiating agents (i.e., alkylating compounds), enhanced in folate deficiency by the mechanism discussed above, would be compounded by an increased persistence of the lesion. Both of these factors (extent and persistence) correlate well with the incidence of tumor development in animals treated with alkylating agents (Pegg and Nicoll, 1976; Kleihues and Margison, 1974; Nicoll *et al.*, 1975).

Finally, the function of the immune system as a defense mechanism against oncogenic viruses and/or newly arising transformed cells should be severely impaired in folate deficiency. The decreased synthesis of nucleotides should prevent the rapid proliferation of sensitized cells needed for an appropriate immune response. A number of studies, reviewed by Nauss and Newberne (1981), indicate a defective cell-mediated immune function, and possibly a reduction in humoral immunity as well, in folate deficiency. Decreased numbers of T cells, decreased cytotoxic activity against foreign transplanted cells, and decreased stimulation of T lymphocytes by phytohemagglutinin have all been found in folate deficient rats.

IV. SUMMARY

In summary, a number of nonmutually exclusive mechanisms seem to operate in folate deficient cells to (1) produce structural chromosomal damage and possible disregulation of gene expression, (2) increase the extent of DNA damage by environmental carcinogens, (3) impede or retard DNA repair, and (4) decrease the immune surveillance against transformed cells and/or oncogenic viruses. We propose that, alone or in combination, these mechanisms facilitate the development of neoplasias in the folate deficient tissues.

REFERENCES

Aizenberg, O. A., Naumova, L. A., and Fradkin, G. E. (1981). Part V. *Genetika (Moscow)* **17**, 996–999.

Allen, R. W., Buchler, B., Ogden, B., Bentley, F. G., and Jung, A. L. (1980). *Pediatr. Res.* **14**, 530.

Andersen, H. A., and Keiding, J. (1977). *Carlsberg Res. Commun.* **42**, 153–161.

Bailey, L. B., Wagner, P. A., Christakis, G. J., Araujo, P. E., Appledorf, H., Davis, C. G., Masteryanni, J., and Dinning, J. S. (1979). *Am. J. Clin. Nutr.* **32**, 2346–2353.

Bailey, L. B., Mahan, C. S., and Dimperio, D. (1980). *Am. J. Clin. Nutr.* **33**, 1997–2001.

Barclay, B. J., and Little, J. G. (1978). *Mol. Gen. Genet* **160**, 33–40.

Benedict, W. F., Banarjee, A., Gardner, A., and Jones, P. A. (1977). *Cancer Res.* **37**, 2202–2208.

Berenblum, I., and Armuth, V. (1977). *Br. J. Cancer* **35**, 615–620.

Blakley, R. L. (1969). "The Biochemistry of Folic Acid and Related Pteridines." Wiley, New York.

Branda, R. F., Moldow, C. F., MacArthur, J. R., Wintrobe, M. M., Anthony, B. K., and Jacob, H. S. (1978). *N. Engl. J. Med.* **298**, 469–475.

Brozmanova, J., and Sedliakova, M. (1980). *J. Gen. Microbiol.* **119**, 527–533.

Buehring, Y. S. S., Poirier, L. A., and Stokstad, E. L. R. (1976). *Cancer Res.* **36**, 2775–2779.

Butterworth, C. E., Jr., Hatch, K. D., Gore, H., Mueller, H., and Krumdieck, C. L. (1982). *Am. J. Clin. Nutr.* **35**, 73–82.

Calabresi, P., and Parks, R. E., Jr. (1980). *In* "The Pharmacological Basis of Therapeutics" (A. G. Gilman, L. S. Goodman, A. Gilman, S. E. Mayer, and K. L. Melmon, eds.), 6th ed., p. 1276. Macmillan, New York.

Chanarin, I. (1979). "The Megaloblastic Anemias," 2nd ed., pp. 332–350. Blackwell, Oxford.

Chung, C. K., Stryker, J. A., Cruse, R., Vannuci, R., and Towfighi, J. (1981).*Cancer* **47**, 2563–2566.

Clemmesen, J., Fuglsang-Frederiksen, V., and Plum, C. M. (1974). *Lancet* **1**, 705–707.

Colman, N. (1977). *Adv. Nutr. Res.* **1**, 77–124.

Comings, D. E., and Riggs, A. D. (1971). *Nature (London)* **233**, 48–50.

Copeland, D. H., and Salmon, W. D. (1946). *Am. J. Pathol.* **22**, 1059–1079.

Das, K. C., and Herbert, V. (1978). *Br. J. Haematol.* **38**, 219–233.

Dormandy, K. M., Waters, A. H., and Molin, D. L. (1963). *Lancet* **1**, 632–635.

Ehrenbard, L. T., and Chaganti, R. S. K. (1981). *Lancet* **2**, 97.

Farber, S., Diamond, L. K., Mercer, R. D., Sylvester, R. F., and Woeff, V. J. (1948). *N. Engl. J. Med.* **238**, 787–793.

Felsenfeld, G., and McGhee, J. (1982). *Nature (London)* **296**, 602–603.

Fisher, E. F., and Caruthers, M. H. (1979). *Nucleic Acids Res.* **7**, 401–416.

Fonatsch, C. (1981). *Hum. Genet.* **59**, 186.

Frei, J. V., and Ritchie, A. C. (1964). *JNCI, J. Natl. Cancer Inst.* **32**, 1213–1220.

Glover, T. W. (1981). *Am. J. Hum. Genet.* **33**, 234–242.

Gold, E., Gordis, L., Tonascia, J., and Szklo, M. (1978). *JNCI, J. Natl. Cancer Inst.* **61**, 1031–1034.

Goulian, M., Bleile, B., and Tseng, B. Y. (1980). *Proc. Natl. Acad. Sci. U.S.A.* **77**, 1956–1960.

Grasbeck, R., Bjorksten, F., and Nyberg, W. (1961). *Nord. Med., NM* **66**, 1343–1348.

Hecht, F., Jacky, P. B., and Sutherland, G. R. (1982). *Am. J. Med. Genet.* **11**, 489–495.

Herbert, V., and Zalusky, R. (1962). *J. Clin. Invest.* **41**, 1263–1276.

Herman, C., Andersen, E., and Videbaek, A. (1980). *Scand. J. Haematol.* **24**, 234–236.

Hertz, R. (1963). *Ann. Intern. Med.* **59**, 931–956.

Hertz, R., Ross, G. T., and Lipsett, M. B. (1963). *Am. J. Obstet. Gynecol.* **86**, 808–814.

Hirata, F., and Axelrod, J. (1980). *Science* **209**, 1082–1090.

Holmes, G. K. T., Stokes, P. L., Sorahan, T. M., Prior, P., Waterhouse, J. A. H., and Cooke, W. T. (1976). *Gut* **17**, 612–619.

Johnson, M. H. (1982). *Nature (London)* **296**, 493–494.

Jones, P. A., Benedict, W. F., Baker, M. S., Mondal, S., Rapp, U., and Heidelberger, C. (1976). *Cancer Res.* **36**, 101–107.

Kafuko, G. W., and Burkitt, D. P. (1970). *Int. J. Cancer* **6**, 1–9.

Kleihues, P., and Margison, G. P. (1974). *JNCI, J. Natl. Cancer Inst.* **53**, 1839–1841.

Krumdieck, C. L., Boots, L. R., Cornwell, P. E., and Butterworth, C. E., Jr. (1975). *Am. J. Clin. Nutr.* **28**, 530–534.

Krumdieck, C. L., Boots, L. R., Cornwell, P. E., and Butterworth, C. E., Jr. (1976). *Am. J. Clin. Nutr.* **29**, 288–294.

Luzatto, L., Falusi, A. O., and Joju, E. A. (1981). *N. Engl. J. Med.* **305**, 1156–1157.

Marquardt, H. (1974). *Cancer Res.* **34**, 1612–1615.

Martinez, I. (1969). *JNCI, J. Natl. Cancer Inst.* **42**, 1069–1094.

Mattei, M. G., Mattei, J. F., Vidal, I., and Giraud, F. (1981). *Hum. Genet.* **59**, 166–169.

Menzies, R. C., Crossen, P. E., Fitzgerald, P. H., and Gunz, F. W. (1966). *Blood* **28**, 581–594.

Mohandas, T., Sparkes, R. S., and Shapiro, L. J. (1981). *Science* **211**, 393–396.

Nauss, K. M., and Newberne, P. M. (1981). *Adv. Exp. Med. Biol.* **135**, 63–91.

Nelson, M. M., Wright, H. V., Asling, C. W., and Evans, H. M. (1955). *J. Nutr.* **56**, 349–369.

Newberne, P. M., Rogers, A. E., and Wogan, G. N. (1968). *J. Nutr.* **94**, 331–343.

Nicoll, J. W., Swann, P. F., and Pegg, A. E. (1975). *Nature (London)* **254**, 261–262.

Noronha, J. M., and Silverman, M. (1962). *Eur. Symp. Vitam. B_{12} Intrinsic Factor, 2nd, 1962* p. 728.

Pegg, A. E., and Nicoll, J. W. (1976). *In* "Screening Tests in Chemical Carcinogenesis" (R. Montesano, H. Bartsch, and H. Tomatis, eds.), pp. 571–590. Lyon.

Pendergrass, T. W., and Hanson, J. W. (1976). *Lancet* **2**, 150.

Peraino, C., Fry, R. J. M., and Staffeldt, E. (1973). *JNCI, J. Natl. Cancer Inst.* **51**, 1349–1350.

Pitot, H. C., and Sirica, A. E. (1980). *Biochim. Biophys. Acta* **605**, 191–215.

Pound, A. W., and Withers, H. R. (1963). *Br. J. Cancer* **17**, 460–470.

Razin, A., and Riggs, A. D. (1980). *Science.* **210**, 604–610.

Richart, R. M., and Barron, B. A. (1969). *Am. J. Obstet. Gynecol.* **105**, 386–393.

Rogers, A. E. (1975). *Cancer Res.* **35**, 2469–2474.

Rogers, A. E. (1977). *Cancer Res.* **37**, 194–199.

Rogers, A. E., and Newberne, P. M. (1973a). *Am. J. Pathol.* **73**, 817–820.

Rogers, A. E., and Newberne, P. M. (1973b). *Nature (London)* **246**, 491–492.

Rogers, A. E., and Newberne, P. M. (1975). *Cancer Res.* **35**, 3427–3431.

Rogers, A. E., Sanchez, O., Feinsod, F. M., and Newberne, P. M. (1974). *Cancer Res.* **34**, 96–99.

Rogers, A. E., Lenhart, G., and Morrison, G. (1980). *Cancer Res.* **40**, 2802–2807.

Ruymann, F. B., Mosijczuk, A. D., and Sayers, R. J. (1977). *JAMA, J. Am. Med. Assoc.* **238**, 2631–2633.

Scherer, E., and Emmelot, P. (1975a). *Eur. J. Cancer* **11**, 145–154.

Scherer, E., and Emmelot, P. (1975b). *Eur. J. Cancer* **11**, 689–696.

Scherer, E., and Emmelot, P. (1976). *Cancer Res.* **36**, 2544–2554.

Scott, J. M., and Weir, D. G. (1981). *Lancet* **2**, 337–340.

Sedwick, W. D., Kutler, M., and Brown, O. E. (1981). *Proc. Natl. Acad. Sci. U.S.A.* **78**, 917–921.

Selby, W. S., and Gallaher, N. D. (1979). *Dig. Dis. Sci.* [N.S.] **24**, 684–688.

Sherman, S., and Roizen, N. (1976). *Lancet* **2**, 517.

Shinozuka, H., Katyal, S. L., and Lombardi, B. (1978). *Int. J. Cancer* **22**, 36–39.

Shklar, G., Cataldo, E., and Fitzgerald, A. L. (1966). *Cancer Res.* **26,** 2218–2224.

Sieber, S. M., and Adamson, R. H. (1975). *Adv. Cancer Res.* **22,** 57–155.

Smith, D. B., and Obbens, E.A.M.T. (1979). *In* "Folic Acid in Neurology, Psychiatry, and Internal Medicine" (M. I. Botez and E. H. Reynolds, eds), p. 267–283. Raven Press, New York.

Steiner, P. E., Camain, R., and Netik, J. (1959). *Cancer Res.* **19,** 567–580.

Strickland, G. T., and Kostinas, J. E. (1970). *Am. J. Trop. Med. Hyg.* **19,** 910–915.

Sutherland, G. R. (1977). *Science* **197,** 265–266.

Sutherland, G. R. (1979). *Am. J. Hum. Genet.* **31,** 125–135.

Thenen, S. W. (1979). *Nutr. Rep. Int.* **19,** 267–274.

Thenen, S. W., and Stokstad, E. L. R. (1973). *J. Nutr.* **103,** 363–370.

Tuma, D. J., Barak, A. J., and Sorrell, M. F. (1975). *Biochem. Pharmacol.* **24,** 1327–1331.

Tye, B. K., Chien, J., Lehman, I. R., Duncan, B. K., and Warner, H. R. (1978). *Proc. Natl. Acad. Sci. U.S.A.* **75,** 233–237.

Velez, H., Restrepo, A., Vitale, J. J., and Hellerstein, E. E. (1966). *Am. J. Clin. Nutr.* **19,** 27–36.

Voorhees, J. J., Janzen, M. K., Harrell, E. R., and Chakrabarti, S. G. (1969). *Arch. Dermatol.* **100,** 269–274.

Whitehead, N., Reyner, F., and Lindenbaum, J. (1973). *JAMA, J. Am. Med. Assoc.* **226,** 1421–1424.

World Health Organization. (1972). "Nutritional Anaemias," Report of a WHO Group of Experts. W. H. O. Tech. Rep. Ser. No. 503. WHO, Geneva.

Ziegler, J. L. (1981). *N. Engl. J. Med.* **305,** 735–745.

15

Choline, Methionine, and Related Factors in Oncogenesis

Paul M. Newberne, Adrianne E. Rogers,† and Kathleen M. Nauss**
*Laboratory of Nutritional Pathology**
Department of Nutrition and Food Science†
Massachusetts Institute of Technology
Cambridge, Massachusetts

I. INTRODUCTION

Lipotropes are an important class of nutrients, major components of which are choline, methionine, vitamin B_{12}, and

247

Nutrition Factors in the Induction
and Maintenance of Malignancy

folic acid. These nutrients are essential to many metabolic processes, especially the synthesis of DNA, nucleoproteins, and membranes, all of which are required for cell proliferation and the maintenance of tissue integrity. The lipotropic nutrients interact extensively with each other and with other nutrients in supply and metabolism of one carbon units.

Choline and folic acid are plentiful in both animal and plant foods, but plants are low in methionine and do not contain vitamin B_{12}. Animal products and microorganisms are the sole dietary sources of vitamin B_{12}.

Among the four nutrients, only vitamin B_{12} is stored in the body for any length of time (from 3 to 6 years after intake of the vitamin ceases). Methionine, an essential amino acid, is not present in its free state, but exists as a structural unit of protein and, in its activated form, S-adenosylmethionine (SAM). It is available from body protein only during the catabolic (breakdown) phase of metabolism. Stores of folic acid last no more than a few months after intake ceases, and choline, as such, lasts only a few days or at most, a few weeks. Like methionine, it can be derived from tissue breakdown, since it is a major component of cell membranes. Thus a dietary deficiency of any or all of these nutrients is a potential continuous threat to health. Diminution of the pool of methyl groups may contribute to susceptibility to many diseases, including cancer.

A significant amount of research has shown that rats fed diets deficient in lipotropes are more susceptible to development of liver cancer induced by a wide variety of natural synthetic carcinogens (Rogers and Newberne, 1980). Lipotrope deficiency influences the hepatic activation or detoxification of xenobiotics including carcinogens, but the direction and magnitude of the effect vary. The deficiency also significantly increases hepatocyte cell division.

Animal studies have demonstrated that lipotrope deficiency leads to impaired immunocompetence; the severity of the impairment depends on the age of the animal and the adequacy of other nutrients in the diet (Nauss and Newberne, 1981). Increased susceptibility to bacterial and parasitic infections has been observed in folate-deficient rats (Kumar and Axelrod, 1978; Williams *et al.*, 1975) and guinea pigs (Thenen, 1978; Haltalin *et al.*, 1970). In offspring of animals fed diets deficient in methionine and choline during gestation and lactation, there are atrophy of lymphoid tissue, diminished response of lymphocytes to mitogens, and increased susceptibility to infectious disease (Newberne and Wilson, 1972; Newberne *et al.*, 1970; Gebhardt and Newberne, 1974).

Thus, animal studies suggest that lipotropes are involved in the activation or deactivation of carcinogens (Campbell *et al.*, 1978; Rogers and

Newberne, 1975) and may alter immunosurveillance for tumor cells (Nauss and Newberne, 1981). These two areas of research related to susceptibility to cancer will be more fully explored following a review of lipotrope deficiency and its influence on the development of cancer in rodents.

II. LIPOTROPE DEFICIENCY, CIRRHOSIS, AND HEPATOCARCINOMA

The lipotrope-deficient model for study of experimental carcinogenesis emerged from studies designed to examine the effects of nutrient interactions on the liver and on other organs and tissues (Allan et al., 1924; György and Goldblatt, 1942; Best et al., 1932; Best and Huntsman, 1932; Bliss, 1982). Rats maintained on choline-deficient diets for long periods of time developed hepatocellular carcinomas, an observation that attracted widespread attention since it was the only case in which omission of a substance from the diet, rather than addition of one, resulted in neoplasia. Hepatocellular carcinoma, associated with choline deficiency, appeared to result when, over time, the deficit of lipotropes produced a series of sequential alterations including fatty liver, parenchymal cell hyperplasia, fibrosis, cirrhosis, and ultimately, liver cancer.

Salmon and colleagues reported a significant incidence of hepatocarcinomas in deficient rats during many years of experimental work (Salmon and Copeland, 1954; Salmon et al., 1954; Schaefer et al., 1950; Salmon and Newberne, 1963). However, after several years it was noted that the incidence of hepatocarcinoma was lower than observed in earlier years even though experimental conditions, including the peanut meal diets, were apparently the same. Various steps in procedures used to induce cirrhosis were examined in great detail, but an explanation for the decreased tumor incidence was not found.

One change that coincided with the decline in hepatocellular tumor incidence was the inclusion in the diets of antimicrobial agents (tetracyclines and sulfonamides) to reduce infectious diseases endemic to the breeding colony. An ameliorating effect of antibiotics on choline deficiency had been cited earlier by György (1954), and the subsequent work of Salmon and Newberne (1962) showed that certain antibiotics did indeed reduce the severity of the acute lesions of choline deficiency. These studies were not of sufficient duration, however, to determine if the antibiotics might influence tumor incidence.

Additional studies confirmed that choline deficiency was associated with a significant incidence of hepatocellular carcinoma in rats. However, in some groups given the same diet supplemented with choline, there also were significant numbers of animals with liver neoplasms (Salmon and Newberne, 1963). This observation raised the question of whether tumor induction required more than the dietary deficiency which led to cirrhosis and concurrent cancer. Subsequent studies indicated that an alcohol-soluble contaminant in the peanut meal diet was responsible for the liver tumors and that deficient rats were more sensitive to the contaminant. A series of investigations suggested that the peanut meal contained the carcinogen. Shortly afterward our laboratory at Massachusetts Institute of Technology (MIT) identified aflatoxins in the peanut meal as the etiologic agents for the hepatocellular carcinoma in choline-deficient rats (Newberne *et al.*, 1964). Furthermore, it was clearly shown, using diets with a protein source exclusively from purified amino acids, that choline deficiency alone did not result in hepatocellular tumors. Fatty, nodular, hyperplastic, cirrhotic livers but no neoplasms resulted from uncomplicated choline deficiency (Newberne *et al.*, 1969). We have continued research in this laboratory on the effects of lipotrope deficiency, other dietary insults, and surgical injury on the susceptibility of the liver to carcinogenesis (Rogers and Newberne, 1980; Newberne *et al.*, 1982; Newberne and Clark, 1982).

This chapter will review the development of hepatic cirrhosis in the rat and the evidence for a greater susceptibility of the deficient liver to chemically induced hepatocarcinogenesis. Further, we shall summarize the evidence demonstrating that choline deficiency alone increases DNA synthesis and hepatocellular turnover with formation of hyperplastic nodules, but that such lesions in rats apparently do not progress to cancer unless a carcinogen is superimposed. Numerous recent publications have reported the interrelationship of choline deficiency, increased cell proliferation, and the development of liver tumors (Abanobi *et al.*, 1982; Newberne and Clark, 1982; Newberne *et al.*, 1966; Rogers and Newberne, 1980).

In contrast to results in the rat, choline deficiency injury to the mouse liver enhances the development of nodules and tumors in the absence of any known carcinogen treatment. Results of theses studies are described elsewhere (Newberne and Clark, 1982; Newberne *et al.*, 1982).

A. Severe Lipotrope Deficiency, Cirrhosis, and Liver Tumors in Rats

A number of strains of outbred and inbred rats have been used for investigations of cirrhosis and its relationship to sensitivity of the liver to carcinogenesis. All strains that have been used are sensitive to the deficiency and its enhancing effects on chemically induced cancer, but there is some variability in degree of sensitivity. Generally, the rats have been fed a choline-free diet (Table I) from weaning until cirrhosis develops, a period of time ranging from 200 to 500 days. In this animal model it is important that the rats be fed the diet continuously from weaning until the study is terminated; starting the diet at a later period does not induce cirrhosis. There often are deaths from the hemorrhagic kidney syndrome induced by choline deficiency between days 8 and 10 following initiation of the dietary treatment; beyond that time the clinical course is uneventful.

The development of cirrhosis proceeds through a series of histologically identifiable changes beginning with fat accumulation, first in the centrilobular zone then throughout the lobules, followed by development of fibrosis, and ultimately cirrhosis (Figs. 1–3). These changes have been documented and illustrated in many publications (Best et al., 1932; Best and Huntsman, 1932; Bliss, 1982; Doll and Peto, 1981; duVigneaud, 1952; Copeland and Salmon, 1946).

Using purified amino acids as a source of protein, in order to preclude the possibility of contamination by carcinogens, in particular aflatoxin,

TABLE I

Diets Used in Lipotrope Studies

	Feed content (gm/kg)			
	Diet 1 control	2 Deficient	3 Control	4 Marginal deficient
Casein	60	60	0	0
Peanut meal	250	250	0	0
Soy protein isolate	0	0	180	182
Corn starch	0	0	236	236
Sucrose	467	470	428	428
Vitamin mix[a]	20	20	18	18
Mineral mix	50	50	45	45
Fat	150	150	90	90
Choline	3	0	3	1
Vitamin B_{12}	50μg	0	50μg	50μg

[a] Vitamin mix complete except for folic acid in folate deficiency studies, and choline and vitamin B_{12} which were added at time of mixing the diet.

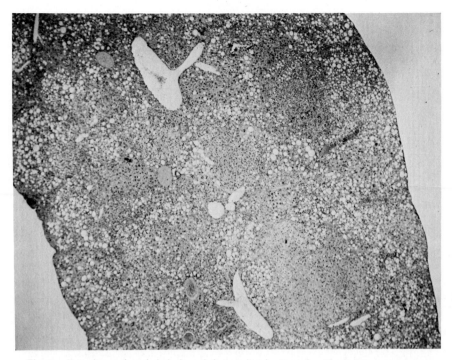

Fig. 1. Fatty liver of rat fed choline-deficient diet for 7 weeks. The lipid accumulation, which began in the centrilobular zone, is distributed fairly uniformly throughout the lobule in the entire lobe. Hematoxylin and eosin. × 40.

we showed that cirrhosis developed in the same way as in livers of rats fed the peanut meal diet, and that none of them progressed to liver carcinoma (Newberne *et al.*, 1969) unless a carcinogen was superimposed. The amino acid mixtures replacing the intact protein were based on the amino acid composition of casein or on amino acid diets previously shown to result in normal growth rate in rats. The livers of the choline-deficient rats had significant lipid accumulation after 10 weeks and fibrosis, progressing to cirrhosis, beginning after 4 months on the diet. Liver lipids reached a maximum of 69% of the dry weight, with triglyceride accounting for the bulk of the increase; cholesterol and phospholipids also significantly increased in the liver. All three of the lipid fractions decreased in the serum of the deficient rats, a characteristic finding in lipotrope deficiency since lipid secretion by the liver is abnormal under these conditions. The chemical and morphological findings in these studies indicated that fatty nutritional cirrhosis, characteristic of choline deficiency and identical to that induced with intact proteins, was induced with the purified L-amino acids diets and, further, that cirrhosis did not progress to carcinoma of the liver. Over the same period we performed experiments that confirmed the increased susceptibility to aflatoxin hepatocarcinogenesis in choline-deficient, cirrhotic rats (Fig. 4) (Table II) (Newberne *et al.*, 1966). We then begin investigations of mechanisms by which the deficiency might influence carcinogenesis.

In the choline-deficient rat (Fig. 5), as liver fat increases, the number of cells labeled by [³H]thymidine also increases (Newberne, *et al.*, 1982). This indicates increased DNA synthesis and suggests increased cell turnover, both of which are essential components of hyperplasia of the liver parenchyma. Other studies in our laboratories (Table III) gave further evidence of a relationship between choline deficiency, fatty liver, and parenchymal cell proliferation. These data taken from work done in collaboration with H. L. Leffert (Salk Institute) indicate that decreased serum very low density lipoprotein (VLDL) content is associated with

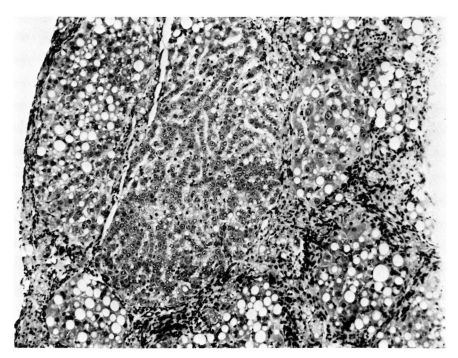

Fig. 2. Liver of rat fed choline-deficient diet for 12 weeks. Fat, fibrosis, and parenchymal cell hyperplasia are characteristic of this stage of liver injury. Hematoxylin and eosin. × 100.

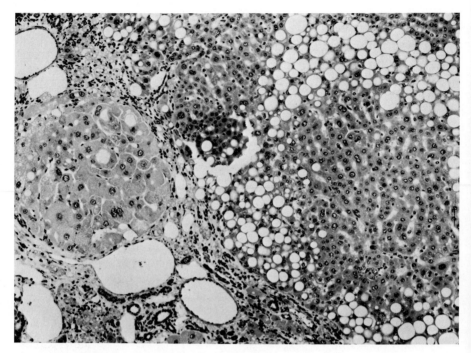

Fig. 3.   Bridging fibrosis, bile duct and vascular hyperplasia, lipid accumulation, nodular hyperplasia of the parenchyma, and varying degree of hepatitis are all represented in this illustration of the cirrhotic liver of a rat fed a choline-deficient diet for 29 weeks. Hematoxylin and eosin. × 200.

increased hepatic DNA synthesis. Partial hepatectomy as well as choline deficiency lower VLDL, and both turn on DNA synthesis and cell proliferation. The results are consistent with the reports of other investigations summarized in a recent paper (Newberne and Thurman, 1981) in which it had been shown clearly that lipids are important to the maintenance and control of cell proliferation.

Chemical induction of hepatocarcinoma is governed in part by the level of DNA synthesis in hepatocytes at the time of carcinogen exposure and also following exposure. Several models have been described and are being used to explore biochemical and morphological aspects of this relationship. It seems likely that it can be used to explain at least part of the enhancement of hepatocarcinogenesis of choline deficiency, but the nature of the effects is unclear.

Shinozuka and colleagues have published on studies that raise questions about the significance of cell division in this relationship. They

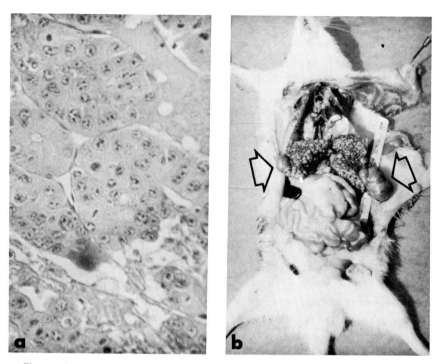

Fig. 4. Liver of rat fed choline-deficient diet and exposed to a carcinogenic level (1 ppm) of aflatoxin B_1 in the diet for 14 months. (a) is typical of the trabecular form of hepatocellular carcinoma associated with aflatoxin and other hepatocellular carcinogens superimposed on the deficient liver. Hematoxylin and eosin. × 400. (b) illustrates the gross appearance of the cirrhotic liver with several nodules (arrows) of liver cancer.

TABLE II

Cirrhosis and Aflatoxin (AFB$_1$) Effects on Liver Tumor Induction in Rats[a]

| | | Liver lesions | |
Treatment	Average days on study	Cirrhosis	Tumors
Control	422 ± 0	0/10	0/10
Cirrhogenic diet	418 ± 85	13/13	0/13
Control diet + AFB$_1$	360 ± 30	0/10	5/10
Cirrhogenic diet + AFB$_1$	426 ± 54	10/10	8/10
Cirrhogenic diet to cirrhosis, then AFB$_1$	390 ± 82	8/9	7/9

[a] From Newberne *et al.* (1966).

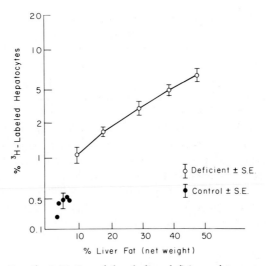

Fig. 5. Following the initiation of the choline deficiency fat accumulates in the liver with time. As fat increases, there is a parallel increase in [³H]thymidine labeling (increased DNA synthesis) and cell proliferation.

found that increase in preneoplastic changes in the deficient liver was not correlated with cell division. The level of cell proliferation in deficient livers was decreased by feeding phenobarbital, but appearance of preneoplastic lesions was unchanged (Shinozuka and Lombardi, 1980; Shinozuka *et al.*, 1982). Second, reducing the amount of fat in the deficient diet reduced the number of preneoplastic lesions without altering hepatocyte hyperplasia. Both alterations of the model must be confirmed in carcinogenesis studies, since the significance of the preneoplastic lesions to liver cell cancer is not clear and a linkage has not been established as yet. The result of the study in which lower fat

TABLE III

Effect of Lipotrope Deficiency on Hepatocyte DNA Synthesis and Serum VLDL in Weanling Rats[a]

Diet	DNA synthesis[b]	Serum VLDL[b]
Control	0.5–4	75
Marginal lipotrope	1–9	50
Low lipotrope	5–20	25

[a] From Newberne and Rogers (1976).
[b] Expressed in arbitrary units as an index of DNA synthesis and concentration of VLDL.

content was fed is particularly interesting, since reduction of dietary fat content reduces the severity of lipotrope deficiency and would be expected to reduce both hepatic fat and DNA synthesis. Neither occurred in this experiment. Further using the same carcinogen, N-nitrosodiethylamine (DEN), we found that lipotrope and lipid effects interacted but in a complex way in final tumor incidence which has not been fully elucidated (Rogers and Newberne, 1980).

Studies conducted earlier in our laboratory on aflatoxin (AFB_1) hepatocarcinogenesis in rats with increased DNA synthesis induced by partial hepatectomy also raised questions about the significance of cell division for carcinogenesis in the lipotrope-deficient model. We found no effect of partial hepatectomy on tumor incidence when the carcinogen AFB_1 was administered at different time points with respect to partial hepatectomy (Rogers et al., 1971).

B. Marginal Deficiency of Lipotropes and Hepatocarcinoma in Rats

In the course of extensive studies conducted with acute and chronic lipotrope deficiencies in rats we observed that it was not necessary to feed a diet sufficiently deficient to induce cirrhosis in order to enhance carcinogenesis. A diet that was only marginal in lipotropes induced fatty liver only (not cirrhosis); it also significantly enhanced the induction of liver cancer by several carcinogens (Rogers and Newberne, 1969). Table IV is a compilation of data from a large series of studies with rats fed marginal lipotrope diets; Fig. 6 illustrates clearly the enhancing effect of marginal diets on three different hepatocarcinogens. Deficient animals developed hepatocarcinoma in higher incidence and after a shorter latent period than animals fed a nutritionally complete diet.

The deficient diets are characterized by high fat content and marginal levels of certain essential amino acids, in addition to their deficiency of lipotropes. The relative importance of these factors in carcinogenesis varies with the carcinogen used to study them. Activity of N-2-fluorenylacetamide (AAF), a carcinogen used in many of the modeling studies cited above, is profoundly affected by choline and methionine but not detectably influenced by dietary fat content, but AFB_1 and DEN results are affected. Tumor induction varies considerably and yield complex results showing effects of lipotropes, amino acids and fat, all of which interact in determining the final tumor data with these carcinogens (Table IV).

In a few cases, lipotrope-deficient diets affected tumor incidence in target organs other than liver. N-nitrosodiethylamine is carcinogenic for

TABLE IV

Chemical Carcinogenesis in Lipotrope Deficiency[a]

	Tumor site	Tumor incidence (%)	
Carcinogen[b]		Control	Deprived
AFB_1	Liver	15	87
DEN	Liver	70	80
DBN	Liver	24	64
	Bladder	84	80
DMN	Liver	28	27
	Kidney	16	3
AAF	Liver	19	41
	Mammary	80	79
FANFT	Bladder	53	61
DMBA	Mammary	48	15
DMH	Colon	86	100

[a] From Rogers and Newberne (1980).
[b] AFB_1, aflatoxin B_1; DEN, *N*-nitrosodiethylamine; DBN, *N*-nitrosodibutylamine; DMN, nitrosodimethylamine; AAF, *N*-2-Fluorenylacetamine; FANFT, *N*-[4-(5-nitro-2-furyl)-2-thiazolyl] formamide; DMBA, 7,12-dimethylbenz[a]anthracene; DMH, 1,2-dimethylhydrazine.

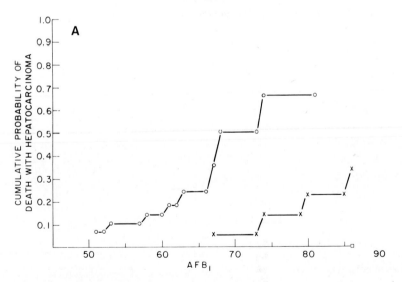

Fig. 6. (A) illustrates the effect of marginal lipotrope diet on hepatocellular carcinoma induced by aflaxtoxin B_1 (AFB_1).

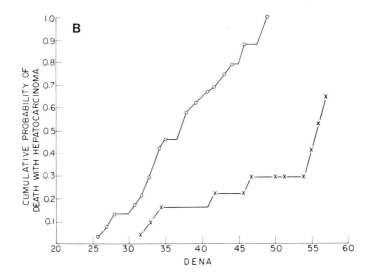

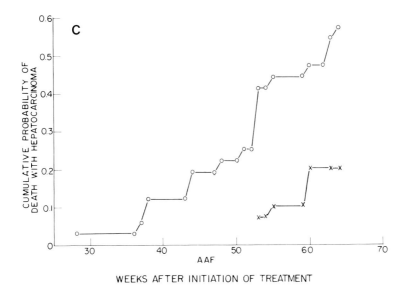

WEEKS AFTER INITIATION OF TREATMENT

Fig. 6. (B) is from a similar study using *N*-nitrosodiethylamine (DEN) as the carcinogen. (C) depicts data from a study using acetylaminofluorene as the carcinogen. In each case the pattern was the same, with tumor appearing earlier and a higher incidence in rats fed the marginal lipotrope diet, compared to animals fed the control diet. x, control, choline supplemented group; ○, marginal lipotrope group.

the esophagus, particularly if it is given in a high dose. Under these conditions it induces tumors earlier in deficient than in control rats. N-nitrosodibutylamine (DBN) induces equally high incidences of tumors in the lung and urinary bladder of control and deficient rats, in contrast to a high incidence of hepatocarcinoma in deficient rats. 1,2-Di-methylhydrazine (DMH) induces a higher incidence of colon tumors in deficient than in control rats, but the effect was associated with the high fat content of the deficient diet and not to the deficiency itself. The effects in the different tissues of the deficiency may be related to activation or deactivation of the carcinogen or its metabolites at the site.

Microsomal oxidase activity of the liver is highly sensitive to lipotrope deficiency, and its decrease may be responsible for modification of carcinogenesis there or at other sites. Poirier and Whitehead (1973) demonstrated that DEN induces tissue folate deficiency even in the presence of adequate dietary folate. Table V contains data abridged from the work of these investigators that illustrate the marked abnormality of folate-dependent histidine metabolism when the animals were exposed to DEN. In support of these observations we found that DEN treatment increased the severity of lipotrope deficiency (Rogers and Newberne, 1980). These data suggest that cellular defects in one-carbon metabolism may be induced by carcinogens as well as by dietary deficiency and may be central to the dietary effects on carcinogenesis.

C. Effects of Lipotrope Deficiency on Xenobiotic Metabolism

Several *in vitro* assays have demonstrated that rats fed the lipotrope-deficient diet have a reduced potential for hepatic metabolism of many carcinogens (Rogers and Newberne, 1980; Suit *et al.*, 1977). There is one exception that will be discussed below. This result, combined with the evidence that such animals are more susceptible than normal animals to hepatic carcinogens, indicates either that the increased susceptibility is not related to carcinogen metabolism or that the balance of the altered metabolism is in favor or activation. The *in vitro* studies have shown increased or decreased activation of carcinogens to bacterial mutagens by livers from deficient rats and no consistent correlation with carcinogenesis. Aflatoxin B_1 and AAF were tested initially by Ames assays using postmitochondrial supernatants prepared from normal or deficient rats livers. Deficient livers were only about 50% as effective as normal livers in producing bacterial mutagens (Suit *et al.*, 1977). The results were confirmed for AFB_1 using the Inductest of Moreau (Suit *et al.*, 1982).

TABLE V

Nitrosodiethylamine (DEN) and Folate Excretion[a]

| | | Urinary FIGLU (moles/100 gm body weight)[b] 95% confidence limits | |
	Mean	Lower	Upper
Control	2.0	1.5	2.6
DEN	11.4	8.8	14.2
DEN + 1.5% DL-methionine	1.8	1.5	2.2
DEN + 1.5% choline chloride	3.5	2.7	4.5

[a] From Poirer and Whitehead (1973).
[b] Mean ± SE.

Following the reports of Roebuck et al. (1981) and of Shinozuka et al. (1978) that 1-azaserine, a pancreatic carcinogen, induced liver as well as pancreatic carcinoma in lipotrope-deficient rats, we examined azaserine activation in the Inductest. This compound, in contrast to the others tested, was activated more readily by livers from deficient rats than from normal rats (Suit et al., 1982). The activation is performed by the cytosol rather than the microsomes and appears to be enzymatic with a partial requirement for NADP and an interaction with glutathione (GSH) (Suit and Rogers, 1983). This is the first example in which we have found a direct correlation between a dietary effect on carcinogenesis and on carcinogen activation in vitro.

There have been indications from in vivo studies that lipotrope deficiency alters carcinogen metabolism. Rats fed the low lipotrope diet are more sensitive to the toxicity of repeated doses of most hepatocarcinogens including AFB_1. They are, however, highly insensitive to toxicity of a single dose of AFB_1 (Rogers and Newberne, 1971). This suggests that there is decreased metabolism of the chemical to its active, toxic form upon first exposure, but induction of metabolism occurs following repeated exposures. This effect was not confirmed however in the bacterial mutagenesis assays (Suit et al., 1977).

It has been established that liver S-adenosylmethionine (SAM) is decreased in lipotrope-deficient rats; but GSH content of liver is not affected (Poirier et al., 1977). The reduction in SAM in rats fed the lipotrope-deficient diet is a direct result of the dietary treatment and has been confirmed by Mikol and Poirier (1981) in rats fed diets deficient in one or more of the lipotropes. S-Adenosylmethionine may influence carcinogenesis by serving as a trap for electrophilic carcinogens or by playing a role in alkylation. It is reduced by feeding the carcinogen, ethionine (Mikol and Poirier, 1981), or certain tumor promoters (Shivapurkar and Poirier, 1982) but not by feeding AAF (Poirier *et al.*, 1977). A reduction in hepatic SAM and of folate (Poirier and Whitehead, 1973) by carcinogens clearly points to a direct interaction occurring in one-carbon metabolism with depletion of SAM (Becker *et al.*, 1981).

Liver microsomal oxidases and NAD–NADH are diminished in rats fed lipotrope-deficient diets (Rogers and Newberne, 1971). The decreased activity of oxidases in liver of deficient rats observed in our laboratory was confirmed in another laboratory, which demonstrated also the diminished content of cytochome P-450 (Campbell, *et al.*, 1978). In the study of Campbell *et al.* (1978) and in the unpublished studies from our laboratory, rats fed the lipotrope-deficient diet bound about the same, or a slightly decreased, amount of AFB_1 to hepatic DNA as did rats fed the control diet. Higher exposure to AFB_1 depressed the binding of AFB_1 to DNA in both control and lipotrope-deficient rats. The assay, like the bacterial assays, therefore indicated no enhancement of AFB_1 activation by the deficiency. More detailed studies of AFB_1-DNA adducts are needed to support the conclusion, however.

The relationship between cirrhosis and liver cell cancer in humans makes the animal model particularly interesting for investigating interactions between diet and cancer. The ongoing hyperplasia of the deficient liver apparently producing a high potential for malignant change may be analogous to hyperplasia of skin and mucous membranes in response to chronic irritation that results also in greater potential for malignancy. The malignant change occurring in cirrhotic liver varies from one part of the world to another, but generally the coexistence is significant, and the risk is high. In most series 60–90% of hepatocarcinomas occur in cirrhotic livers, while the incidence of cirrhosis in the population tends to be about 10% (MacSween and Scott, 1973; MacSween, 1974). In western countries, including the United States, chronic alcoholism seems to be the most common condition associated with the genesis of both cirrhosis and liver cell cancer. The choline deficiency rat liver model for cirrhosis is histologically similar to alcoholic cirrhosis in human patients and, as such, provides a convenient means for exploring mechanisms for development of cirrhosis and hepatocellular carcinoma in humans.

D. Lipotropes and Immunocompetence

Hematopoetic cells, lymphoreticular tissues, and tumors that arise from them are sensitive to alterations in methyl group metabolism. This is the basis for antimetabolic chemotherapy of tumors arising in such tissues. Rapid cell turnover creates a need for methyl groups over and above the normal requirement, a condition characteristic of neoplastic tissues. The rapid cell turnover may result in cells with increased susceptibility to alkylating or other agents or conditions which modify the genetic material of the cell.

Recent studies from our laboratory have revealed that a number of animal species deprived of one or more of the major lipotropes have diminished immunocompetence. A few illustrations will be provided here.

E.   Folic Acid

Several studies have demonstrated impaired humoral and cell-mediated immunity in folate-deficient humans and animals (Nauss and Newberne, 1981) (Table VI). A number of investigators have observed that guinea pigs are particularly susceptible to infectious disease in the deficiency state (Haltalin et al., 1970). Morbidity following Shigella flexneria infection in three groups of Hartley strain guinea pigs, fed either a control natural ingredient diet, or semi-synthetic folate deficient or sup-

TABLE VI

Effects of Folate Deficiency on Immune Function

I.   Human studies
    A.   Depressed peripheral lymphocyte response to PHA
    B.   No change in neutrophil function
    C.   Increased incidence of folate deficiency in patients with hyperplastic candidosis
    D.   Depressed delayed cutaneous hypersensitivity
II.   Animal studies
    A.   Guinea pig
        1.   Decreased WBC
        2.   Increased susceptibility to Shigella infection
    B.   Rats
        1.   Decreased leukocytes and granulocytes
        2.   Decreased hemagglutination titers
        3.   Decreased number of antibody forming cells
        4.   Decreased number of T cells
            a.   Depressed cytoxicity
            b.   Depressed splenic PHA response
            c.   Decreased delayed cutaneous hypersensitivity
        5.   Increased susceptibility to parasitic infection
    C.   Chickens
        1.   Decreased bacterial agglutination titers
        2.   Increased susceptibility to viral infection

---

plemented diets was 0%, 89%, and 17% respectively. There was a marked leukopenia the day after challenge with the organism; the increased susceptibility to infection could be reversed if the animals were supplemented with folic acid only a short time prior to exposure.

Table VII illustrates typical results of studies conducted in our laboratories at MIT. Weanling Sprague-Dawley rats kept on a folate-deficient diet for 3 months had depressed numbers of T cells in the spleen and in the peripheral blood. Furthermore, the cytotoxic activity of splenic lymphocytes of folate-deficient animals, exposed to Brown Norway rat thymocytes, was diminished significantly from a percentage killing of 29.1 ± 3.7 in controls, to 5.2 ± 1.5 in the folate-deficient animals. Furthermore, there was a decrease in sensitivity to stimulation by the T cell mitogen, phytohemagglutinin (PHA). In other studies with the same animal model, it was observed that *in vivo* measurement of cell-mediated immune function, using skin test sensitivity to intradermal PHA injection, was depressed in the deficient animals.

The experiments referred to above and others with similar results established clearly that there was a significant defect in young animals maintained on a folate-deficient diet from weaning. Rats fed a diet deficient in folate from 1 month of age through 1 year and examined sequentially for transformation response of lymphocytes from the thymus and lymph nodes to a variety of mitogens exhibited a clear defect in response. The maximal response to mitogenic stimulation occurred in young animals about 7 weeks of age, 3 weeks after initiation of the diet, a postnatal period in the life of the rat when there is rapid growth and

TABLE VII

Folic Acid Deficiency in Rats[a]

Immune parameter tested	Control	Folate deficient
Delayed hypersensitivity (skin test response to PHA)	3.8 ± 0.4[b]	1.6 ± 0.4
Lymphocyte-mediated cytotoxicity (% killing)	29.1 ± 3.7[c]	5.2 ± 1.5
Spleen transformation (PHA response)	19,398 ± 1014[d]	4263 ± 579
[^{3}H]Uridine labeling of T cells		
Spleen	70 ± 2.4[e]	42 ± 1.9
Thymus	82 ± 1.5	73 ± 2.0
Blood	67 ± 1.7	44 ± 2.8

[a] From Williams *et al.* (1975).

[b] Histological grading based on degree of mononuclear cell infiltration: 0, no response; 4, severe response.

[c] Results expressed as mean ± SE.

[d] Results expressed as cpm ± SE.

[e] Results expressed as percent cells labeled.

development of total body and of the lymphatic system. During this period, even a short-term folate deprivation caused a depressed mitogen transformation response. With aging there was a decrease in the amount of [³H]thymidine incorporated into lymphocytes of deprived animals; they also demonstrated a reduction in the stimulation index of lymphocytes. However, after 12 months there were no significant differences between the control and experimental groups. These observations indicated that after 1 year the lymphatic system had in some way adjusted to the deficiency, possibly by recovery from the initial lesion or, alternatively, the type(s) of lymphocytes sensitive to folate deficiency disappeared during the aging process.

Folate deficiency is one of the common deficits found in protein–energy malnutrition in developing countries and in some subsets of populations of developed countries (i.e., women taking oral contraceptives, patients treated with anticonvulsants). Yet it has rarely been singled out for study in human clinical trials to determine its specific effects on immunity. Studies from our laboratory have shown a number of interesting correlates of cell-mediated immunity and megaloblastic anemia in human patients due to nutritional folate deficiency (Gross *et al.*, 1975). These studies involved cell-mediated immune response in 23 Bantu patients in South Africa, with normal levels of serum iron and vitamin B_{12}, except for two subgroups studied in regard to iron deficiency and combined folate–iron deficiency. Cellular immunity was investigated using a dinitrochlorobenzene (DNCB) skin test and peripheral lymphocyte response to PHA stimulation. Table VIII illustrates some of the results of these studies. These data show that prior to treatment there was a highly significant depression in skin reaction to DNCB in the deficient groups, compared to the group with pure iron deficiency or to control groups. Following folate supplementation, 80% of the patients in the first three groups had a positive skin test within about 3 weeks. The PHA response in the peripheral lymphocytes was one-third of the control or of the pure iron-deficient subjects. However it returned to normal values in from 7 to 14 days following therapy. A deficiency of vitamin B_{12} was ruled out in these patients by a negative Schilling test, which involves administration of a loading dose of the vitamin. These data clearly indicate a profound effect of folate deficiency on immunocompetence of human patients.

F. Vitamin B_{12}

There are certain disadvantages associated with the use of laboratory experimental animals in the study of vitamin B_{12} deficiency, primarily because pigs, rats, and other laboratory animals do not develop a clear-

TABLE VIII

Dinitrochlorobenzene (DNCB) Skin Test and PHA Response before Treatment in Folic Acid-Deficient, Iron-Deficient, and Control Patients[a]

Group[b]	Degree of DNCB skin test reaction (No. of patients)			PHA stimulation of lymphocytes[b] (dpm)	Unstimulated lymphocytes[c] (dpm)
	0	+	++		
Folate deficient (nonobstetric)	11	0	0	8,800+3600 (3,091–13,995)	510 (219–1202)
Folate deficient (obstetric)	6	6	1	6,800±2900 (3,691–12,323)	480 (176–1250)
Folate and iron deficient	5	0	0	6,000±3280 (3,527–10,049)	330 (130–501)
Iron deficient	0	2	3	23,300±5470 (15,005–28,896)	390 (162–672)
Control	1	4	8	26,340±5680 (18,740–33,725)	370 (130–719)

[a] From Gross *et al.* (1975).
[b] Uptake of [³H]thymidine; results are expressed in disintegrations per minute (dpm); mean ± SD and range.
[c] Uptake of [³H]thymidine by lymphocytes in presence of saline; results are expressed as disintegrations per minute (dpm); mean ± SE; and range.

cut megaloblastic anemia when fed a vitamin B_{12}-deficient diet. Megaloblastic anemia is not observed even though levels of serum vitamin B_{12}, methylmaloynyl-CoA mutase activities, and tissue coenzyme levels associated with vitamin B_{12} may be significantly decreased. This probably explains why there is very little in the literature relative to vitamin B_{12} deficiency and its relation to immunocompetence per se. In rats, vitamin B_{12} can have long-term effects when the deficit is imposed in early life (Newberne and Young, 1973).

Studies relative to immunocompetence and vitamin B_{12} deficiency in human patients are few in number, except in cases of autoimmune phenomena associated with pernicious anemia. It has been shown that peripheral lymphocytes from patients with pernicious anemia are sensitized to a variety of gastric antigens (Tai and McGuigan, 1969). Using the leukocyte migration test, other workers have demonstrated *in vitro* a delayed hypersensitivity to these antigens (Finlayson *et al.*, 1972; Goldstone *et al.*, 1973; MacCuish *et al.*, 1974). The mean transformation response, measured by [³H]thymidine uptake by peripheral lymphocytes from patients with pernicious anemia, was significantly lower than that of controls. Autoradiographic studies on four pernicious anemia patients and three controls indicated no difference in the degree of blast transformation, but the extent of labeling was higher in controls. Moreover, there were no significant differences in the percentages of B and T lymphocytes measured by immunofluorescence and the rosette techniques, respectively.

G. Methionine and Choline

There are conflicting reports on the effect of methionine deficiency on immunocompetence in experimental animals, part of which can be explained on the basis of differences in species, age at time of initiation of the experimental diet, and other factors. Table IX lists the effects of methionine on immune function drawn from literature references and from work conducted in our own laboratories.

Kenney et al. (1970) reported that although the addition of methionine to a soybean protein diet improved weight gain, it resulted in a depression in hemolysin titers following sheep red blood cell (SRBC) injection. Soybean is low in methionine and has no vitamin B_{12}. Methionine depri-

TABLE IX

Effect of Methionine on Immune Function

Dietary treatment	Species	Reported effect	Reference
Methionine deficient	Rat Monkey	No effect on primary or secondary antibody response	Gershoff et al. (1968) Gill and Gershoff (1967)
Methionine deficient	Chickens	No effect on resistance to Salmonella gallinarum infection	Hill (1979)
Marginal methionine–cystine	Mice	Depressed humoral immune response, no change in cytotoxicity	Jose and Good (1973)
Marginal methionine–choline	Rats during gestation and weaning	Increased susceptibility to infection, decreased CMI,[a] decreased lymphoid organ development	Newberne et al. (1970), Newberne and Wilson (1972), Gebhardt and Newberne (1974), Williams et al. (1975, 1979)

[a] CMI, cell-mediated immunity.

vation had little if any effect on primary or secondary responses to a synthetic polypeptide in rats or in monkeys (Gill and Gershoff, 1967). Still other studies have shown different requirements for humoral and cellular immune response in mice fed diets low in methionine (Jose and Good, 1973) and chicks low in methionine (Hill, 1979).

We have observed, in a series of studies, that the effect of a specific nutrient deficiency on the immune system is dependent on a number of factors, including the age of the animal, the length of time it is fed the experimental diet, the adequacy of other nutrients, and the time at which the immune system is challenged. It is important that these parameters be defined. For example, Table X illustrates effects of lipotrope deprivation at different periods of the pre- and perinatal period on the response of offspring to the stress of infection. Clearly, the prenatal period is a time where the immune system of the developing embryo and fetus is subject to profound effects of deprivation, and these effects have long-range influences on immunocompetence later in life. As with any study about the interactions of nutrients and environmental compounds, the complexity is enormous.

Lipotropes are intimately involved with lipid metabolism and in maintaining the integrity of the immune system (Newberne and Thurman,

TABLE X

Effect of Lipotropes on Response of Rats to Infection with *Salmonella typhimurium* 3 Months Postweaning

Dietary treatment		Average weight at infection (gm)	Percent mortality[a]
Gestation and lactation	Postweaning		
Marginal methionine–choline − B_{12}	Marginal methionine–choline − B_{12}	233 ± 6	100
Marginal methionine–choline − B_{12}	Control	240 ± 8	100
Marginal methionine–choline + B_{12}	Marginal methionine–choline + B_{12}	248 ± 5	91
Marginal methionine–choline + B_{12}	Control	285 ± 7	90
B_{12} Deficient	B_{12} Deficient	260 ± 3	71
B_{12} Deficient	Control	308 ± 4	35
Control	Control	303 ± 4	25

[a] Thirty days postinfection.

1981). Lipids are in some way related to immunocompetency (Table XI), and the accumulating body of evidence in this regard offers some exciting possibilities. We have observed in studies with rats that unsaturated fats depress the response of lymphocytes to the mitogen PHA. Moreover, individuals with the immunosuppression from chemotherapy or from ingestion of certain classes of drugs are at greater risk for development of a primary cancer or the development of a second type of tumor at another site.

III. DISCUSSION

We do not know the mechanism by which lipotropes exert their influence on carcinogenesis. We have postulated, however, that the effect of a lipotrope deficiency is exerted early in the carcinogenesis process. Most of our studies have been directed toward detecting dietary effects on carcinogen metabolism, hepatocyte turnover, and indicators of carcinogen interaction with hepatocytes, such as the induction of hyperplastic foci and secretion of α-fetoprotein. More recently, immunocompetence as it may relate to cancer induction has been of interest. While a direct linkage is not currently obvious between lipotropes, chemical activation/deactivation, immunocompetence, and cancer, the observations are highly suggestive for interactions. It is clear from data presented in this chapter that lipotrope deficiency results in diminished immunocompetence, altered xenobiotic metabolism, and increased risk for

TABLE XI

Lipids and the Immune System[a]

Agent/condition	Effects
Host infection	Ketosis
	Protein synthesis decreases
Obesity	Cell-mediated immunity decreases
	Polymorphonuclear bacterial killing decreases
Plasma lipoproteins	Lymphocytes inhibited by LDL; surface receptors influenced; LDL maturation of T lymphocytes: killer or suppressor
25-Hydroxycholesterol	HMG-CoA reductase; immunosuppression linked?
Cholesterol	Oxidized derivatives immunosuppressive; T lymphocytes require it for cytotoxic activity

[a] From Newberne and Thurman (1981).

chemically induced cancer of a number of sites. The challenge now is to identify the linkage, if such exists, and to determine the mechanisms by which susceptibility to carcinogens is modified.

NOTE ADDED IN PROOF

Following the preparation of this chapter we have had personal communications from Lionel Poirier, of the National Cancer Institute, and Emmanuel Farber, of the University of Toronto, that each of them has observed hepatocellular carcinomas in rats given a choline-devoid diet without added carcinogen. If these observations can be confirmed, they coincide with the observations of Salmon *et al.* (1954) and with our observations in mice reported elsewhere (Newberne *et al.*, 1982). Our attempts to produce tumors in rats with choline-devoid diets only have not been successful.

REFERENCES

Abanobi, S. E., Lombardi, B., and Shinozuka, H. (1982). *Cancer Res.* **42**, 412–415.
Allan, F. N., Bowie, D. J., MacLeod, J. J. R., and Robinson, W. L. (1924). *Br. J. Exp. Pathol.* **5**, 75–83.
Becker, R. A. Barrows, L. R., and Shank, R. C. (1981). *Carcinogenesis* **2**, 1181–1188.
Best, C. H., and Huntsman, M. L. (1932). *J. Physiol (London)* **75**, 405–412.
Best, C. H., Hershey, J. M., and Huntsman, M. E. (1932). *J. Physiol. (London)* **75**, 56–66.
Bliss, M. (1982). "The Discovery of Insulin." Univ. of Chicago Press, Chicago, Illinois.
Campbell, T. C., Hayes, J. R., and Newberne, P. (1978). *Cancer Res.* **38**, 4569–4573.
Copeland, D. H., and Salmon, W. D. (1946). *Am. J. Pathol.* **22**, 1059–1081.
Doll, R., and Peto, R. (1981). *JNCI, J. Natl. Cancer Inst.* **66**, 1191–1308.
duVigneaud, V. A. (1952). Trail of Research in Sulfur Chemistry and Metabolism and Related Fields." Cornell Univ. Press, Ithaca, New York.
Finlayson, D., Fauconate, N. H., and Krohm, K. (1972). *Dig. Dis.* **17**, 631–638.
Gebhardt, B. M., and Newberne, P. M. (1974). *Immunology* **26**, 489–495.
Gershoff, S. N., Gill, T., Sinionian, S. J., and Steinberg, A. I. (1968). *J. Nutr.* **95**, 184–189.
Gill, T. J., and Gershoff, S. N. (1967). *J. Immunol.* **99**, 883–893.
Goldstone, A. H., Calder, E. A., Barnes, E. W., and Irvine, W. J. (1973). *Clin. Exp. Immunol.* **14**, 501–508.
Gross, R. L., Reid, J. V. O., Newberne, P. M., Burgess, B., Marston, R., and Hift, W. (1975). *Am. J. Clin. Nutr.* **28**, 225–232.
György, P. (1954). *Ann. N.Y. Acad. Sci.* **57**, 925–931.
György, P., and Goldblatt, H. (1942). *J. Exp. Med.* **75**, 355–362.
Haltalin, K. C., Nelson, J. D., and Whitman, E. B. (1970). *J. Infect. Dis.* **121**, 275–283.
Hill, C. H. (1979). *Fed. Proc. Fed. Am. Soc. Exp. Biol.* **38**, 2129–2133.
Jose, D. J., and Good, R. A. (1973). *J. Exp. Med.* **137**, 1–9.
Kenney, N. A., McGee, J. L., and Pascual, F. (1970). *J. Nutr.* **100**, 1063–1072.
Kumar, M., and Axelrod, A. E. (1978). *Proc. Soc. Exp. Biol. Med.* **157**, 421–423.
MacCuish, A. C., Urbaniak, S. J., Goldstone, A. H., and Irvine, W. J. (1974). *Blood* **44**, 849–855.
MacSween, R. N. M. (1974). *J. Clin. Pathol.* **27**, 669–682.
MacSween, R. N. M., and Scott, A. R. (1973). *J. Clin. Pathol.* **26**, 936–942.

Mikol, Y. B., and Poirier, L. S. (1981). *Cancer Lett.* **13,** 195–201.

Nauss, K. N., and Newberne, P. M. (1981). *In* "Diet and Resistance to Disease" (M. Phillips and A. Batz, eds.), pp. 63–91. Plenum, New York.

Newberne, P. M., and Clark, A. J. (1982). *Toxicologist* **1,** 63.

Newberne, P. M., and Rogers, A. E. (1976). *In* "Fundamentals in Cancer Prevention" (P. N. Magee, S. Takayama, T. Sugimura, and T. Matsushima, eds.), pp. 15–40. University Park Press, Baltimore, Maryland.

Newberne, P. M., and Thurman, G. B. (1981). *Cancer Res.* **41,** 3803–3805.

Newberne, P. M., and Wilson, R. B. (1972). *Nutr. Rep. Int.* **5,** 151–158.

Newberne, P. M., and Young, V. R. (1973). *Nature (London)* **242,** 263–265.

Newberne, P. M., Carlton, W. W., and Wogan, G. N. (1964). *Pathol. Vet.* **1,** 105–132.

Newberne, P. M., Harrington, D. H., and Wogan, G. N. (1966). *Lab. Invest.* **15,** 962–969.

Newberne, P. M., Rogers, A. E., Bailey, C., and Young, V. R. (1969). *Cancer Res.* **29,** 230–235.

Newberne, P. M., Wilson, R. B., and Williams, G. (1970). *Br. J. Exp. Pathol.* **51,** 231–235.

Newberne, P. M., deCamargo, J. L. V., and Clark, A. (1982). *Toxicol. Pathol.* **10,** 95–106.

Poirier, L. A., and Whitehead, V. M. (1973). *Cancer Res.* **33,** 383–388.

Poirier, L. A., Grantham, P. H., and Rogers, A. E. (1977). *Cancer Res.* **37,** 744–748.

Roebuck, B. D., Yager, J. D., and Longnecker, D. S. (1981). *Cancer Res.* **41,** 888–893.

Rogers, A. E., and Newberne, P. M. (1969). *Cancer Res.* **29,** 1965–1972.

Rogers, A. E., and Newberne, P. M. (1971). *Toxicol. Appl. Pharmacol.* **20,** 113–121.

Rogers, A. E., and Newberne, P. M. (1975). *Cancer Res.* **35,** 3427–3431.

Rogers, A. E., and Newberne, P. M. (1980). *Nutr. Cancer* **2,** 104–112.

Rogers, A. E., Kula, N. S., and Newberne, P. M. (1971). *Cancer Res.* **31,** 491–495.

Salmon, W. D., and Copeland, D. H. (1954). *Ann. N.Y. Acad. Sci.* **57,** 664–667.

Salmon, W. D., and Newberne, P. M. (1962). *J. Nutr.* **76,** 483–491.

Salmon, W. D., and Newberne, P. M. (1963). *Cancer Res.* **23,** 571–575.

Salmon, W. D., Copeland, D. H., and Burns, M. J. (1954). *JNCI, J. Natl. Cancer Inst.* **15,** 1549–1568.

Schaefer, A. E., Copeland, D. H., Salmon, W. D., and Hale, O. M. (1950). *Cancer Res.* **10,** 786–792.

Shinozuka, H., and Lombardi, B. (1980). *Cancer Res.* **40,** 3846–3849.

Shinozuka, H., Katyal, S. L., and Lombardi, B. (1978). *Int. J. Cancer* **22,** 36–39.

Shinozuka, S., Takahashi, S., Lombardi, B., and Abanobi, S. E. (1982). *Cancer Lett.* **16,** 48–55.

Shivapurkar, N., and Poirier, L. A. (1982). *Carcinogenesis* **3,** 589–591.

Suit, J. L., and Rogers, A. E. (1983). In preparation.

Suit, J. L., Rogers, A. E., and Jettin, N. E. (1977). *Mutat. Res.* **46,** 312–323.

Suit, J. L., Cruz, B., Roebuck, B. D., and Rogers, A. E. (1982). *Toxicologist* **2,** 123.

Tai, C., and McGuigan, J. E. (1969). *Blood* **34,** 63–71.

Thenen, S. W. (1978). *J. Nutr.* **108,** 836–842.

Williams, E. A. J., Gross, R. L., and Newberne, P. M. (1975). *Nutr. Rep. Int.* **12,** 137–148.

Williams, E. A. J., Gebhardt, B. N., Morton, B., and Newberne, P. M. (1979). *Am. J. Clin. Nutr.* **32,** 1214–1223.

16

The Inhibition of Some Cancers and the Promotion of Others by Folic Acid, Vitamin B_{12}, and Their Antagonists

Victor Herbert

Hematology and Nutrition Laboratory
Veterans Administration Medical Center
Bronx, New York
and
State University of New York Downstate Medical Center
Brooklyn, New York

I. INTRODUCTION

Newberne (Chapter 15, this volume) has reviewed the role of the lipotropes folate, vitamin B_{12}, methionine, and choline in immune function and modulation of immune response. Krumdieck (Chapter 14, this volume) has reviewed what is known about the role of folate deficiency in carcinogenesis.

Nutrition Factors in the Induction
and Maintenance of Malignancy

To start at the end, I should like to suggest the hypothesis that deficiency of folate or vitamin B_{12}, or any other cause of failure to methylate DNA and/or RNA, can activate malignancy by hypomethylation of oncogenes, and that methylating oncogenes can inhibit malignancy by making them dormant. This concept for DNA is similar to that of "relaxed control" of RNA synthesis. Borek *et al.* (1954), who were among the earliest to note methylated RNA, had noted three decades ago that when an organism auxotrophic for methionine is deprived of methionine, it loses its ability to suppress synthesis of RNA, which then is synthesized more rapidly; we speculated that vitamin B_{12} or folate deficiency could produce such "relaxed control" (Herbert, 1965). It is probable that folate and vitamin B_{12} and their antagonists are involved in the control of gene expression because hypomethylation of their DNA may "switch on" normal genes and methylation may switch them off (Ley *et al.*, 1982). It is not much of a leap to suggest that hypomethylation of the DNA and/or RNA of oncogenes would switch them on (i.e., activate them), and methylation would switch them off. Perhaps some of the second cancers that develop after successful antimetabolic chemotherapy are due to the same chemotherapy that directly destroys an active cancer, demethylating an oncogene of a dormant cancer.

II. FOLATE DEFICIENCY

Some years ago, Heller and his associates (1963) observed that folate deficiency increased normal hemoglobin production in a patient with sickle cell trait; since higher normal hemoglobin means lower sickle cell hemoglobin, this was a desirable phenomenon. Treatment with folic acid produced the undesirable result of lowering the normal hemoglobin. In an unpublished case study, we confirmed that observation and proposed to several workers in the field of hemoglobinopathies exploration of the effect of methotrexate on normal hemoglobin production. We did not get an enthusiastic response, and so did not follow up on it, but Heller did follow up his original observation with a recent spectacular outcome.

Recognizing that the primary role of folate is in transferring one-carbon units, one of which is the methyl unit, Heller and others focused in on cytidine, one of the four bases in the genetic code, and the one which is most heavily methylated (the other sometimes methylated base is guanine). In 1982, they presented dramatic evidence (Ley *et al.*, 1982; Benz, 1982) that 5-azacytidine selectively activates the gene for fetal hemoglobin synthesis in patients with β-thalassemia and sickle cell disease. It apparently does this by being incorporated as cytidine into the gene for hemoglobin, and, because its 5 position is blocked, the cytidine cannot take on the methyl group made available in folate- (and vitamin B$_{12}$-) dependent reactions, and is not methylated. Failure to methylate the cytidine of the gene for fetal hemoglobin prevents it from becoming dormant, and it is activated to produce fetal hemoglobin. Whether or not the bases that make up the genetic code are methylated or not methylated plays a major role in gene expression (Jones and Taylor, 1980; Compere and Palmiter, 1981). Normally, 4 to 5% of cystosine residues in human DNA are methylated (Tolstoshev et al., 1981). We need to learn whether oncogene expression can similarly be prevented by increasing ordinarily vitamin B$_{12}$-dependent and folate-dependent one-carbon transfer to the genetic code of the oncogene. Carrying a cancer gene may not be a problem if we can prevent that gene from expressing itself by methylating it.

The B vitamin, folic acid, was isolated in pure form in 1943 when Stokstad purified pteroylglutamic acid (PGA) and Pfiffner and associates crystallized folate from liver (Herbert, 1975). Within a year, working at Mount Sinai Hospital in New York City, Leuchtenberger and associates (Leuchtenberger et al., 1944; Leuchtenberger and Leuchtenberger, Chapter 9, this volume) reported that a form of this vitamin, called "folic acid concentrate," [later known to be oxidized folate triglutamate (teropterin)] inhibited the growth of transplanted sarcoma 180 in mice. This material and similar crystalline oxidized triglutamate known as "fermentation L. casei factor" produced complete regression of single spontaneous breast cancers in mice (Leuchtenberger et al., 1945). Today, that work raises the question: Does oxidized folate triglutamate methylate sarcoma 180 and mouse breast cancer oncogenes? Her first paper stated that Pollack et al. (1942) had reported that fermentation L. casei factor [which was folic acid in triglutamate form (Farber et al., 1947)] was present in humans and rat cancers at higher levels than inositol and at much higher levels than biotin or pyridoxine.

Laszlo and Leuchtenberger (1943) had reported that inositol, then believed to be a B vitamin for humans but more recently shown to be a B vitamin only for some bacteria, since it is synthesized adequately by humans (Food and Nutrition Board, 1980), inhibited animal tumor growth, but other B vitamins (except vitamin B$_{12}$, which was yet to be discovered) did not. Here, too, today's question is: Can inositol methylate oncogenes?

Lewisohn et al. (1946) reported that oxidized folate monoglutamate ("liver L. casei factor" from Lederle Laboratory) not only did not inhibit spontaneous breast cancers in mice, but actually produced a more rapid growth of the primary tumors and a significant increase in lung metastases. Here was evidence that one of the monoglutamate forms of the vitamin promoted tumor growth, but one of the triglutamate forms of the same vitamin inhibited the growth of the same tumor. Today, this raises the question: Can oxidized folate monoglutamate inhibit methylation of oncogenes, thereby allowing their expression, and can the triglutamates do the opposite? This is not far-fetched, since there is substantial evidence that folate triglutamates are frequently more active than monoglutamates in methylation in man (Chanarin, 1979; Food and Nutrition Board, 1977).

Folate triglutamate has a much greater affinity than folate monoglutamate for milk folate binding protein (Colman and Herbert, 1980b), which appears to be a folate delivery protein (Colman et al., 1981).

For many years, workers have been exploring the question of whether one form of a vitamin can be a growth promoter, by acting as a coenzyme, while another form of the same vitamin could attach to the same apoenzyme or other ligand, such as a vitamin-transporting protein, and then jam the machinery, just as a key with a tooth missing can fit into a lock, but then not turn. The answer to that question is clearly yes. Different forms and major parts of the same basic vitamin structure, i.e., analogs and cogeners, both exist in nature and are synthesizable, and some of them are antagonists, or antivitamins, which can be created from vitamins by only slightly warping their structure.

Farber et al. (1947) reported from Harvard giving pteroyltriglutamic acid (teropterin) and pteroyldiglutamic acid (diopterin), both synthesized by Y. SubbaRow and his associates at Lederle Laboratories, to 90 patients with various malignancies, noting that "in general, adult patients experienced improvement in energy, appetite, sense of well being . . . might be ascribed to improved morale resulting from frequent visits, more medical attention . . ." they also reported inconstant temporary decreases in size of metastases in some tumors and degeneration and necrosis in others.

The apocryphal story is that Farber was also giving folic acid (the oxidized, stable pharmaceutical form of the vitamin) to children with lymphoproliferative malignancies (lymphocytic leukemia and lymphoma) until one of his residents collected sufficient data to suggest that the children receiving this new vitamin were dying faster than those children not receiving it. This observation allegedly led Farber to ask the Lederle people to create a warped folic acid molecule which would interfere with folate metabolism in the malignant cells, and this was done by adding an NH_2 group, thereby creating aminopterin. A second alteration, methylation in the 10-position, created methotrexate, still one of our most potent anticancer agents, particularly effective against childhood lymphoproliferative disorders and trophoblastic malignancies.

There is considerable evidence that rapidly growing neoplastic tissue consumes folate at so rapid a rate that folate deficiency megaloblastosis can occur in the host cells (Herbert, 1959b; Chanarin, 1979). There is also evidence that tumor growth may be slowed by vitamin B$_{12}$ deficiency, whether that deficiency results from inadequate absorption or from elevated levels in serum of a vitamin B$_{12}$ binder that does not deliver the vitamin to tumor tissue (Corcino et al., 1971) but to the liver in a calcium-dependent fashion (Herbert, 1958, 1959b; Herbert and Spaet, 1958; Allen, 1975; Beck, 1982). Interestingly, granulocytes and liver are a major source of serum binding proteins for both vitamin B$_{12}$ and folic acid (Herbert and Colman, 1980), and malignancies of granulocytes and liver may partly control themselves by releasing into the serum large amounts of binders for vitamin B$_{12}$ and folic acid that bind those vitamins and thereby prevent delivery to, and nourishment of, the tumor.

Oxidized folate (such as pteroylglutamic acid, the stable pharmaceutical form of the vitamin) is metabolically not useful, and may even be neurotoxic; we had noted the structural similarity of folic acid to Dilantin (Herbert and Zalusky, 1962), and it can produce seizures in patients with epilepsy by blocking the protective action of Dilantin, as Butterworth's group has shown (Ch'ien et al., 1975). Folic acid and Dilantin compete for intestinal absorption (Gerson et al., 1972), and probably also at the brain cell, where Dilantin may interfere with ATPase, as in the gut (Hepner et al., 1970). There appears to be a one-way transport system to remove noxious oxidized folates from the nervous system, and a one-way transport system to deliver useful reduced folate into the nervous system (Colman and Herbert, 1980a). We recently used this information to treat successfully with folinic acid a child with congenital folate malabsorption unresponsive to folic acid (Poncz et al., 1981a,b).

Similarly, there may be a one-way transport system to remove noxious vitamin B$_{12}$ analogs from the body, as Allen (1975) had suggested and as we reported earlier this year (Kanazawa et al., 1983), and a transport system to deliver helpful forms of the vitamin to normal tissues, as we first reported for human serum delivery of vitamin B$_{12}$ to liver (Herbert and Spaet, 1958).

These transport systems have different affinities for different forms of vitamin B$_{12}$ and folic acid, and different delivery ability for helpful and noxious forms of the vitamins with respect to different normal cells, and possibly also tumor cells. Sutherland (Chapter 5, this volume) has indicated that folate deficiency produces fragile chromosomes. In this connection, we should note that Das noted that folate therapy will not correct folate deficiency in circulating human lymphocytes for up to 1–2 months after the start of therapy (Das and Herbert, 1978), whereas it is corrected in bone marrow cells within 6 hours after the start of folate therapy. Thus fragile chromosomes might persist in lymphocytes for 1 or 2 months after the beginning of replacement therapy for folate deficiency. This is because circulating lymphocytes are impervious to nutrients such as the B vitamins until they are triggered to make DNA by a virus or lectin (Colman and Herbert, 1978).

Vitamin B_{12} does not appear to be metabolically useful in its stable pharmaceutical form, cyanocobalamin. The cyanide must be removed before it can function. Hydroxocobalamin can block vitamin B_{12} metabolism by competing with adenosylcobalamin for the binding site on the adenosylcobalamin-dependent enzyme methyl malonyl-CoA mutase (Willard and Rosenberg, 1979). Conversely, the oncogenic potential of absorbed cyanide from cassava and other foods (Herbert, 1981) may be muted by inactivation of the cyanide by hydroxocobalamin, a metabolically active form of vitamin B_{12}. Indeed, anesthesiologists have used massive doses of hydroxocobalamin to reverse cyanide toxicity by soaking up the cyanide from the nitroprusside used in open-heart operations (Cottrell et al., 1978).

Butterworth noted that naturally occurring folate analogs such as pteroic acid may be lethal for rats (Butterworth, 1969) and can displace folate from human tissues and flush it out in the urine (Johns and Plenderleith, 1963). We need to know if there is a folate analog that will selectively flush folate or vitamin B_{12} out of tumor tissue or selectively deliver folate or vitamin B_{12} to tumor tissue. Can it be done with pteroic acid, followed by folate rescue?

There is evidence that human serum, Dilantin, or methotrexate will inhibit pteroyl monoglutamate and methyl tetrahydrofolate uptake by human bone marrow cells in vitro, but 2-deoxyglucose, an antagonist of glucose, will enhance such uptake (Tisman and Herbert, 1971). One wonders whether simultaneous administration of folate and 2-deoxyglucose would be more harmful to tumor cells than to normal ones.

Another intriguing finding is that a patient with that blood malignancy known as DiGugliemo syndrome had a rise in serum folate from 23 to 245 ng/ml and a fall in urine formiminoglutamate from 410 to 23 mg/12 hours after 10 days of 750 μg daily of coenzyme B_{12}, but no other improvement (Herbert and Sullivan, 1964).

A folate-free diet was given for more than 4 months to seven patients with disseminated cancers with no clinical benefit. The folate levels in tumor, liver, and blood all declined at the same rate (Gailani et al., 1970).

On the other hand, Whitehead *et al.* (1973) observed the disappearance of megaloblastosis in cervical epithelial cells with folate therapy of women taking oral contraceptives, and Butterworth *et al.* (1982) reported improvement in apparent cervical dysplasia in oral contraceptive users when treated with folic acid. Longo *et al.* (1975) had noted human selective folate deficiency in the lymphocyte cell line after 4 months of oral contraceptives, and we suspect lymphocytes and cervical epithelium may be similarly selectively deprived. The first report of selective folate deficiency in one cell line and not another was our 1962 production of dietary folate deficiency in a volunteer, whose intestinal biopsy showed normal epithelial cells when his bone marrow had become megalobalastic (Herbert, 1962).

III. VITAMIN B$_{12}$

Turning to vitamin B$_{12}$, shortly after Minot and Murphy reported that liver therapy cured pernicious anemia, for which they won the Nobel Prize, Minot reported the development of a malignancy (polycythemia vera) occurring immediately after the start of treatment for pernicious anemia. There were a number of subsequent intermittent reports of myeloproliferative disorders associated with therapy for pernicious anemia with liver extract, and subsequently with pure vitamin B$_{12}$ after it was isolated in 1948 and proved to be the active principle in liver therapy of pernicious anemia (Corcino *et al.*, 1971).

In 1958, we began to use warped vitamin B$_{12}$ molecules (the anilide and ethylamide of vitamin B$_{12}$, synthesized by E. Lester Smith of Glaxo Laboratories) in the treatment of myelogenous leukemia refractory to all other therapy (Herbert, 1959a). One woman to whom we gave the anilide of vitamin B$_{12}$ appeared to go into a complete remission, with her bone marrow aspirate changing from florid myelogenous leukemia to a fibrotic picture. However, she continued to have a few leukemic cells in her peripheral blood. When she died of pneumonia 6 months later, we found her marrow largely fibrotic. We never published the case in detail because it is impossible in one case to separate cause and effect from coincidence, and our supplies of analogs dried up when Lester Smith retired.

Bodian (1959) at the Great Ormond Street Hospital for Sick Children in London reported that megadoses of vitamin B$_{12}$ produced remission in neuroblastoma in children, but Sawitsky and Desposito (1965) did not confirm this in 103 children. Bodian believed that megadoses of vitamin

B_{12} produced maturation of the tumor, but spontaneous maturation and spontaneous remission can occur in neuroblastoma with no therapy.

Day et al. (1950) and Ostryanina (1972) reported that vitamin B_{12} enhanced the carcinogenic effect of p-dimethylaminoazobenzene and three other carcinogens in rats consuming a methionine-deficient diet. Conversely, Rogers and Newberne (1975) reported that chemically induced tumors of the liver, colon, and esophagus were enhanced by diets deficient in folic acid, vitamin B_{12}, choline, and methionine.

Folic acid and vitamin B_{12} can prove useful in those tumors that grow better as more of these vitamins are supplied, because the tumor cells can be stimulated into the DNA synthesis phase in which a number of cancer chemotherapy agents exert their deadly effects, and those agents can be used in a sequence right after folic acid and/or vitamin B_{12}.

Apparent analogs of vitamin B_{12} appear to be ubiquitous, being present in human serum (Kolhouse et al., 1978), human cells (Kanazawa and Herbert, 1983), human bile (Kanazawa et al., 1983), multivitamin pills (Herbert et al., 1982; Kondo et al., 1982), and a wide variety of microorganisms (Dolphin, 1982). Two analogs from multivitamin pills have been reported to block vitamin B_{12} metabolism in normal human cells in vitro (Kondo et al., 1982). The highest known pill content of analog of vitamin B_{12} is in the health food fad pill Spirulina (Herbert and Drivas, 1982). Such analogs require study for their ability to block vitamin B_{12} metabolism in both normal and malignant cells. The human body seems anxious to get rid of vitamin B_{12} analogs and appears to have a system for their constant removal (Kanazawa and Herbert, 1983).

One of the new areas of vitamin B_{12} research relates to the fact that the anesthetic gas, nitrous oxide, can produce acute vitamin B_{12} deficiency, as first made clear from Mollin's laboratory in London by Amess et al. (1978). We recently reported that nitrous oxide produces an over 95% reduction in liver vitamin B_{12} in the fruit bat (van der Westhuyzen et al., 1982a), and we suspect the same could occur in any tissue on similar exposure. Scott and Weir, in Dublin (1981), and Metz' group in South Africa (van der Westhuyzen et al., 1982b) showed that methionine can prevent the nerve damage of nitrous oxide-induced vitamin B_{12} deficiency in primates and the fruit bat, respectively. Chanarin suggests that formyl folate monoglutamate, with its formate derived from methylthioribose, is the preferred substrate for the polyglutamate forms of folate that normal cells preferentially use (Perry et al., 1982). Studies of the effects of nitrous oxide on tumors in experimental animals, without versus with methionine "rescue" of normal cells, will be of great interest.

Difference in ability of normal versus tumor cells in taking up various nutrients and antinutrients are being sought in efforts to kill tumor cells selectively. Normal cells treated with nitrous oxide to destroy vitamin B$_{12}$ are better "rescued" by methionine than by S-adenosyl methionine, even though S-adenosyl methionine is the active form, because methionine much more readily crosses normal cell walls (Perry *et al.*, 1982). We need to study the relative ability of these two "rescue" agents to cross tumor versus normal cell walls.

Because folic acid and vitamin B$_{12}$ are intimately related to the synthesis of DNA, lack of either damages DNA synthesis. The primary damage is to *de novo* DNA synthesis, with the result that there may be a secondary increment in salvage DNA synthesis. In those tumors in which synthesis of DNA by the salvage pathway is relatively greater than in normal cells, as compared to the *de novo* pathway of DNA synthesis, it is theoretically possible that folic acid and/or vitamin B$_{12}$, by enhancing *de novo* DNA synthesis, could be relatively more helpful to normal than to tumor cells, and relatively more harmful to certain tumor cells.

IV. SUPPRESSION TESTING

Some years ago, we developed the deoxyuridine (dU) suppression test to measure deficiencies of both vitamin B$_{12}$ and folate in terms of the slowing of DNA synthesis produced by either deficiency, expanding it from the Killman experiment, which measured only vitamin B$_{12}$ deficiency (Killman, 1964). In a sense, Killman's laboratory created a unicycle, and our laboratory then created a bicycle (Metz *et al.*, 1968).

The immediate precursors of cellular DNA synthesis are dATP, dGTP, dCTP, and dTTP. In most mammalian cells, *de novo* synthesis of thymidylate (dTMP) from deoxyuridylate (dUMP) is a rate-limiting step and requires 5,10-methylene tetrahydrofolate as a coenzyme (Friedkin, 1963). However, the incorporation of preformed thymidine (TdR) into replicating cells provides a "salvage pathway" of dTMP synthesis (Feinendegen *et al.*, 1961). Killman (1964) reported that excess of deoxyuridine (dU) added to culture of normal bone marrow suppressed the incorporation of [^{3}H]TdR into DNA, but failed to do so in bone marrow of patients with vitamin B$_{12}$- and folate-deficient megaloblastic anemia. It was also shown that this defect (impaired "dU suppression" of [^{3}H]TdR incorporation into DNA) was partially corrected by added vitamin B$_{12}$ in the bone marrow cultures of vitamin B$_{12}$-deficient, but not folate-deficient, patients; it was almost completely corrected by large doses of folic acid (PteGlu) and smaller doses of folinic acid (5-formyl tetrahydrofolate) in both types of deficiencies; 5-methyl tetrahydrofolate corrected only folate deficiency. Further, the corrective effect of either vitamin was prevented by the folate antagonist methotrexate. The main folate coenzyme in plasma, 5-methyl tetrahydrofolate, which has been shown to "pile up" in the plasma of patients with vitamin B_{12} deficiency, corrected the abnormal dU suppression in folate-deficient marrows but failed to do so in vitamin B_{12}-deficient marrows, unless vitamin B_{12} was also added to the *in vitro* system. Essentially similar abnormalities in DNA synthesis were found to occur in PHA-stimulated lymphocytes of patients with vitamin B_{12}- and folate-deficient megaloblastic anemia (Das and Hoffbrand, 1970). These findings indicated that abnormal dU suppression of [^{3}H-TdR incorporation into DNA in deficiency of vitamin B_{12} and/or folate was due to impaired *de novo* synthesis of thymine-DNA (impaired conversion of deoxyuridylate to thymidylate) because of reduced availability of the pertinent folate coenzyme, 5,10-methylenetetrahydrofolate (Metz *et al.*, 1968; Das and Hoffbrand, 1970).

The two alternative pathways of thymine-DNA synthesis, the *de novo* and the salvage pathways, are interrelated by a common end product, thymidine triphosphate (dTTP), which exerts a regulatory influence on both pathways by a feedback inhibition, and presumably thereby maintains a balanced synthesis of cellular DNA. It would be expected that, just as nonradioactive dU added to cell cultures in excess inhibits the incorporation of radioactive thymidine ([^{3}H]TdR) into DNA (the "dU suppression test") (Killman, 1964; Metz *et al.*, 1968), nonradioactive TdR in excess would cause a reciprocal inhibition of incorporation of radioactive deoxyuridine ([^{3}H]dU) into DNA (i.e., a "thymidine suppression test"). In a preliminary report, we showed that excess of TdR added to PHA-stimulated lymphocyte cultures inhibited the incorporation into DNA of subsequently added [^{3}H]dU (Das and Herbert, 1976), but a seemingly contrary claim (without data) was made by Beck (1975). We subsequently (Das *et al.*, 1980) described the results of such "thymidine suppression tests" in short-term suspension cultures on bone marrow and PHA-activated lymphocytes. These studies indicate that there is, in fact, a reciprocity of the *de novo* and salvage pathways in the regulation of thymine-DNA synthesis in both cell systems. This supported the theoretical concept of the dU suppression test in defining biochemical megaloblastosis caused by deficiency or inhibition of folate and vitamin B_{12}. Beck subsequently reversed his position and published data supporting ours (Pelliniemi and Beck, 1980), but mentioned neither our data nor his prior contrary position, even though our data was presented at a meeting he attended early in 1979 (Das and Herbert, 1979) and had also been previewed in 1978 (Herbert, 1978).

Since some but not other patients with cancer have tumor shrinkage on therapy with massive doses of thymidine (Chiuten *et al.*, 1979; Woodcock *et al.*, 1979), it is possible that patients who will respond can be separated prospectively from those who will not by determining the reciprocity or lack thereof of the salvage and *de novo* pathways of thymine-DNA synthesis in the tumor, using *in vitro* "deoxyuridine suppression tests" and "thymidine suppression tests" (Das *et al.*, 1980).

It should be noted that in our routine "dU suppression tests" we now use hydroxocobalamin instead of cyanocobalamin, as recommended by van der Weyden *et al.* (1973) and Zittoun *et al.* (1978a,b), since it is better taken up by the cells, as is coenzyme B$_{12}$ (Herbert and Sullivan, 1964). We also eliminate the PteGlu control and use only the methyl folate control to identify folate deficiency, for reasons first noted by Metz *et al.* (1968). Zittoun *et al.* (1978b) indicated they have unpublished similar data to ours indicating decreased incorporation of either labeled thymidine or labeled deoxyuridine after preincubation with the unlabeled other material.

The possibility that "dU suppression tests" and "thymidine suppression tests" involve repression and derepression of a number of biochemical pathways indicated in Fig. 2 of Das *et al.* (1978) does not reduce the value of these tests to diagnose biochemical megaloblastosis. In fact, using appropriate radioactive substrates and drug inhibitors, these tests would be of great value in working out the internal machinery of positive and negative controls of DNA synthesis in normal and malignant cells.

V. 5-METHYLCYTIDINE AND MALIGNANCY

Strong and Matsunaga (1975) reported an inverse dose-response effect of 5-methylcytidine (5mC) on the development of spontaneous mammary malignancies in mice, with small doses retarding and large doses enhancing tumor development. Theiss (1980) reported small doses of 5mC inhibited urethane-induced lung tumors in mice. Did these findings relate to methylation control of oncogene expression? As an approach to this question, our laboratory, in collaboration with Dr. Ludwik Gross and his staff, carried out a series of pilot studies in the first six months of 1983 to determine whether 5mC, at similar small or large doses, would affect the development of presumably RNA-virus-induced transplanted L2C (Gross, 1970, 1983) leukemia–lymphoma in guinea pigs. Ordinarily, overt leukemia–lymphoma appears in such recipients approximately 21 days after subcutaneous injection of donor leukemia cells. Guinea pig leukemia–lymphoma appears to be an animal model for human leuke-mia–lymphoma of RNA-virus etiology (Gallo and Wong-Staal, 1982). With one exception, we found that neither a series of small nor of large injections of 5mC significantly affected the time of development or se-verity of leukemia–lymphoma, regardless of whether the injections were started weeks before or with the injection of tumor cells. The exception was one group of guinea pigs who, after 5mC, developed overt leukemia–lymphoma in one week instead of three; this experi-ment was not reproducible on a subsequent attempt to repeat it, and the one unusual result was therefore believed to be human error in that experiment. An extensive literature indicates that preformed 5mC does not get into DNA or RNA (Borek, 1981; Borek et al., 1983), and our study would tend to support that position. We have no explanation for the results of Strong and Matsunaga (1975) or of Theiss (1980), although it should be noted that they worked respectively with a spontaneously developing malignancy and a urethane-induced lung tumor, and we worked with a malignancy produced by graft from donor to recipient. The possibility that 5mC may yet play a role in regulation control of viral disease, including oncogenic virus-produced disease, remains open, since Guntaka et al. (1979) reported that 5mC may reduce virus release from cells, and some 5mC (and other methylated bases) is present in the RNA we eat in our food, digest in our intestine, and presumably then absorb as free bases. The excretion by cancer patients of elevated levels of certain methylated bases in their urine and the quantitation of such bases as a measure of degree of tumor activity (Borek, 1981; Heldman et al., 1983; Borek et al., 1983) further suggests that the subject is not closed.

NOTE ADDED IN PROOF

Not only the quality (i.e., the chemical content of nutrients and other ingredients) but also the quantity (i.e., the caloric content) of food may have a decisive effect on the development of spontaneous leukemia and lymphoma (Gross, 1983, pp. 281, 317, 418). Caloric food reduction reduces considerably the incidence of spontaneous leukemia, lym-phoma, and mammary carcinoma in mice (Gross, 1983).

REFERENCES

Allen, R. H. (1975). Prog. Hematol. **9,** 57.

Amess, J. A. L., Burman, J. F., Nancekievill, D. G., and Mollin, D. L. (1978). Lancet **2,** 339–342.

Beck, W. S. (1975). In "Cobalamin: Biochemistry, and Pathophysiology" (B. M. Babior, ed.), pp. 403–450. Wiley, New York.

Beck, W. S. (1982), *In* "B$_{12}$" (D. Dolphin, ed.), Vol. 2, pp. 1–30. Wiley, New York.

Benz, E. J. (1982). *N. Engl. J. Med.* **307,** 1515–1516.

Bodian, M. (1959). *Pediatr. Clin. North Am.* **6,** 449.

Borek, E. (1981). *Cancer Detect. Prev.* **4,** 185–191.

Borek, E., Ryan, A., and Rockenbach, J. (1954). *Fed. Proc.* **13,** 184.

Borek, E., Sharma, O. K., and Waalkes, T. P. (1983). "New Applications of Urinary Nucleoside Markers. Recent Results in Cancer Research." Springer-Verlag, Berlin and Heidelberg.

Butterworth, C. E. (1969). *In* "Malabsorption" (R. H. Girdwood and N. A. Smith, eds.), pp. 237–247. Williams & Wilkins, Baltimore, Maryland.

Butterworth, C. E., Hatch, K. D., Gore, H., Mueller, H., and Krumdieck, C. L. (1982). *Am. J. Clin. Nutr.* **35,** 73–82.

Chanarin, I. (1979). "The Megaloblastic Anemias," 2nd ed. Blackwell, Oxford.

Ch'ien, L. T., Krumdieck, C. L., Scott, C. W., Jr., and Butterworth, C. E. (1975). *Am. J. Clin. Nutr.* **28,** 21–58.

Chiuten, D. F., Wiernik, P. H., Zaharko, D. S., and Edwards, L. (1979). *Am. Assoc. Cancer Res. Annu. Meet. Abstracts,* **20,** 76. Abstr. 305.

Colman, N., and Herbert, V. (1978). *Blood* **52,** Suppl. 1, 132.

Colman, N., and Herbert, V. (1980a). *In* "Biochemistry of Brain" (S. Kumar, ed.), pp. 103–125. Pergamon, Oxford.

Colman, N., and Herbert, V. (1980b). *Clin. Res.* **28,** 491A.

Colman, N., Hettiarachchy, N., and Herbert, V. (1981). *Science* **211,** 1427–1429.

Compere, S. J., and Palmiter, R. D. (1981). *Cell* **25,** 233–240.

Corcino, J., Zalusky, R., Greenberg, M., and Herbert, V. (1971). *Br. J. Haematol.* **20,** 511–520.

Cottrell, J. E., Casthely, P., Brodie, J. D., Patel, K., Klein, A., and Turndorf, H. (1978). *N. Engl. J. Med.* **298,** 809–811.

Das, K. C., and Herbert, V. (1976). *Clin. Hematol.* **5,** 697–725.

Das, K. C., and Herbert, V. (1978). *Br. J. Haematol.* **38,** 219–233.

Das, K. C., and Herbert, V. (1979). *In* "Vitamin B$_{12}$: Proceedings of the Third European Symposium" (B. Zagalak and W. Friedrich, eds.), pp. 881–887. de Gruyter, Berlin.

Das, K. C., and Hoffbrand, A. V. (1970). *Br. J. Haematol.* **19,** 459–468.

Das, K. C., Manusselis, C., and Herbert, V. (1980). *Br. J. Haematol.* **44,** 61–63.

Das, K. C., Herbert, V., Colman, N., and Longo, D. (1978). *Br. J. Haematol.* **39,** 357–375.

Day, P. L., Payne, L. D., and Dinning, J. S. (1950). *Proc. Soc. Exp. Biol. Med.* **74,** 854.

Dolphin, D., ed. (1982). "B$_{12}$," Vols. I and II. Wiley, New York.

Farber, S., Cutler, E. C., Hawkins, J. W., Harrison, J. H., Peirce, E. C., and Lenz, C. G. (1947). *Science* **106,** 619–621.

Feinendegen, L. E., Bond, V. P., and Painter, R. B. (1961). *Exp. Cell Res.* **22,** 381–405.

Food and Nutrition Board (1977). In "Folic Acid: Biochemistry and Physiology in Relation to the Human Nutrition Requirement." Nat. Acad. Sci., Washington, D.C.

Food and Nutrition Board (1980). "Recommended Dietary Allowances." Nat. Acad. Sci., Washington, D.C.

Friedkin, M. (1963). *Annu. Rev. Biochem.* **32,** 185–214.

Gailani, S. C., Carey, R. W., Holland, J. R., and O'Malley, J. A. (1970). *Cancer Res.* **30,** 327–333.

Gallo, R. E., and Wong-Staal, F. (1982). *Blood* **60,** 545–557.

Gerson, C. D., Hepner, G. W., Brown, N., Cohen, N., Herbert, V., and Janowitz, H. D. (1972). *Gastroenterology* **63,** 353–357.

Guntaka, R. V., Katz, R. A., Weiner, A. J., and Widman, M. M. (1979). *J. Virol.* **29,** 475–482.

Gross, L. (1970). "Oncogenic Viruses," 2nd ed., pp. 611–619, Pergamon, New York.

Gross, L. (1983). "Oncogenic Viruses," 3rd ed., Vol. 1, pp. 636–662, Pergamon, New York.

Heldman, D. A., Grever, M. R., and Trewyn, R. W. (1983). Blood 61, 291–296.

Heller, P., Yakulis, V. J., Epstein, R. B., and Friedland, S. (1963). Blood 21, 479–483.

Hepner, G. W., Aledort, L. M., Gerson, C. D., Cohen, N., Herbert, V., and Janowitz, H. D. (1970). Clin. Res. 18, 382.

Herbert, V., (1958). Proc. Soc. Exp. Biol. Med. 97, 668–691.

Herbert, V. (1959a). Am. J. Clin. Nutr. 7, 433–443.

Herbert, V. (1959b). "The Megaloblastic Anemias." Grune & Stratton, New York.

Herbert, V. (1962). Trans. Assoc. Am. Physicians 75, 307–320.

Herbert, V. (1965). "Disease-a-Month." Yearbook Med. Publ., New York.

Herbert, V. (1975). In "The Pharmacological Basis of Therapeutics" (L. S. Goodman and A. Gilman, eds.), 5th ed., pp. 1324–1349. Macmillan, New York.

Herbert, V. (1978). Cong. Int. Soc. Haematol., Congr. Int. Soc. Blood Transf., 17th, 1978 p. 426.

Herbert, V. (1981). Nutrition Cultism: Facts and Fictions." George F. Stickley Company, Philadelphia, Pennsylvania.

Herbert, V., and Colman, N. (1980). In "Lithium Effects on Granulopoiesis and Immune Function" (A. H. Rossof and W. A. Robinsins, eds.), pp. 61–78. Plenum, New York.

Herbert, V., and Drivas, G. (1982). JAMA, J. Am. Med. Assoc. 248, 3096.

Herbert, V., and Spaet, T. H. (1958). Am. J. Physiol. 195, 194–196.

Herbert, V., and Sullivan, L. W. (1964). Ann. N.Y. Acad. Sci. 112, 855–870.

Herbert, V., and Zalusky, R. (1962). J. Clin. Invest. 42, 1134–1138.

Herbert, V., Drivas, G., Foscaldi, R., Manusselis, C., Colman, N., Kanazawa, S., Das, K., Gelernt, M., Herzlich, B., and Jennings, J. (1982). N. Engl. J. Med. 307, 255–256.

Johns, D. G., and Plenderlieth, I. H. (1963). Biochem. Pharmacol. 12, 1071.

Jones, P. A., and Taylor, S. M. (1980). Cell 20, 85–93.

Kanazawa, S., and Herbert, V. (1983). Am. J. Clin. Nutr. 37, 774–777.

Kanazawa, S., Herbert V., Herzlich, B., Drivas, G., and Manusselis, C. (1983). Lancet 1, 707–708.

Killman, S. A. (1964). Acta Med. Scand. 175, 483–488.

Kolhouse, J. F., Kondo, H., Allen, N. C., Podell, E., and Allen, R. H. (1978). N. Engl. J. Med. 299, 785–792.

Kondo, H., Binder, M. J., Kolhouse, J. F., Smythe, W. R., Podell, E. R., and Allen, R. H. (1982). J. Clin. Invest. 70, 889–898.

Laszlo, D., and Leuchtenberg, C. (1943). Science 97, 515.

Leuchtenberger, C., Lewisohn, R., Laszlo, D., and Leuchtenberger, R. (1944). Proc. Soc. Exp. Biol. Med. 55, 204–205.

Leuchtenberger, C., Leuchtenberger, R., Laszlo, D., and Lewisohn R. (1945). Science 101, 46.

Lewisohn, R., Leuchtenberger, C., Leuchtenberger, R., and Keresztesy, J. C. (1946). Science 104, 436.

Ley, T. J., DeSimone, J., Anagnou, N. P., Keller, G. H., Humphries, R. K., Turner, P. H., Young, N. S., Heller, P., and Neinhuis, A. W. (1982). N. Engl. J. Med. 307, 1469–1476.

Longo, D. L., Colman, N., and Herbert, V. (1975). Clin. Res. 23, 403A.

Metz, J., Kelly, A., Swett, V. C., Waxman, S., and Herbert, V. (1968). Br. J. Haematol. 14, 575–592.

Ostryanina, A. D. (1972). Vopr. Pitan. 3, 25–29.

Pelliniemi, T. T., and Beck, W. S. (1980). J. Clin. Invest. 165, 449–450.

Perry, J., Deacon, P., Lumb, M., and Chanarin, I. (1982). *Blood* **60**, Suppl. 1, 31a.

Pollack, M. A., Taylor, A., and Williams, R. J. (1942). *In* "Studies on B Vitamins in Human, Bat and Mouse Neoplasms," pp. 4237–4256. University of Texas Publications.

Poncz, M., Colman, N., Herbert, V., Schwartz, E., and Cohen, A. R. (1981a). *J. Pediatr.* **98,** 76–79.

Poncz, M., Colman, N., Herbert, V., Schwartz, E., and Cohen, A. R. (1981b). *J. Pediatr.* **99,** 828–829.

Rogers, A. E., and Newberne, P. M. (1975). *Cancer Res.* **35**, 3427.

Sawitsky, A., and Desposito, F. (1964). *J. Pediatr.* **67,** 99.

Scott, J. M., and Weir, D. G. (1981). *Lancet* **2,** 337–340.

Strong, L. C., and Matsunaga, H. (1975). *Cytobios* **12,** 13–18.

Theiss, J. C. (1980). *Cytobios* **29,** 159–163.

Tisman, G., and Herbert, V. (1971). *Clin. Res.* **19,** 433.

Tolstoshev, P., Berg, R. A., Rennard, S. I., Bradley, K. H., Trapnell, B. C., and Crystal, R. G. (1981). *J. Biol. Chem.* **256,** 3135–3140.

van der Westhuyzen, J., Fernandes-Costa, F., Metz, J., Kanazawa, S., Drivas, G., and Herbert, V. (1982a). *Proc. Soc. Exp. Biol. Med.* **171,** 88–91.

van der Westhuyzen, J., Fernandes-Costa, F., and Metz, J. (1982b). *Int. Congr., ISH-ISBT, 1982* Abstracts, p. 237.

van der Weyden, M. B., Cooper, M., and Firkin, B. G. (1973). *Blood* **41,** 299–308.

Whitehead, N., Reyner, F., and Lindenbaum, J. (1973). *JAMA, J. Am. Med. Assoc.* **226,** 1421–4.

Willard, H. R., and Rosenberg, L. E. (1979). *Clin. Res.* **27,** 508A.

Woodcock, T., Damin, L., O'Hehir, M., Hansen, H., Andreef, M., and Young, C. (1979). *Abstr., Am. Assoc. Cancer Res., Annu. Meet.* p. 357.

Zittoun, J., Marquet, J., and Zittoun, R. (1978a). *Blood* **51,** 119–128.

Zittoun, J., Marquet, J., and Zittoun, R. (1978b). *Congr. Int. Soc. Haematol. Congr. Int. Soc. Blood Transf., 17th, 1978* Abstracts, p. 428.

17

Low Vitamin C Intake as a Risk for Cervical Dysplasia

Sylvia Wassertheil-Smoller

Department of Community Health
Division of Epidemiology and Biostatistics
Albert Einstein College of Medicine
Bronx, New York

I. INTRODUCTION

The 1982 report of the National Research Council on Diet, Nutrition, and Cancer exemplifies the increasing interest in the role of nutrition in the etiology and potential for prevention of cancer. The National Cancer Institute commissioned the National Research council to evaluate the current evidence pertaining to nutrition and the incidence of cancer, to develop dietary recommendations for the public, and to formulate a series of recommendations for future research.

Reading the report, one can appreciate how complex an area this is, how difficult the methodology, and how little is

Nutrition Factors in the Induction
and Maintenance of Malignancy

conclusively known about the relationship of specific nutrients to specific cancers. Nevertheless, epidemiologic and laboratory evidence is beginning to accumulate that cancers of most major sites are influenced by dietary patterns, although the mechanisms are not altogether clear. Thus, the National Research Council (1982) was able to make interim dietary recommendations, "both consistent with good nutritional practices and likely to reduce the risk of cancer." Among these recommendations was an emphasis on the importance of including fruits and vegetables in the daily diet—foods rich in vitamin C. The study described below contributed to the evidence leading to that recommendation.

We have done a case-control study to investigate the relationships of certain nutrients to cervical dysplasia (Wassertheil-Smoller et al., 1981; Romney et al., 1981). We were particularly interested in vitamin A, but found, unexpectedly, that a lower reported intake of vitamin C increased the risk of dysplasia. Cervical dysplasia is generally accepted as a precursor to cervical cancer, progressing over time to more severe dysplasia, to carcinoma in situ, and potentially to invasive carcinoma. While the dysplasia can undergo complete regression, its identification requires close follow-up of the patient and provides the opportunity to assess the association of nutritional intake with risk..

II. CASE-CONTROL STUDY OF NUTRITION AND CERVICAL DYSPLASIA

A. Design

The design of the study is shown in Fig. 1. Cases were recruited from among women who came to a free walk-in Papanicolaou (Pap) screening clinic or to the medical screening clinic at the Bronx Municipal Hospital Center. A patient was considered to be a case if she had one positive Pap smear or two consecutive suspicious Pap smears. A patient was considered a control if she had two negative Pap smears and a negative colposcopic examination and no prior gynecologic disease. The project nutritionist, blinded to the Pap smear results, obtained a 24-hour recall from the patient and provided detailed instructions for completing a 3-day food record, which was to include consecutively 2 weekdays and 1 weekend day. All 3-day food records were subsequently clarified by the nutritionist and with the patient, then coded and processed by the Computerized Nutrient Analysis System at the Albert Einstein College of Medicine. The Computerized Nutrient Analysis System provides 71 nu-

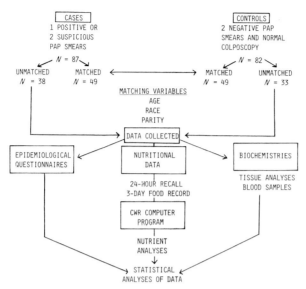

Fig. 1. Nutrition and cervical cancer study design.

trient components of dietary intake, estimated from a data base that contains over 2500 different food items, with nutrient composition derived from the USDA food composition tables, as well as additional commercial items. Not all food items have information on all 71 nutrients.

B. Results

Eighty-seven cases and 82 controls were recruited and included a subset of 49 cases and controls who were matched for age, race, and parity. The cases were considerably younger than the controls; 91% of them were under the age of 45, presumably premenopausal, while only 55% of the controls were under 45. Cases also had a greater proportion of black women than the controls (54% compared to 34.1% of the controls) and they also tended to have a lower income with 46.6% having income at welfare levels compared to 24.4% of the controls. Total numbers of pregnancies were similar in both groups (Table I). The matched subset of cases and controls were comparable in age, race, and income, as well as the total number of pregnancies.

Our primary hypothesis in this study was that a lower dietary intake of vitamin A was associated with a higher risk of cervical dysplasia. However, after careful consideration of plausible biological relationships

TABLE I

Demographic Comparisons between Controls and Cases in the Unmatched Group of Patients

	Unmatched group	
	Controls $N = 82$	Cases $N = 87$
Age (years)		
15–44	54.5	90.8
45–75	45.5	9.2
Race/ethnicity		
Black	34.1	54.0
White	50.0	25.3
Other	15.9	20.7
Total number of pregnancies		
0	1.3	3.5
1–4	74.3	76.6
5 or more	24.5	19.9
Income		
<$5000	24.4	46.6
>$5000	75.6	53.4

between other nutrient items and dysplasia, we selected 18 nutrients out of the 71 available from the computer analysis for more detailed examination. These selected nutrients included vitamin C. Table II displays the mean values per day as estimated by the 3-day food record. Estimates from the 3-day food records were generally higher than those from the 24-hour recall and are considered more stable, thus, these are used in the future discussion, although the results reported for the 3-day food record data held for the 24-hour recalls as well. Only β-carotene and vitamin C showed a significantly lower intake among the cases than the controls ($p < 0.01$), with a mean vitamin C intake for controls being 107 mg and for cases 79.6 mg. A more practical way of looking at this, however, might be in terms of the Recommended Daily Allowance, which is 60 mg for vitamin C. Figure 2 shows 23% of the cases compared to 4% of the controls had daily intakes of vitamin C less than 50% of RDA. This relationship yields an odds ratio of 6.8 as an estimate of relative risk, meaning that women whose daily intake is less than 30 mg run approximately a sevenfold increase in risk of cervical dysplasia compared to women who have intakes above that value. The 95% confidence interval for this odds ratio is between 1.9 and 24.7 (Schlesselman, 1982). Women whose daily intake is less than 150% of RDA (90 mg) have approximately 2.5 times the risk of women whose intake is above 150% of RDA, with 61% of the cases and 38 percent of the controls having daily intakes below 90 mg of vitamin C. The 95% confidence interval for this odds ratio runs between 1.3 and 5.0. Similar results were obtained when women with mild or moderate dysplasia were omitted from the analysis, and only women with severe dysplasia or carcinoma *in situ* were compared to the controls.

An obvious question to ask is whether this result is due to the greater proportion of women with low income in the case group than in the control group, since we know that low socioeconomic level is associated with higher risk of cervical dysplasia. Since vitamin C intake is confounded with income (i.e., a greater proportion of low income women had low vitamin C intake and a greater proportion of cases were low income women) we examined vitamin C within income level. Figure 3 shows that among women with low incomes, the proportion of cases with low vitamin C intake is more than three times greater than for controls (35% versus 11%) and among women with higher incomes, the

TABLE II

Mean Values of Selected Nutrients from the 3-Day Food Record

Nutrients	Mean values 3-day food record/day	
	Controls	Cases
Calories	1611	1621
Protein (gm)	65.6	68.0
Fat (gm)	68.2	70.9
Carbohydrates (gm)	175	168
Refined carbohydrates (gm)	33.2	41.8
Saturated fat (gm)	21.0	22.2
Cholesterol (mg)	266.0	307.3
Vitamin A (IU)	4565	3906
β-Carotene (IU)	2984[a]	2018
Vitamin C (mg)	107[a]	79.6
Sodium (mg)	1719	1929
Potassium (mg)	2096	1881
Zinc (mg)	5.85	5.88
Total tocopherol (IU)	9.12	10.7
α-tocopherol (IU)	2.29	2.42
Pyridoxal (B6) (mg)	549	540
Folic acid (mg)	.06	.06
Iron (mg)	10.7	10.8

[a] $p < .01$.

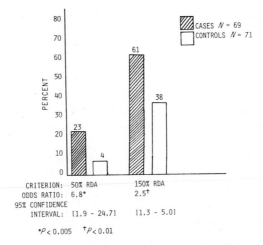

Fig. 2. Percent of patients below criterion for daily intake of vitamin C. Women with less than 50% of RDA intake of vitamin C have a 6.8 times greater risk of cervical dysplasia than women with intake greater than 50% RDA. Women with intake less than 150% RDA have 2.5 times the risk of cervical dysplasia compared to women with intake greater than 50% RDA.

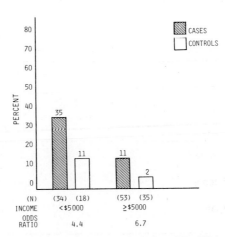

Fig. 3. Percent of patients with daily intake below 50% RDA of vitamin C. Women with annual income less than $5000 who have an intake of vitamin C less than 50% of RDA have a risk of cervical dysplasia 4.4 times that for women who have intakes above 50% of RDA. For women with incomes above $5000, the risk for women with intake less than 50% of RDA is 6.7 times that for women with intake above 50% of RDA.

proportion of cases with low vitamin C is approximately six times greater for cases than for controls (11 versus 2%). A look at the odds ratios indicates that women with a low vitamin C intake run a substantially greater risk of cervical dysplasia than women with higher vitamin C intakes, regardless of income status. These results are not statistically significant, probably due to the small sample size in the subgroups.

However, to assess the impact of vitamin C intake it is necessary to control for variables that have been found to be related to cervical cancer. We confirmed the findings of others that sexual history plays a role in this disease. Table III shows that 55% of the controls versus 87% of the cases were below 19 years of age at their first sexual intercourse, and cases were also more likely to have greater sexual frequency than controls. Variables reflecting such history were controlled for in the multiple logistic analyses. Many models were fitted; however, one that gave a reasonable partition of the population into quintiles of risk included as independent variables age, age at first sexual contact, sexual frequency, and vitamin C.

The probability of severe dysplasia or carcinoma *in situ* is equal to $1/(1 + e^{-k})$ where k is a regression function. The estimates of the regression coefficients are shown in Table IV. These regression coefficients can be used to calculate the odds ratio. From these calculations it can be seen that there is a 9% increase in risk per each year of age younger, a 17% in risk per year younger at first sexual intercourse, a 3% increase in risk per

TABLE III

Selected Epidemiological Variables from the Sexual History

	Unmatched (%)		Matched (%)	
	Control range of N^a 77 to 82	Study range of N^a 82 to 87	Control $N = 49$	Study $N = 49$
Age of first sexual contact 19 years	55.0	87.1[b]	70.2	85.4
Sexual frequency 5 times/ month or more	34.6	69.0[b]	45.0	69.0[c]
Age at first menstruation (11 years)	17.1	36.6[d]	18.4	30.6

[a] Range in N is due to difficulties in eliciting complete sexual histories from all participants.
[b] $p < 0.001$.
[c] $p < 0.01$.
[d] $p < 0.05$.

TABLE IV

Multiple Logistic Analysis

$$P = \frac{1}{1 + e^{-K}} \quad K = B_O + \Sigma B_i X_i$$

(severe dysplasia or carcinoma *in situ*)

$$P = \frac{1}{1 + e^{-(5.8874 - 0.0866[\text{age}] - 0.161[\text{age at 1st sex}] + 0.0068[\text{sex freq}] - 0.0098[\text{vit C}])}}$$

Variable	Increase in risk	Unit
Age	9%	Per year younger
Age at first sex	17%	Per year younger
Sexual frequency	3%	Per increase of 1 per week
Vitamin C	10%	Per 10 mg decrease

Odds ratio $= e^{[\Sigma B_i(X_i^* - X_i)]}$
of individual X^* compared to X

increase of once per week in sexual frequency, and a 10% increase in risk for each 10 mg decrease of daily vitamin C intake. A more dramatic way to illustrate this is to look at the examples of the effect of different variables on relative risk of severe dysplasia or carcinoma *in situ* as shown in Fig. 4. Woman 1 and woman 2 differ only in age. The effect of age when comparing a 25-year-old woman to a 60-year-old woman is a 20-fold increase in risk for the younger woman. Comparing woman 1 to woman 3 shows the effect of age at first sexual intercourse. The woman who began her sexual activity at age 16 is 4.26 times at greater risk than the woman who began at age 25. Comparing woman 1 to woman 3 shows the effect of current sexual frequency. Comparing woman 1 to woman 5 shows the effect of low vitamin C intake. The woman with daily intake of 10 mg has 17 times the risk of a woman comparable on the other variables but having an intake of 300 mg of vitamin C. One might be tempted to conclude that sexually active women could protect themselves by taking more vitamin C. We certainly hesitate to make such a conclusion without further studies to corroborate these findings. Nevertheless, they are suggestive.

III. STABILITY OF VITAMIN C INTAKE

Two important questions naturally arise concerning inferences to be made from this study: (1) Is current vitamin C reflective of past vitamin

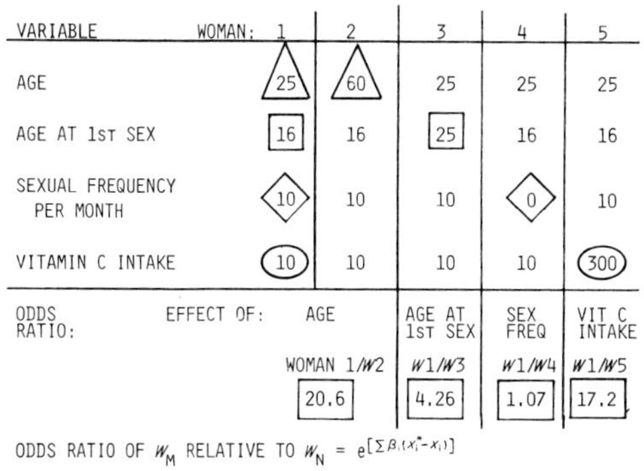

VARIABLE	WOMAN: 1	2	3	4	5
AGE	25	60	25	25	25
AGE AT 1ST SEX	16	16	25	16	16
SEXUAL FREQUENCY PER MONTH	10	10	10	0	10
VITAMIN C INTAKE	10	10	10	10	300

ODDS RATIO: EFFECT OF:	AGE		AGE AT 1ST SEX	SEX FREQ	VIT C INTAKE
	WOMAN 1/W2		W1/W3	W1/W4	W1/W5
	20.6		4.26	1.07	17.2

ODDS RATIO OF W_M RELATIVE TO W_N = $e^{[\Sigma \beta_i (x_i' - x_i)]}$

Fig. 4. Effect of different variables on relative risk of cervical dysplasia or carcinoma *in situ.*

C intake and (2) is vitamin C highly correlated with another nutrient which is the factor responsible for decreasing the risk of cervical dysplasia? With regard to the question of the stability of vitamin C intake over time, we have data from a study on diet and hypertension (Wasser-theil-Smoller *et al.,* 1982). In the Dietary Intervention Study of Hypertension, the objective was to see whether patients' blood pressure could be maintained under control without drugs but through dietary intervention. Patients were randomly assigned to a salt restriction intervention group, a weight reduction intervention group, or a control group who would receive no dietary intervention. Three-day food records were collected from participants at the baseline of the study, at 8 weeks, at 32 weeks, at 56 weeks. This was a collaborative study including Jackson, Mississippi; Birmingham, Alabama; and Bronx, New York. Thus, the patients represent a broad spectrum of socioeconomic status, racial distribution, and regional dietary customs. Analysis of the 3-day food records from the control group, then, provides us with estimates of variability in vitamin C intake over time. Table V shows that the mean intake for the 121 control group patients for the 12 days spread over 56 weeks did not vary substantially. The mean vitamin C intake for the first 3-day food record collected at baseline was 112 mg, while the mean at the 56-week food record collection was 118 mg. In general, the intake on the third day was slightly higher than the intake on the first 2 days.

In answer to the second question concerning the correlation of vitamin C with other nutrients examined in this study see Table VI. Vitamin C correlates with an *r* of 0.26 with vitamin A, 0.24 with β-carotene, and 0.35 with folic acid, nutrients which have been associated with carcinogenesis. Such correlations highlight one of the problems of studying the relationships between specific nutrients and cancer. It is very difficult, if not impossible, to tease out the role of a single nutrient

TABLE V

Means for Vitamin C[a] over Time[b]

Day	Baseline	Day	8 Weeks	Day	32 Weeks	Day	56 Weeks	Average
1	105	4	108	7	106	10	111	107
2	105	5	101	8	117	11	120	111
3	127	6	112	9	122	12	122	121
Average	112		107		115		118	113

[a] Measured in milligrams.
[b] 121 patients from Dietary Intervention Study of Hypertension.

as being the responsible factor from among other nutrients with which it is correlated.

IV.   DISCUSSION

The association of vitamin C in cancer has been reported for gastric cancer (Higginson, 1966; Haenszel and Wissler, 1975; Bjelke, 1975;

TABLE VI

Correlations between Vitamin C and Other Nutrients $N = 142$

Nutrient	Vitamin C
Total calories	0.06
Total protein	0.18
Total fat	−0.05
Total carbohydrates	0.20
Refined carbohydrates	−0.17
Total saturated fat	−0.09
Cholesterol	0.04
Total vitamin A	0.26
Vitamin C	1.00
β-Carotene	0.24
Sodium	−0.05
Potassium	0.53
Zinc	0.16
Total tocopherol	−0.11
α-Tocopherol	−0.02
Pyridoxal (B₆)	0.29
Folic acid	0.35
Iron	0.29

Kolonel *et al.*, 1982) and esophogeal cancer (Mettlin *et al.*, 1981; Cook-Mozaffari, 1979), as well as for laryngeal cancer (Cook-Mozaffari *et al.*, 1979), and laboratory studies support a role of vitamin C in inhibiting carcinogens (Graham *et al.*, 1981; Ivankovic *et al.*, 1974; Mirvish *et al.*, 1972). Nevertheless, epidemiologic data are not extensive and are generally based on inferences of vitamin C intake from consumption of foods known to contain high levels of the vitamin, but which also contain other nutrients that may play a role.

Among the difficulties in studying a relatively rare disease with a relatively long lag time between induction and clinical manifestation is that prospective studies require many subjects, a long observation period, and a great deal of money. Case-control studies, on the other hand, offer an opportunity for estimating relative risk and investigating hypothesized associations, while controlling for confounding variables, at a much lower cost in a much shorter period of time. Thus, they usually precede the large scale prospective studies that may be ultimately necessary to establish a stronger link in the chain of evidence implicating a particular factor in the etiology of a disease.

The implication of vitamin C in cancer has come from correlational or case-control studies. It would appear that a fruitful area for future research would include more case-control studies on a large population samples using food records as the source of estimation of vitamin C intake, studying the interrelationships among other nutrients intakes, and assessing the physiological status of vitamin C from blood serum. If the suggestive results of our study and other studies implicating vitamin C are confirmed in these expanded case-control designs, then further investigations with prospective designs will become important. If the prospective studies, which observe exposed and nonexposed individuals to determine the relative rates of development of disease in the two groups, confirm the case-control studies, it will then be necessary to focus on the potential for prevention of cervical cancer for women at higher risk due to other correlated variables. It is possible that supplementary vitamin C intake can be useful in prevention. Data from the United States Department of Agriculture's 1977–1978 Nationwide Food Consumption survey indicated that vitamin C was one of the three vitamins and three minerals which may be problem nutrients for a number of sex–age groups in the United States. It was estimated that 20 to 40% of all women in the United States have vitamin C intakes below 70% of RDA.

Given the relatively sparse but increasing body of evidence that vitamin C may be protective for certain cancers, what about the interim dietary recommendations of the National Research Council?

The usefulness of interim recommendations in the absence of conclusive supporting data can be demonstrated by examining the situation with regard to risk factors for cardiovascular disease. It was long known that elevated blood pressure, high levels of serum cholesterol, and cigarette smoking were associated with cardiovascular deaths, but before evidence that reversal of these risk factors would reduce risk was firmly established, groups concerned with public health were mounting vigorous campaigns against smoking, were educating and encouraging the public and health professionals to lower blood pressure, and were advocating a "prudent diet" which would lower serum cholesterol. These public health measures resulted in declining death rates in the 1970s from strokes and heart attacks, reversing a rising trend in the 1960s. It appears in the area of diet and cancer we may be at the same stage as we were in heart disease a decade ago.

ACKNOWLEDGMENTS

In addition to Dr. Sylvia Wassertheil-Smoller, collaborators in the study of dietary vitamin C and cervical dysplasia were Dr. S. Romney, Dr. J. Wylie-Rosett, Dr. C. Duttagupta, Dr. P. Palan, Ms. S. Slagle, Ms. G. Miller, and Mr. D. Lucido, all at the Albert Einstein College of Medicine.

Collaborators in the study of dietary intervention and hypertension were Dr. H. Langford of the University of Mississippi, Dr. M. D. Blaufox, Albert Einstein College of Medicine, Dr. A. Oberman of the University of Alabama in Birmingham, and Dr. M. Hawkins and Ms. C. Babcock of Houston, Texas.

REFERENCES

Benedict, W. F., Wheatley, W. L., and Jones, P. A. (1980). *Cancer Res.* **40,** 2796–2801.
Bjelke, E. (1975). *Int. J. Cancer* **15,** 561–565.
Cook-Mozaffari, P. (1979). *Nutr. Cancer* **1**(2), 51–60.
Cook-Mozaffari, P., Azordegan, F., Day, N. E., Ressicaud, A., Sabaic, A. B. (1979). *Br. J. Cancer* **39,** 293–309.
Graham, S., Mettlin, C., Marshall, J., Priore, R., Rzepica, T., and Shedd, D. (1981). *Am. J. Epidemiol.* **11,** 675–680.
Haenszel, S. L., and Wissler, R. W. (1975). *Cancer Res.* **35,** 3452–3459.
Higginson, J. (1966). *JNCI, J. Natl. Cancer Inst.* **37,** 527–545.
Ivankovic, S., *et al.* (1974). *In* "N-Nitroso Compounds in the Environment" (P. Bogovski and E. A. Walker, eds.), pp. 101–102. Lyon, France.
Kolonel, L. N., Normura, A. M. Y., Hirohata, T., Hankin, J. H., and Hinds, M. W. (1982). *Am. J. Clin. Nutr.* **34,** 2478–2485.
Mettlin, C., Graham, S., Priore, R., Marshall, J., and Swanson, M. (1981). *Nutr. Cancer* **2,** 143–147.
Mirvish, S. S., Walcave, L., Eagen, M., and Shubik, P. (1972). *Science* **177,** 65–68.

National Research Council (1982). "Diet, Nutrition, and Cancer." Nat. Acad. Press, Washington, D.C.

Romney, S., Palan, P. R., Duttagupta, C., Wassentheil-Smoller, S., Wylie, J., Miller, G., Slagle, N., S., and Lucido, D., (1981). *Am. J. Obstet. Gynecol.* **141**, 890–894.

Schlesselman, J. L. (1982). "Case-Control Studies." Oxford Univ. Press, London and New York.

Wassertheil-Smoller, S., Romney, S. L., Wylie-Roset J., Slagle S., Miller G., Lucido, D., Duttagupta, C., and Palan, P. R. (1981). *Am. J. Epidemiol.* **114**, 714–724.

Wassertheil-Smoller, S., Langford, H., Blaufox, M. P., Oberman, A., Babcock, C., and Hotchkiss, J. (1982). *Clin. Sci.* **63**, 423s–425s.

Index

A

Absorption, folate, 277
Acetylaminofluorene, 259
Acetyl-CoA carboxylase, 78
Actinic keratoses, 207
Adenosine monophosphate, 125
Adenosine triphosphatase, 277
Adenosine triphosphate, 125, 128
Adenosine triphosphate citrate lyase, 78
Adenosylcobalamin, 278
S-Adenosylmethionine, 237, 248
  lipotrope deficiency and, 261–262
  methionine rescue, 281
Adenoviruses, 39, 43, 44
Adrenal glands
  C3HBA tumor effects, 172–173
  radiation and, 189, 192
  vitamin A and, 172–173, 184
Aflatoxins
  in choline-deficient cirrhotic rats, 253
  lipotropes and, 230–231, 259, 261
  and liver tumor induction, 250, 255
Africa, 13
Agricultural communities, lymphomas in, 21–22
Alcohol dehydrogenase, 151
Alcoholism, and liver disease, 262
Alkylating agents, cell turnover and, 263
Alkylation, S-adenosylmethionine and, 262
Allograft rejection, vitamin A and β-carotene and, 170
Amino acids
  cell culture media, 37, 52, 57
  purified, 251–252

Aminopterin
  and chromosomes, 227–228
  development of, 275–276
  and folate, 225–226
Ammonia, fiber and, 6
AMP, and phase absorption, 125
Analogs, vitamin, 276
  folate, 278
  vitamin B$_{12}$, 277, 278, 279, 280
Anemias, see also Pernicious anemia
  aplastic, 102–103
  Fanconi, 109
  megaloblastic, 102, 265–266, 281
Anesthesia, vitamin A and, 184
Aniline dyes, 213
Antibiotics
  in cell culture, 34
  and choline deficiency, 249
Anticonvulsants, and folate, 233–234, 235, 265
Antigens
  Epstein-Barr virus, 15–16
  gastric, 266
  and lymphomagenesis, 24
  viral infections and, 40
  virus-transformed cells, 44–45
Antimetabolites, and folate, 225–226
Antisera, baseplate, and phage activity, 124
Antivitamins, 276
Aplastic anemia, folate uptake deficiency and, 102–103
Appendicitis, 2, 3, 5
Aromatic hydrocarbons, 221
Ascorbate, see Vitamin C
ATP, 125, 128